RETINITIS PIGMENTOSA

RETINITIS
PIGMENTOSA

JOHN R. HECKENLIVELY, M.D.

Associate Professor, Jules Stein Eye Institute
UCLA Center for the Health Sciences, Los Angeles
Harbor-UCLA Medical Center, Torrance, California

WITH TWELVE CONTRIBUTORS

 J.B. LIPPINCOTT COMPANY   Philadelphia

London • Mexico City • New York • St. Louis • São Paulo • Sydney

Acquisitions Editor: Lisette Bralow
Sponsoring Editor: Sanford J. Robinson
Manuscript Editor: Helen Ewan
Indexer: Barbara Littlewood
Design Director: Tracy Baldwin
Design Coordinator: Don Shenkle
Designer: Adrianne Onderdonk Dudden
Cover Design: Anita R. Curry
Production Manager: Kathleen P. Dunn
Production Coordinator: Caren Erlichman
Compositor: Ruttle, Shaw & Wetherill, Inc.
Printer/Binder: Mandarin Offset

Library of Congress Cataloging-in-Publication Data

Heckenlively, John R.
    Retinitis pigmentosa.

    Includes bibliographies and index.
    1. Retinitis pigmentosa. I. Title. [DNLM:
1. Retinitis Pigmentosa. WW 270 H448r]
RE661.R45H43 1988   617.7'3   87-3328
ISBN 0-397-50656-2

The authors and publisher have exerted every effort to ensure that testing
procedures set forth in this text are in accord with current recommendations and
practice at the time of publication. However, in view of ongoing research,
changes in government regulations, and the constant flow of information relating
to techniques, the reader is urged to check the manufacturer's information for any
change in indications and for added warnings and precautions. This is particularly
important when using a new or infrequently employed procedure.

To Mary Alice Wilcox and Chris Ernst

Contributors

Alan C. Bird, M.B., M.D. FRCS
Professor of Clinical Ophthalmology
Moorfields Eye Hospital
London, England

Joann A. Boughman, Ph.D.
Associate Professor
Division of Human Genetics
University of Maryland School of Medicine
Baltimore, Maryland

Ronald E. Carr, M.D.
Professor of Ophthalmology
New York University
New York, New York

Don S. Ellis, M.D.
Department of Ophthalmology
Pacific Medical Center
San Francisco, California

Scott G. Foxman, M.D.
Clinical Instructor in Ophthalmology
Scheie Eye Institute
University of Pennsylvania
Philadelphia, Pennsylvania

Lorraine H. Friedman, M.A.
Medical Genetics Counsellor
Jules Stein Eye Institute
Los Angeles, California

Nancy G. Kennaway, Ph.D.
Associate Professor
Division of Medical Genetics
University of Oregon School of Medicine
Portland, Oregon

Howard R. Krauss, M.D.
Assistant Clinical Professor
Jules Stein Eye Institute
UCLA School of Medicine
Los Angeles, California

Toni G. Marcy, M.D.
Medical Consultant
LA Blind Childrens Center
Los Angles, California

John Marshall, Ph.D.
Sembal Professor of Experimental Ophthalmology
Institute of Ophthalmology
London, England

Janet Silver, M.PHIL., FBCO, FBIM
Principal Ophthalmic Optician
Moorfields Eye Hospital
London, England

Richard G. Weleber, M.D.
Associate Professor of Ophthalmology
University of Oregon
School of Medicine
Portland, Oregon

Foreword

By the time this book is printed, I may have no vision left to read the precious words written on the following pages; and so with this thought, I ask you, the reader, to consider these printed words carefully, and to read with great passion, even at the times that you may care not to, for the gift of reading is the most precious gift of all, given to you by the sense that is the most precious of all—your own eyes.

I have walked through the years of impending darkness with the agony that goes along with the loss of sight. My childhood was spent in the bewilderment of being night blind, yet reading with 20/20 vision during the day. My youth and young adult life were spent trying to understand clumsy behavior because of my eye disease, retinitis pigmentosa.

When my sons were diagnosed as having inherited RP, it aroused in me great pain, sorrow, and anger. These emotions have led me through the years fighting for awareness, education, and research for retinal degenerative diseases. Though I have accomplished much in these 12 years, nothing pleases me more than the development and publication of this, the first textbook on retinitis pigmentosa. At last RP has been given the dignity of having a textbook about the disease that affects hundreds of thousands or people, not just myself and my family as I thought so many years ago.

We ask that God grant the reader the wisdom and scientific resources to find the answers somewhere within these pages to end the diseases that have created a community of "sighted-blind" individuals.

Helen J. Harris
President and Founder
RP International
Woodlawn Hills, California

After reviewing the contents of this book, I cannot help but reminisce back to the days when I first learned the meaning of retinitis pigmentosa. In 1971, when two of my children were diagnosed with RP, very limited research was being done, and many ophthalmologists were unfamiliar with the problem.

Today the situation has changed considerably. When the RP Foundation Fighting Blindness established its first multidisciplined research center in 1971, it did not envision that it would support 13 centers in the U.S. and England before 1986. Although retinitis pigmentosa may not be household words as yet, significant inroads in awareness have been made in the scientific and lay communities. Several research books on RP have been published, as well as this important reference on clinical evaluations and observations. I am deeply gratified by the outstanding progress made in 15 years.

However, the needs are still great. Ophthalmologists must use standardized techniques as described herein to evaluate and classify patients properly. This text makes an invaluable contribution because it can be used as a reference for ophthalmologists and researchers working with retinal degenerative diseases.

The sensitivity in the handling of RP patients is another area in need of improvement. We would recommend that doctors should advise patients that research is being conducted and refer them to the foundation for additional information.

Today there is hope where once there was none. If ophthalmologists and researchers become more aware that they are working with people, not just with diseases, much will be gained. This book represents a giant step in the right direction. There are answers to the mysteries of RP, Usher's syndromes, and other retinal degenerative diseases, and together we will work toward a brighter tomorrow for all affected by these sight-stealers.

Bernard Berman, President
RP Foundation Fighting Blindness
Baltimore, Maryland

Preface

Our understanding of the disease retinitis pigmentosa (RP) has made great progress since Donders first formulated the term in 1855. That label, while not well chosen, since there is no evidence of true inflammation in hereditary retinitis pigmentosa, has persevered despite attempts to use other diagnostic terms such as tapetoretinal degeneration (another term that is unaccurate, since humans do not have a tapetum). Nettleship, Usher, and Bell, from 1910 to 1920 in various reports, defined the hereditary types of retinitis pigmentosa. The advent of indirect ophthalmoscopy in the 1960s allowed ophthalmologists to find early cases; the age of molecular genetics was heralded in 1984 with Bhattacharya and colleagues mapping the X-linked recessive retinitis pigmentosa gene to Xp11 on the short arm of the X-chromosome.

Until recently, research into retinitis pigmentosa was handicapped by a lack of understanding of the many forms of hereditary pigmentary retinopathy, and heterogenous retinitis pigmentosa groups were investigated with generally fruitless results, in part because each type of retinitis pigmentosa was expected to have unique findings and etiology. Clinical classification of retinal disease is imperfect, but until we have the necessary tools, such as disease-specific DNA probes and microbiochemical assays for known retinitis pigmentosa biochemical pathway defects, so that the types of retinitis pigmentosa can be distinguished, it is unlikely that effective therapies can be devised to counter the degenerative mechanisms of these diseases.

It is my hope that this attempt to organize this large set of diseases will lead to an increasingly better understanding and classification based on the pathogenesis rather than the clinical expression of the gene effect. It is important that we develop a common nomenclature in dealing with these sets of diseases, otherwise communication among researchers and clinicians is handicapped. Likewise, communication between clinician and the patient must be enhanced, which will doubtless be aided by the increased availability of information about these various disorders.

One of the rewards of writing a book is having the opportunity to acknowledge those persons who have helped in its creation, either directly or through support of the author's career. Much credit must be given to my parents and family, who have inspired me to undergo the rigors of medical education and academic pursuits.

There are many wonderful friends and mentors who have expended time and energy to help my education, whom I would like to thank; Jonathan Wirtschafter, M.D., my residency chairman who help me acquire early skills in the field of retinal dystrophy and provided me the opportunity to run the visual physiology lab during residency; Bradley Straatsma, M.D., my present chairman, who has strongly supported my academic and research efforts; Allan (Buzz) Kreiger, M.D., Chief of Vitreoretinal Disease at the Jules Stein Eye Institute, who patiently taught me vitreoretinal surgical skills; Jerome T. Pearlman, M.D., Professor of Ophthalmology at Jules Stein, now deceased, who graciously shared his knowledge of retinitis pigmentosa and inspired all around him with his gentleness and depth of character; Thomas Ogden, M.D., Ph.D., who first taught me ocular electrophysiology; Williams Hoyt, M.D., who took in a raw medical student and opened up the horizons and mysteries of ophthalmology as well as instilling methodology; Dean Hope Lowry at the University of Colorado Medical School, Thomas Sherman, Ph.D., at Oberlin College, who opened the horizons of Science; Victor McKusick, M.D., "Mr. Genetics" whose energy for sorting out genetic diseases is truly phenomenal; Alex E. Krill, M.D., whom I never knew personally, but a giant who continues to inspired those persons in the field of retinal dystrophy.

Special recognition should be given to the efforts of clinical and basic science colleagues who have helped to develop knowledge of RP over the last 20 years: Gus Aguirre, V.M.D., Professor Desmond Archer, Professor Geoffrey Arden, S.S. Bhattacharya, Ph.D., Eliot Berson, M.D., Professor Alan Bird, Pro-

fessor Dean Bok, Joann Boughman, Ph.D., Ronald Carr, M.D., Gerry Chader, Ph.D., Professor August Deutman, Chris Ernst, Ph.D., Professor Debora Farber, Daniel Finklestein, M.D., Professor Jules François, Gerald Fishman, M.D., Peter Gouras, M.D., Professor Michael Hall, Professor Harold Henkes, Paul Henkind, M.D., Ph.D., Tatsuo Hirose, M.D., Joe Hollyfield, Ph.D., Marcelle Jay, Ph.D., Barrie Jay, M.D., Matthew LaVail, Ph.D., Richard Lewis, M.D., Michael Marmor, M.D., Professor John Marshall, Professor Robert Massof, Professor Saul Merin, Professor Günter Neimeyer, Ronald Pruett, M.D., Professor Harris Ripps, Thomas H. Roderick, Ph.D., Michael Sandberg, Ph.D., Professor Irwin Siegel, Professor Roy Steinberg, Professor GHM van Lith, and Richard Weleber, M.D., to name a few.

In the last 10 years, knowledge of retinitis pigmentosa has taken a leap forward because of efforts by the National RP Foundation and in particular Mr. Ben Berman, Alan Laties, M.D., and others who have built recognition of the disease and have encouraged research efforts by funding hundreds of RP research projects around the world.

A special thanks must go to Mrs. Helen Harris, President, and the Board of Directors of RP International, for their generous support in underwriting the color production in this book, an act which greatly enhances the educational impact of the text and also helped to keep the book price more economical.

Finally, I would like to thank my friend Sherwin Isenberg, M.D., Chief of Ophthalmology, and S. Eric Wilson, Chairman, Department of Surgery at Harbor-UCLA Medical Center, for their strong support, Mrs. Alamada Barrett for assistance in editing, Ms. Margaret Kowalczyk for medical illustrations, Ms. Nicki Chang and Mrs. Lorraine Friedman for pedigrees, Mr. Jay Sands, Mr. Dennis Thayer, Ms. Audrey Friedman, and Mr. Charlie Martin for their photographic skills, and particularly my hard-working secretary, Mrs. Jill Oversier, who has patiently assisted me in many projects, as well as being a mainstay for countless RP patients.

John R. Heckenlively, M.D.

Contents

RETINITIS
PIGMENTOSA

1

Retinitis Pigmentosa
JOHN R. HECKENLIVELY

INTRODUCTION

Retinitis pigmentosa (RP) is the name commonly given to a group of heredofamilial diseases characterized by progressive visual field loss, night blindness, and abnormal or nonrecordable electroretinogram (ERG). This broad definition encompasses a large number of primary (ocular only) and secondary (other organ or systemic involvement) diseases. Over the years, various diagnostic criteria have been employed in an effort to provide better understanding of the diseases known as RP; at times, definitions were too restrictive, excluding patients who presented with signs and symptoms similar to those of other RP patients, but who often had atypical features. Some researchers avoided wrestling with the problem of setting definitions by having almost no criteria beyond the patient's having a pigmentary retinopathy in order to make the diagnosis of RP, often reporting isolated cases in which no hereditary pattern could be found.

DEFINITION OF RP

RP has been defined in a number of ways; one such definition is that it is a set of hereditary disorders that diffusely and primarily affect photoreceptor and pigment epithelial function.[1] Even this broad definition tends to exclude those frequently found RP patients in whom no family history can be found; it is commonly assumed, but not proven, that patients with a negative family history have genetically determined disease, such as diseases transmitted by autosomal recessive inheritance. Some patients with pigmentary retinopathy as a sequelae from previous retinal inflammatory disease are often diagnosed as having RP retinitis pigmentosa because they present with similar signs and symptoms. Frequently, it is difficult or impossible to definitely distinguish these "pseudo-RP" patients from hereditary forms. As specific biochemical, histopathological, and/or genetic markers for each form of RP become available, problems in classification of RP will be resolved.

HISTORICAL BACKGROUND

Donders is generally credited with first describing "retinitis pigmentosa" in 1855 and 1857,[2,3] although there were early observations of familial complicated night blindness by Ovelgun in 1744[4] as well as reports of poor vision and pigmented lesions in the retina by Schon in 1828[5] and Von Ammon in 1838[6]; subsequently, various authors have attempted to suggest, without great success, other names for the disease. The term "retinitis" is a misnomer, since there is little evidence of inflammation on histopathology. In 1916, Leber introduced the commonly used term "tapeto-retinal degeneration." Other terms which have been used for RP include primary pigmentary degeneration, dystrophia retinae pigmentosa, abiotrophia retinae pigmentosa, and hemeralopic retinosis.[7]

In 1858, von Graefe demonstrated the hereditary nature of the disease to which he gave the name of pigmentary degeneration.[8] Liebreich in 1861 emphasized the importance of consanguinity in association with pigmentary retinopathy.[9] The hereditary nature of RP was well documented by Nettleship in 1908 when he published the results of family studies in RP based on 976 families.[10] Usher (1914) published 40 detailed family trees further confirming the hereditary nature of these diseases.[11] A comprehensive study of all the known reported cases of RP was made by Julia Bell in 1922.[12]

In 1945, Karpe demonstrated that there was an abnormal to nonrecordable ERG response in patients with pigmentary retinopathy and that this electrophysiological response occurred in many patients before the appearance of clinical or ophthalmoscopic changes.[13] With the advent of setting conditions in ERG testing so that cone and rod responses could be examined separately, Gouras and Carr found that in early cases of dominant RP, patients had a markedly reduced scotopic (rod) ERG while the photopic (cone) ERG was relatively normal.[14] Because of investigations by Carr, Gouras, Berson, and Krill, showing that preferential rod damage occurred more than cone damage in early cases, the term "rod-cone" dystrophy came to be synonymous with RP, in fact, to the point where, for some clini-

cians, only a nonrecordable ERG or an abnormal ERG in the rod-cone pattern (see ERG section, Chapter 5) was considered consistent with the diagnosis of RP. Berson, Gouras, and Gunkel published an article in 1968 on progressive cone-rod dystrophy whose ERG pattern was not generally regarded as being related to RP because of atypical features. However, Heckenlively in 1981 published 20 cases of RP from all three main inheritance types meeting all standard definitions of RP in which the cone-rod pattern was present on the ERG.[15] Interestingly, these RP patients were not night-blind until the visual field was less than 10°.

At the same time, Massoff and Finkelstein published psychophysical data which suggested a similar grouping. They reported two basic types of RP degenerative patterns: one in which there was diffuse rod disease (type I RP) and the other in which both rods and cones were affected (type II RP).[16] It currently appears that the psychophysical schemes generally correlate with the ERG designations of rod-cone and cone-rod, though there are occasionally exceptions to this rule.

"SPLITTING" VERSUS "LUMPING"

Researchers in the field of RP have been confronted with the problem of how to adequately diagnose and classify a group of patients who generally have the same symptomatology and clinical findings. Over the years, various approaches have been taken to cope with this confusing array of diseases. Because there is no specific diagnostic biochemical or pathohistological marker for any type of primary RP, a few researchers have chosen to "lump" RP patients together without a serious attempt to separate them by other means.

The role of heredity is widely acknowledged as a significant determinant, and most studies have attempted to divide RP populations by inheritance. Further subdivision has been tried with limited success, but such methods as the ERG and receptor sensitivity studies do not have pathophysiological collaboration that these methods are capable of diagnosing specific types of RP.

However, unless there is an attempt to "split" the

RP types, many biochemical and clinical studies of RP are not likely to make much sense; but incorrectly split, these studies also will be nonsense.

A COMMON DEGENERATIVE PATHWAY

One of the main problems in distinguishing the various types of RP on clinical examination is that there is a commonality to the fundus findings. Most patients demonstrate pigment deposition in the retina, often in walls of sclerosed retinal vessels giving a characteristic "bone spicule" pattern. The retinal deterioration taking place is intrinsic to the disease process and does not appear to be related directly to the pigment deposition process, which is a secondary effect. Whether the pigment contributes to the deterioration of retinal function is not known. Localized retinal pigment deposition is commonly seen in processes that injure or destroy the retinal pigment epithelium (RPE) layer, and the RP pigmentary pattern can be regarded as a common degenerative pathway for a number of different acquired and hereditary retinal degenerations.

TYPICAL CLINICAL FINDINGS

While there is great variability among RP patients, if a stereotypical picture were to be drawn, the typical RP patient complains of night blindness dating from childhood years, with noticeable symptoms of visual field loss dating from the late twenties. The patient would complain of severe visual disability with tubular fields and severe night blindness in the forties and would have little or no functional vision by sixty to seventy. In later stages, flashes or rolling waves of light are a common occurrence. The duration of the disease is somewhat dependent on the age of onset and the severity of the type of RP. Slightly less than half of RP patients will develop cataracts, usually in advanced stages of the disease, and some will do well with cataract extraction.

The most characteristic ophthalmoscopic findings in the hereditary pigmentary degenerations are depigmentation or atrophy of the RPE, pigment deposition in the retina, and narrowing of the retinal arterioles. The pigmentary disturbance often takes the form of clumps and strands of black pigment, occurring most prominently in the periphery and often in a perivascular pattern due to pigment within vessel walls. Bone corpuscular-like arrangements of pigment are common, but small, irregular clumps and spots of pigment may be seen almost as often. In many cases those areas of the fundus not involved wtih pigmentary deposition show a moth-eaten appearance or a salt-and-pepper scattering of pigment.

TABLE 1-1
PRIMARY FORMS OF RP

Rod-cone Degenerations*

Autosomal dominant†
Autosomal recessive
X-linked recessive†‡
Retinitis punctata albescens
Preserved para-arteriolar retinal pigment epithelium (PPRPE)†
Choroideremia†
Simplex/multiplex forms

Cone-rod Degeneration*

Autosomal dominant†
Autosomal recessive
X-linked recessive†‡
Simplex/multiplex forms

Congenital Onset

Leber's amaurosis congenita, typical form†
Congenital RP with macular colobomata†
Juvenile Leber's amaurosis**
Autosomal dominant form (rare)†

* Nonspecific pigmentary retinopathy in which there is no unique morphological change in the fundus and onset is not congenital. "Rod-cone" or "cone-rod" refers to the pattern seen on the ERG, or to cases in which dark adaptometry or spectral sensitivity testing is diagnostic.

† These forms of RP appear to be distinct genetic entities; forms unmarked may or may not be single diseases, and there is a possibility of several genetic diseases being included as one listing.

‡ Whether rod-cone and cone-rod X-linked RP are determined by one and the same or different genes is not known at publication time. Linkage analysis studies demonstrate the same locus for both.

** Leber also described a group of children who had visual symptoms or signs after 6 months of age but before age 2 (discussed in Chapter 7).

Histological studies of RP retinas suggest that the source of the pigment is the RPE rather than the choroid.

Occasionally the retina has a refractile, nearly edematous appearance, which with time develops more characteristic degenerative changes. Wrinkling of the inner limiting membrane is common. As the RPE atrophies or depigments, the choroidal vessels may become more prominent. Some patients show atrophy of the RPE without depigmentation. Fortunately, in most patients the macular region is more resistant to the disease process, and central vision is usually relatively preserved even into advanced stages in most patients.

For years the optic nerve was reported as having "waxy pallor," reflecting the widespread use of the direct ophthalmoscope in diagnosing more advanced cases. With the use of the indirect ophthalmoscope, earlier cases are found, and frequently the optic nerve is pink, though it may not appear completely normal. The disc substance may appear "waxy" or clouded, perhaps from epipapillary membrane formation. Small disc vessel beading is common, and the cup-to-disc ratio is abnormally small in most patients.

CLASSIFICATION OF RP

RP as well as other hereditary retinal and choroidal diseases have been classified by a number of different approaches; usually the fundus pattern (morphological appearance) and the inheritance pattern are correlated with the results of electrophysiological/psychophysical tests such as the ERG, electro-ocu-logram (EOG), dark adaptation test (DA), and visual field. These results are compared with the patterns seen in established disease entities for the most accurate diagnosis. Frequently, the clinical appearance and test results clearly establish the diagnosis, but because many retinal diseases have similar fundus appearances or clinical presentations, it may be necessary to observe the clinical course of the disease over many years and to examine other affected family members in order to finalize the diagnosis. Frequently, a specific diagnosis is not possible even after extensive testing and pedigree analysis.

RP can be divided into two large groups: primary RP in which the disease process is confined to the eyes, with no other systemic manifestation; and secondary RP, in which the pigmented retinal degeneration is associated with single or mutliple organ system disease. A list of primary forms of RP can be found in Tables 1-1 and 2-6. The most common secondary forms of disease with associated RP, such as Usher's syndrome, Bardet-Biedl syndrome, abetalipoproteinemia, and Senior-Loken syndrome, will be covered in some detail while other secondary forms will be briefly reviewed. A chapter on gyrate atrophy is included since these patients fulfill standard definitions of secondary RP, though clearly enough is known about this disease that it should be distinguished by a distinct diagnostic name.

UCLA RP REGISTRY

Both published and unpublished data based on studies of over 900 RP patients in the UCLA RP Registry will be presented in this text.

REFERENCES

1. Marmor MF et al: Retinitis pigmentosa; A symposium on terminology and methods of examination. Ophthalmology 90:126–131, 1983
2. Donders FC: Beiträge zur pathologischen Anatomie des Auges. Graefes Arch Clin Exp Ophthalmol 1(II):106–l18, 1855; 3(I):139–165, 1857
3. Donders FC: Torpeur de la rétine congénital e héréditarie. Ann Ocul (Paris) 34:270–273, 1855
4. Ovelgün. Nyctalopia haerediotria. Acta Physico Med (Nuremburg) 7:76-77 obs. 28, 1744
5. Schon M: Handbuch der pathologischen Anatomie des menschlichen Auges, p 202. Hamburg, 1828 [Vinken]
6. Von Ammon FA: Klinische Darstellungen der Krankheiten unds Bildungsfehler des menschlichen Auges, vol l. Berlin, G Reimer, 1838 [Vinken]
7. Botermans CHG: Primary pigmentary retinal degeneration and its association with neurological diseases. In Vinken PJ, Bruyn GW (eds): Neuroretinal Degenerations, vol 13, p 148. Amsterdam, North-Holland Publishing Co, 1972
8. von Graefe A: Exceptionnelles Verhalten des Gesichtsfeldes bei Pigmententartung der Netzhaut. Graefes Arch Clin Exp Ophthalmol 4(II):250–253, 1858 [Franceschetti]
9. Liebreich R: Abkunft aus Ehen unter Blutsverwandstenals Grund von Retinitis pigmentosa. Dtsch Klin 1:53–55, 1861 [Franceschetti]
10. Nettleship E: On retinitis pigmentosa and allied diseases.

Roy Lond Ophthal Hosp Rep 17(I):1–56; (II):151–166; (III):333–427, 1907/1908 [Franceschetti]

11. Usher CH: On the inheritance of retinitis pigmentosa with notes of cases. Roy Lond Ophthal Hosp Rep 19:1930–2036, 1914

12. Bell J: Retinitis pigmentosa and allied diseases. In Pearson K: Treasury of Human Inheritance, vol II, part I. Cambridge University Press, 1922

13. Karpe G: The basis of clinical electroretinography. Acta Ophthal (Kbh) 24(suppl):1–118, 1945

14. Gouras P, Carr RE: Electrophysiological studies in early retinitis pigmentosa. Arch Ophthalmol 72:104–l10, 1964

15. Heckenlively JR, Martin DA, Rosales TO: Telangiectasia and optic atrophy in cone-rod degenerations. Arch Ophthalmol 99:1981–1991, 1981

16. Massof RW, Finkelstein D: Subclassifications of retinitis pigmentosa from two-color scotopic static perimetry. Doc Ophthalmol Proc Series 26:219–225, 1981

2

The Diagnosis and Classification of Retinitis Pigmentosa

JOHN R. HECKENLIVELY

The diagnosis of retinitis pigmentosa (RP) traditionally was based on the clinical examination, in which the affected patient has a history of night blindness, symptoms referrable to visual field loss, and pigmentary retinopathy. A tangent visual field examination confirmed the diagnosis and was used to follow the patient. If a positive family history was obtained, the diagnosis was felt to be conclusive. Since the advent of electroretinographic testing in the 1950s, making possible the objective documentation of retinal abnormalites, other physiological and psychophysical tests have been developed for better defining the various types of hereditary and nonhereditary retinal degenerations.

TESTING FOR RP

Four main tests, the electroretinogram (ERG), visual fields, best corrected visual acuity, and pedigree analysis, are used clinically in the diagnosis and management of RP. However, the clinical history and other tests give important supplementary information which is useful in classifying the types of RP and in

understanding the effects of the disease process. These tests include the dark adaptation test, the electro-oculogram (EOG), fluorescein angiography, and color vision testing. Aspects of refractive and visual acuity changes, and their use in management and diagnosis of RP are discussed in Chapters 5 and 6; visual fields in RP are covered in Chapter 3.

Several research procedures that appear promising for better classifying RP types include spectral sensitivity testing, flicker studies, and fundus reflectometry.

THE ELECTRORETINOGRAM

The ERG is a response evoked from the retina by a flash of light and is usually recorded from the corneal surface by a contact lens electrode or gold foil electrodes. Eyelid skin electrodes are occasionally used in children but may not give tracings as reproducible or of as good quality as those obtained using corneal electrodes. A Ganzfeld stimulus device which gives a broad illumination is the preferred method of presenting the flash for most laboratories.

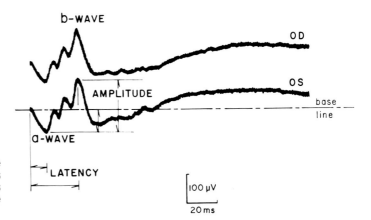

FIG. 2-1. Photopic ERG, typical waveform of the cone system in which the first negative wave is called the a-wave, and the positive peak is termed the b-wave. Oscillatory potentials can be seen in the ascending b-wave.

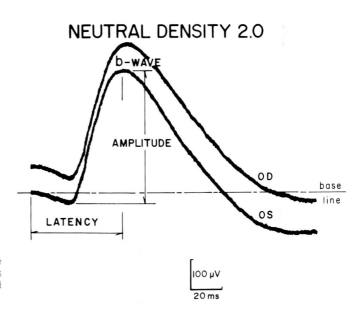

FIG. 2-2. Scotopic ERG, typical waveform of the rod system. Neutral density filters reduce the stimulus flash intensity below cone threshold. Rod-mediated ERG waveforms have almost no a-wave.

The ERG response, as recorded in the standard clinical setting, is biphasic, with the first negative downward peak called an "a" wave, and the next positive upward peak called a "b" wave (**Fig. 2-1**). The a-wave represents repolarization of photoreceptor cells, while the b-wave is derived from cells in the bipolar region of the middle retina. Under special conditions with the use of salt-bridge electrodes and direct current (DC) amplification, a late positive "c-wave" can be recorded about 2 to 3 seconds after the light flash. This response is an indicator of the health of the retinal pigment epithelium (RPE). The DC-ERG is difficult to use clinically: it requires maximum patient cooperation because it is uncomfortable and eye movement easily causes artifacts on tracings. Patients find that the standard ERG is a relatively easy experience involving minimal discomfort.

When performed in the light-adapted state, the test is called a *photopic* or cone-mediated ERG, since it measures the function of the cone system (**Fig. 2-1**). To obtain a photopic response, the background conditions must be lighted so that the rods are bleached out and thus will not respond to the flash stimulus. To measure the rod system response, the patient is dark-adapted for at least 30 minutes, and a dim blue or white flash below cone threshold is given (**Fig. 2-2**). This technique gives a rod-mediated signal. Both the rod and cone systems can be stimulated by using a bright flash in the dark-adapted state (**Fig. 2-3**).

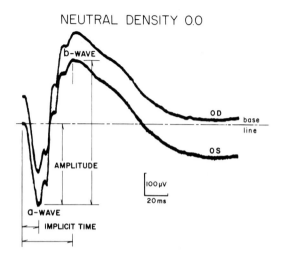

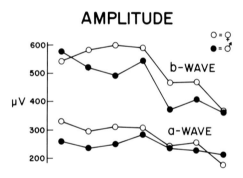

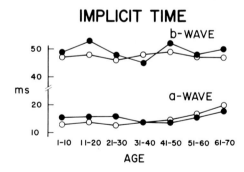

FIG. 2-3. Dark-adapted bright flash ERG represents the signal from both rods and cones in response to a bright flash. There is a large a-wave and b-wave as well as oscillatory potentials in the ascending b-wave. An example of gender and age differences in amplitudes and implicit times is graphed below. (Reproduced by permission, Dr. W. Junk, Publishers, Documenta Ophthalmologica Proceeding Series 31:140, 1982)

The photopic (cone-mediated) and scotopic (rod-mediated) waveforms are quite distinctive; the photopic ERG has smaller a- and b-wave amplitudes, approximately 46 to 70 microvolts* for the a-wave and 120 to 193 microvolts* for the b-wave (**Fig. 2-1**). The photopic implicit times are faster than in dark-adapted ERGs, with the b-wave peak time normally ranging from 31 to 35 milliseconds* for a photopic ERG compared with 72 to 92 milliseconds* for the rod-mediated ERG. The shapes of the waveforms change with test conditions.

Rod-mediated ERGs have virtually no a-wave, while the b-wave amplitude is about two to three times larger than the photopic ERG, averaging 367 microvolts* (**Fig. 2-2**). In the bright flash dark-adapted ERG, both a- and b-waves are larger than either the photopic or scotopic ERGs (**Fig. 2-3**). Flickering bright light of increasing frequency can be used to test the responsiveness of the cone system, which normally responds up to 70 cycles a second. Rods are capable of responding up to about 8 cycles a second.

The bright flash dark-adapted ERG waveform has not been used diagnostically in classifying RP types; the classification system presented in this text is based on the relative damage to the rod and cone systems as demonstrated in photopic (cone-mediated) and scotopic (rod-mediated) tracings as well as psychophysical testing. However, since the bright flash dark-adapted test condition along with the flicker test maximally stimulates the retina, they may provide the only recordable waves when the photopic and scotopic single-flash ERGs are nonrecordable.

The type of ERG test condition often can be predicted from analyzing the shape of the waveform. An ERG which occurs fairly rapidly with both an a- and b-wave with smaller amplitudes is likely to be a photopic ERG tested with a flash in light-adapted conditions. Likewise, an ERG waveform which has no a-wave but a large b-wave is a rod-mediated ERG. Consequently, a waveform labeled "scotopic," dem-

---

*Accurate interpretation of ERG normal values is highly dependent on setting standardized testing protocols; while normal laboratory values will vary from laboratory to laboratory, waveforms and implicit times will be similar if testing protocols are similar.

onstrating a large a-wave, is *not* a rod-isolated ERG, since higher intensities which stimulate cones were used, evoking an a-wave in the dark-adapted patient.

Because the ERG is so responsive to changes in test conditions, it is extremely important to set up a standardized testing protocol and to establish normal controls under identical conditions for every test. Separate control values should be established by *gender* and *age* group, since ERG amplitudes and implicit times vary by these parameters; females have larger amplitudes and shorter implicit times as compared with age-matched males (**Fig.** *2-3 bottom*). Even the slightest change in the protocol can give significant changes in ERG values.[1]

The ERG is a recording of a mass response of the outer and middle retinal layers and does *not* correlate with visual acuity, which is a function of macular health. The macula area contributes at most 10% to 15% to the cone ERG response, so that a large photopic loss cannot be attributed to macular damage alone.[2]

In examining 215 RP patients of all types at UCLA we found that at least one component was recordable in 41% (89/215) of patients. There was a significant difference in recordability between patients with cone-rod degeneration and those with rod-cone degeneration. The specific data can be found in Chapter 5, Clinical Characteristics of RP.

Development of the ERG for RP Testing

In 1945, Karpe reported that the ERG was absent in patients with RP, and from that point the ERG evolved to become an important test in the diagnosis of RP.[3] However, within a decade, Bjork and Karpe in 1951,[4] Armington and Schwab in 1954,[5] and Franceschetti and Dieterle in 1957[6] established that not all RP patients had nonrecordable ERGs and that the response was proportional to the severity of the disease. In 1956, Henkes, van der Tweel, and van der Gon[7] found activity in previously nonrecordable ERGs by using selective frequency amplification. In 1961, Armington, Gouras, Tepas, and Gunkel reported the use of computer averaging to enhance RP ERGs that were extinguished by single flash technique.[8] At times, the response may be as small as .05 to 1.0 microvolts, but under standardized conditions

computer averaging may be a useful objective test for monitoring in clinical trials of medications or other means of intervention.[9] Since computer averaging is more uncomfortable for the patient, requiring multiple sustained flashes of light, it is not as commonly used as single-flash testing. However, most RP patients tolerate ERG testing without serious complaint or discomfort.

Electroretinographic Classification of RP

It is known from histopathology that in typical RP rods are affected more than cones; this preferential loss can also be demonstrated on electoretinographic testing. In these patients, the rod-mediated ERG is much more severely affected than the cone-mediated ERG and has been termed a "rod-cone" degenerative pattern.[10]

Some patients present with progressive visual field loss and a history of no or late-onset night blindness. However, they have recordable ERGs in which the cone-mediated ERG is more severely affected than the rod-mediated ERG; this has been termed a "cone-rod" response (**Fig. 2-4**).[11] Psychophysically, rod-cone degeneration patients demonstrate diffuse rod loss, while cone-rod patients usually show areas of preservation of rod and cone function.

In looking for the rod-cone and cone-rod patterns, the cone and rod b-wave amplitudes are evaluated; if the photopic b-wave is larger than the scotopic b-wave amplitude and both are abnormal, the

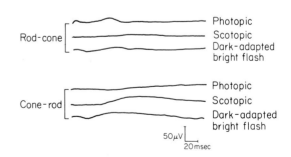

FIG. 2-4. Comparison of rod-cone to cone-rod electroretinographic patterns in two different patients with RP in which the waveforms are still recordable. The first named term is worse affected; thus a patient with a rod-cone pattern has a rod ERG b-wave which is smaller than the cone ERG b-wave amplitude.

patient has a rod-cone degeneration. If the scotopic b-wave amplitude is larger than the photopic b-wave amplitude and both are abnormal, a cone-rod pattern is present. The first term listed, cone or rod, denotes the system which is more severely affected.

In cases where the ERG is extinguished or the photopic and scotopic b-wave amplitudes are nearly the same, the dark adaptation test is helpful in separating the two patterns; cone-rod patients are not markedly night-blind until the visual field is less than 10°.

In cases where the ERG is nonrecordable, the visual field is less than 10°, and the dark adaptation test shows severe night blindness, it may not be possible to classify the patient into either the rod-cone or cone-rod category. A few patients will give a history of late onset night blindness which is suggestive of the cone-rod pattern of disease, and, conversely, many patients will have severe night blindness from early childhood, and the rod-cone pattern retinal degenerative pattern is assumed though not proven. Many patients with advanced disease may present with such a vague history that neither rod-cone nor cone-rod degenerative patterns can be determined.

The time that the a-wave and b-wave amplitudes take to reach their peak, or the implicit time, has also been the subject of investigation. Berson, Gouras, and Hoff evaluated the ERG responses in patients with chorioretinal scars and compared the results in patients with various types of hereditary RP, cone degeneration, and congenital stationary night blindness.[12] They found that patients with chorioretinal scars had decreases in ERG a- and b-wave amplitudes, but the implicit times were normal. In the hereditary panretinal degenerations, progressive amplitude reduction often leads to delays in the implicit time; specifically, these investigators reported delayed photopic implicit times in patients with dominant RP with reduced penetrance,[13,14] autosomal recessive RP,[15] and X-linked recessive RP.[16] However, the implicit-time story will have to be further evaluated with consideration for the age and visual field of the patient at the time of testing (severity of disease), in order to tell if specific types of RP correlate with specific changes in ERG implicit times.

While many carriers of X-linked RP can be identified on fundus examination or may even have symptoms of night blindness, many younger carriers, often in the child-bearing years, may appear normal. However, Berson and co-workers found that virtually all carriers could be distinguished by abnormalities in the bright flash dark-adapted mixed cone and rod response, or by delayed implicit times during bright flash flicker.[17] In a survey of X-linked RP, Arden and associates found that only half of their obligate carriers demonstrated these abnormalities on ERG testing.[18]

The Early Receptor Potential

The early receptor potential (ERP) of the ERG, the initial signal in the first 2 milliseconds of the response representing the photochemical events in the outer segments, has been evaluated in X-linked RP by Berson and Goldstein.[19] They found that in an affected male the ERP was 20% of normal, while the X-linked carriers had a 50% reduction even though their electroretinographic amplitudes were within normal limits. The ERP is a research procedure used to evaluate receptor function; however, it is not used in the standard clinical setting, since the test is performed with an extra-bright flash in the dark-adapted state, which is difficult for patients to tolerate.

THE ELECTRO-OCULOGRAM

The EOG measures a standing potential which exists between the front and back of the eye and has been demonstrated to be generated by the RPE.[20] The test is set up by placing skin electrodes medially and laterally to each canthus; after preadaptation with a bright light, the patient looks alternately between two points 20° apart first in the dark and then in the light, typically 12 to 15 minutes for each segment. As the patient looks between the two points, a square-wave signal is generated (**Fig. 2-5**). The amplitude of this signal changes with light adaptation so that in a normal patient the amplitude is twice as big in the light-adapted state as in the dark. Usually, the test is reported as an *Arden ratio* by dividing the largest light-adapted amplitude by the smallest dark-adapted value and multiplying by 100.[21] While each clinical electrophysiology laboratory has to establish its own

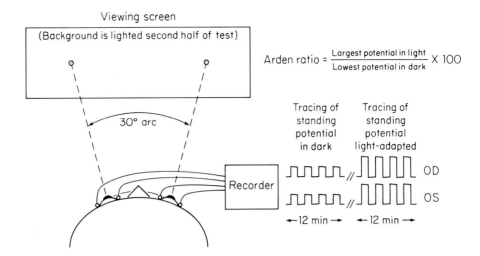

FIG. 2-5. EOG test measures a standing potential generated by the RPE. Skin electrodes are placed at the inner and outer canthus of each eye. The test is first performed in the dark over 12–15 minutes with the patient periodically looking between two dim red lights 30° apart; then the test is repeated with the background brightly lighted. The amplitude of the largest light potential is compared to that of the smallest dark potential (light peak to dark trough) and multiplied by 100 (Arden ratio).

normal range of Arden values, they typically range from 175% to 220%. Rod-cone patients typically demonstrated Arden ratios of 100% to 120%, while cone-rod patients commonly have higher values, ranging from 130% to 150%. Advanced RP patients of either rod-cone or cone-rod type are typically near 100%.

The EOG has not proven to be as helpful diagnostically in RP as it has in other conditions such as Best's disease, since it tends to duplicate information obtained from the ERG and dark adaptation tests. Generally, the EOG is an auxilliary test for RP patients although it will give diagnostic information in cases where the patient refuses an ERG. It can also help to distinguish between rod-cone and cone-rod degenerative patterns if the patient does not have advanced disease.

DARK ADAPTATION TEST

The dark adaptation test measures the threshold of sensitivity of the retina to a spot of light after the patient is placed in the dark. Some laboratories standardize the test by initially giving a light bleach and by using cycloplegia to eliminate potential variability

caused by accommodation. This is a subjective test requiring reasonable patient cooperation. As the patient fixates on a centrally placed, dim red target in the dark, a test spot is presented, commonly 12° above fixation. Many dark adaptometers allow the spot to be placed anywhere in the visual field. The intensity of the spot is varied until the value is identified where the patient just can perceive the light. This intensity threshold is noted on special graph paper that is attached to a timer on the machine and advances throughout the test. Threshold readings are generally measured every 1 to 2 minutes. A characteristic cone-rod break can be seen at 9 to 11 minutes when rod sensitivity becomes more prominent. At about 40 minutes, the curve reaches an asymptote (**Fig. 2-6**). Maximum sensitivity is normally achieved by 40 minutes, although in some RP patients slow improvement in sensitivity has been documented over several hours of testing.[22]

Krill and co-workers demonstrated that normally there is an absolute threshold defect in the inferior retina compared with the superior retina, which they attributed to the effects of "faulty closure of the embryonic fissure."[23] This view was supported by the finding of the highest thresholds in the inferior vertical meridian. These data are quite relevant to

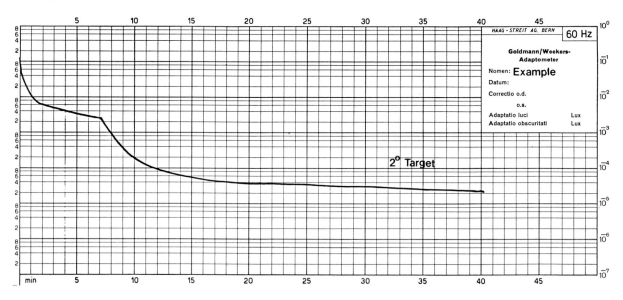

FIG. 2-6. Dark-adaptation curve in which the patient's threshold perception to a point of light is measured in the dark over time. After about 7–10 minutes of dark adaptation, the greater sensitivity of the rods becomes apparent, and a "cone-rod" break is said to occur. Most normal patients have reached their maximum rod sensitivity by 40 minutes in the dark.

the clinical situation, since many RP patients show differences in amount of pigmentary deposition as well as visual field changes, between the inferior and superior halves of the retina, and basic embryologically derived differences would help to explain this asymmetrical behavior. Another prominent theory for the cause of decreased inferior retinal function is chronic increased exposure to sunlight.

Performing a full-dark adaptation curve is time-consuming for both technician and patient, and basic information can be obtained in this group of patients by obtaining a *final rod threshold* at several retinal locations. In this screening maneuver, readings of sensitivity are taken only after the patient has been dark-adapted for 40 minutes. Rod-cone degeneration patients typically have a final rod threshold of 3.50 log units or greater, while cone-rod degeneration patients typically have final rod thresholds of 2.00 log units or less unless their visual field is less than 10°, in which case they show greater elevations in sensitivity. Measuring the final rod threshold after 40 minutes of dark adaptation is a good screening procedure for assessing night vision.

It may come as a surprise to realize that many RP patients in early to middle stages of their disease are not night-blind, but studies as early as 1971 by Wein-

stein demonstrated that a number of RP patients have normal dark adaptation studies.[24,25] While the majority of RP patients are night-blind, both normal and prolonged times for dark adaptation have been demonstrated in a number of patients.[22] RP patients with measurable prolonged dark adaptation may represent a group with dysfunction of rhodopsin metabolism; fundus reflectometry is currently being used in conjunction with dark adaptation studies to explore this possibility.

The subjective age of onset of night blindness has been reported to be useful in evaluating the risk of inheriting RP.[24] Typically, Mendelian inheritance patterns are used to counsel patients, but in some patients the risk can be further assessed by using Bayesian methods of probability based on whether the person in question is experiencing night blindness.[26] For instance, an 18-year-old woman whose mother had autosomal dominant RP would normally have a 50% risk of inheriting the disease, but because she had no night blindness at age 18, under Bayesian calculation she would have about an 88% chance of not having inherited the disease. As data showing various RP characteristics by RP type become available for analysis, these principles can be better applied to individual cases.

Any panretinal disease, including inflammatory insults to the retina which cause rod damage, may result in night blindness quantifiable by the dark adaptation test.

SPECTRAL SENSITIVITY TESTING

Zeavin and Wald in 1956 reported the use of a specially adapted perimeter in which threshold profiles were measured along vertical and horizontal meridians in dark-adapted RP patients with orange and blue stimulus spots.[27] These colors were chosen because in the normal dark-adapted eye cones are more sensitive to orange than to blue, and rods are more sensitive to blue than to orange. Using different colors therefore allows for the measurement of retinal function of rods and cones across the retina. These authors correlated their results with the visual field in three patients with dominant rod-cone degeneration, but no classification of disease was performed.

Massof and Finkelstein in 1981 pursued this technique further, reporting that there were two basic degenerative mechanisms present, consistent within pedigrees, which they could separate on the basis of sensitivity profiles.[28,29] Those patients characterized by diffuse loss of rod sensitivity, which they called Group 1, report night blindness from infancy or childhood. Those patients characterized by regional combined loss of rod and cone sensitivity, which they called Group 2, report adulthood onset of night blindness. They found these two patterns in autosomal dominant, autosomal recessive, and simplex RP.

Ernst and co-workers further explored this technique by developing an automated static perimeter using light-emitting diodes with blue-green and red stimuli.[30] The advantage over using the Tübinger perimeter in which the test is manually performed is that patients can be more rapidly tested and their performances evaluated by computer analysis.

Using the automated two-color static perimeter, Lyness, Ernst, and colleagues[31] surveyed 104 patients from 44 pedigrees with autosomal dominant RP. Their studies suggested two genetic subgroups, one characterized by the loss of rod function, which was diffuse and severe. In the other group, there was loss of rod and cone function, which was regional.

Similarly, they found that the diffuse rod loss group did not have rod ERGs but had cone b-waves greater than 20 microvolts (i.e., rod-cone degeneration). Their regional loss patients had both maximum rod and cone b-waves greater than 20 microvolts, but their report, because of its psychophysical orientation, did not compare the photopic and scotopic responses to each other; consequently, it is not possible to tell whether their patients had the cone-rod electroretinographic pattern, although the data certainly suggest this. Members of the diffuse rod dysfunction group have the onset of night blindness by age 10, while the regional loss group did not note night blindness until after the age of 20, similar to the pattern found in rod-cone and cone-rod degeneration, respectively. Many of their patients could not be classified because they had advanced disease.

PSYCHOPHYSICAL FLICKER TESTING

Tyler, Ernst, and Lyness reported photopic psychophysical flicker high-frequency sensitivity losses in simplex and multiplex RP,[32] and other studies by this group in X-linked heterozygote carriers of RP demonstrate abnormalities in modulation thresholds, with an usual peak in the 10-to-20-hertz region, which eventually may be useful in detecting X-linked carriers of RP.[33]

COLOR VISION TESTING

Many retinal degenerations affect the cones, giving color vision abnormalities. Since the mechanism of color vision is not well understood, it is not clear what significance, if any, should be placed on color vision abnormalities. This area of testing is further confused by the variety of tests available, including pseudo-isochromatic plates, Ishihara plates, Farnsworth-Munsell 15- and 100-hue tests, and the Nagel anomaloscope.[34–36] The most common color vision abnormality seen in RP is a tritanomalous change (blue-yellow axis), though deuteranomalous and even protanomalous changes are occasionally seen.[37] Fishman and colleagues examined 67 patients with various types of RP for color vision defects.[38] They found that when an atrophic macular lesion was present or if the visual acuity was less than 20/30, no patient had normal color vision. When no foveal lesion was present, autosomal dominant patients tested better in comparison with autosomal recessive and X-linked recessive patients. RP patients with cystoid macular edema tested better than patients with foveal lesions. They concluded that the Farnsworth-Munsell 100-hue test is a more sensitive test in RP patients than the Nagel anomaloscope.

Heckenlively evaluated color vision abnormalities in cone-rod forms of RP of all inheritance types; of 40 eyes, 37 had abnormal error scores on the Farnsworth-Munsell 100-hue test, even though the average visual acuity was 20/30.[39] Tritanomalous defects were the most common on testing.

Serial color vision studies over the natural history of the various types of RP have not been published, although there are many case reports available documenting color vision abnormalities in RP patients.

FLUORESCEIN ANGIOGRAPHY AND FUNDUS PHOTOGRAPHY

Fluorescein angiography and fundus photography have proven to be valuable clinical research tools and at times have been useful in management of RP. However, whether these procedures should be used routinely in a nonresearch setting is not clear, and depends on the rationale and method of practice of the clinician ordering the tests. While light toxicity has never been demonstrated from these procedures, a rare RP patient will complain bitterly that it may take as long as 6 weeks for his prephotography vision to return. However, most RP patients have no problem with these procedures. No RP patient at UCLA has demonstrated any identifiable loss from the procedure.

Fundus photography is useful for documenting the baseline appearance of the patient so that any subsequent fundus changes can be easily identified. Patients often will have questions regarding progression, or retinal changes from the disease may be clarified by the availability of fundus photographs. Because there are differences in retinal degenerative patterns, fundus documentation may eventually prove useful in retrospective identification of specific RP types or degenerative mechanisms. Occasionally, the management of complications associated with pigmentary retinopathy, such as Coats' reaction, retinal neovascularization, or cystoid macular edema, are aided by fundus photography and fluorescein angiography.

The fluorescein angiogram is particularly helpful in identifying cases in which the diagnosis of choroideremia is being considered (see Type III, Chapter 10), and is helpful in confirming the presence of cystoid macular edema. As a research tool the fluorescein angiogram has been useful in identifying retinal, choroidal, and disc telangiectasia, alterations in retinal vessels, generalized retinal edema, and patterns of damage to the RPE, whether localized or diffuse. A discussion of clinical findings of fluorescein angiography in RP can be found in Chapter 5.

Pedigree Analysis

JOHN R. HECKENLIVELY
JOANN A. BOUGHMAN
LORRAINE H. FRIEDMAN

The genetic aspects of RP and allied disorders are very important to the diagnosis, evaluation, and provision of service for patients. RP is a heterogeneous group of disorders, with multiple genetic forms having been described within the three main Mendelian inheritance patterns. Although RP patients are considered by definition to have a genetic disorder, the mode of inheritance often is not easily recognized. The classification of patients by genetic type is essential not only for appropriate counseling but also for identification of homogeneous groups of RP patients. In the past a number of clinical and biochemical investigations of RP patients were performed without attention to inheritance or the studies were performed in patients where the inheritance pattern had not been determined. This approach has often provided confusing results since it is difficult to determine pathophysiologic mechanisms when looking at a mixture of different diseases.

Principles of classic Mendelian genetics should be followed in properly evaluating patients with hereditary retinal degenerations. Patients and their families should be carefully questioned in a search for other affected family members. It is *not* sufficient to ask simply whether anyone else in the family is affected; a pedigree should be drawn with each family member identified and considered for the possibility of having the disease (**Fig.** 2-7). When careful consideration is given to each family member, a surprising number of reportedly affected family members (by historical symptoms or blindness) may be found, whereas nothing more than a negative family history may be obtained through casual questioning.

Once the family tree is obtained, it may be possible to identify a Mendelian inheritance pattern, or it may be that the pedigree will clearly be inadequate because the patient does not know his family history. When this occurs, the patient is asked to check with other family members who can assist him in filling in the information. In some cases, particularly when

family members are spread widely, it may take several visits before the inheritance pattern clarifies; occasionally, further information or investigations within a family will change the inheritance pattern to which a family originally may have been assigned.

MENDELIAN GENETICS

Since Mendel first recorded specific segregation patterns of traits in his pea plants, the field of genetics has expanded greatly. One of the basic axioms in genetics has been the use of Mendelian inheritance patterns to better understand the etiology of a large number of diseases; McKusick's *Catalogue of Mendelian Inheritance in Man,*[40] with a listing of more than 3368 genetic diseases inherited in the autosomal dominant, autosomal recessive, and X-linked patterns, attests to the usefulness of this approach. While finding a Mendelian inheritance pattern does not disclose the pathogenesis of a disease, it has served as a reliable way of classifying and separating similar-appearing disease states and has proven invaluable for genetic counseling.

The following section will briefly cover Mendelian

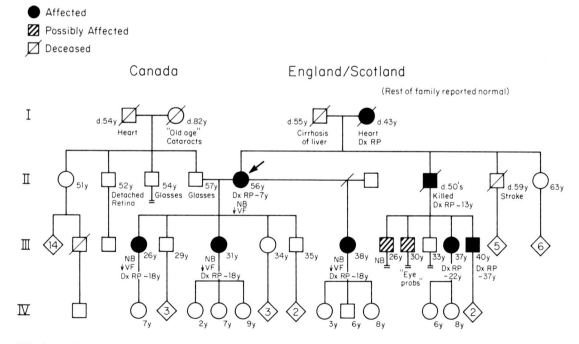

FIG. 2-7. Typical working pedigree of a family with autosomal dominant RP. Propositus is marked with an arrow. There are three known generations of affected individuals. Males are represented by boxes, females by circles; diamonds are used when the gender is unknown or for combining offspring where their status is unknown. Hatching is used in individuals whose history is vague but suggestive that they have the same disease as the propositus.

inheritance, as it is critical in the classification of RP, but the reader may wish to consult genetics texts for detailed explanations of the following mechanisms.

AUTOSOMAL DOMINANT INHERITANCE

Genetic traits are transmitted from generation to generation by genes, or groups of base pairs on DNA strands, which express themselves through various mechanisms as body components or functions. Autosomal dominant genes may show full expression of the trait or disease with only one copy of the gene present. There is a 50% chance of that particular dominant gene being passed to any offspring of the individual. A summary of the criteria for autosomal dominant inheritance can be found in Table 2-1. An example of an autosomal dominant RP pedigree is demonstrated in **Figure 2-8**.

Autosomal dominant diseases may have variable expressivity, that is, some affected patients may show milder signs of the disease or trait. Occasionally, a person with the gene may not show the disease at all, which is called nonpenetrance; an example of two individuals who demonstrate nonpenetrance of the autosomal dominant RP gene is shown in the pedigree in **Figure 2-9**. Conclusive evidence of au-

TABLE 2-1

DISTINGUISHING CHARACTERISTICS OF DOMINANT INHERITANCE

1. Trait is transmitted by affected person to 50% of the off-spring.
2. Unaffected persons do not transmit trait to their children.
3. Both sexes are affected equally on the average.
4. Trait appears in every generation.

tosomal dominant inheritance requires the demonstration of the disease in three successive generations, with both sexes showing equal effects of the disease. Male-to-male transmission is further proof that the pedigree is autosomal dominant and not an X-linked recessive family in which carriers are severely affected (Table 2-1).

AUTOSOMAL RECESSIVE INHERITANCE

In autosomal recessive inheritance, two copies of an identical gene must be present (in a double dose) in order for the trait or disease to manifest itself. In

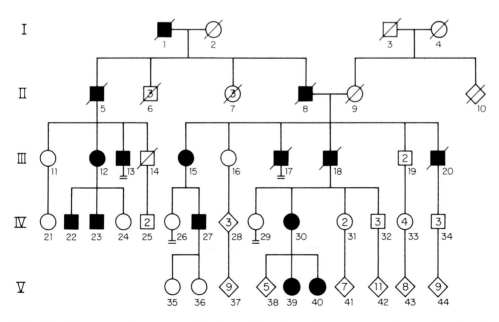

FIG. 2-8. Five-generation autosomal dominant RP pedigree; there are several examples of male to male transmission.

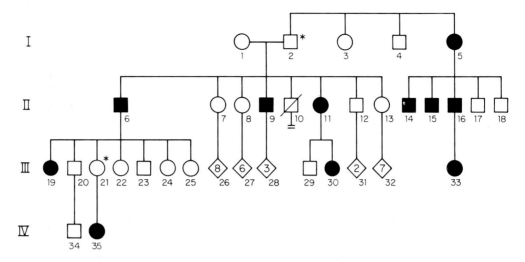

FIG. 2-9. Pedigree, autosomal dominant RP with incomplete penetrance of the gene. Three-generation pedigree of autosomal dominant RP; individuals I-2 and III-21 *(asterisks)* carry the gene since they have affected children although they show no sign of the disease.

some disorders, autosomal recessive carriers with one abnormal gene will have measurable changes or a subclinical disease state, but in general most autosomal recessive carriers are asymptomatic without measurable changes. Matings between relatives (consanguinity) is more commonly noted among parents of individuals with autosomal recessive diseases than in the general population. Consanguinity increases the probability that two individuals carry the same recessive genes. An example of a pedigree in which autosomal recessive inheritance in RP is demonstrated may be found in **Figure 2-10.**

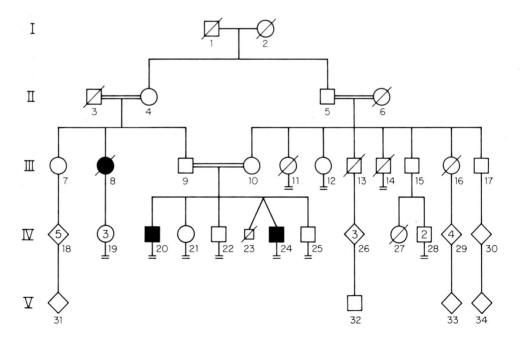

FIG. 2-10. Autosomal recessive pedigree in which there are several examples of affected individuals in different generations of both genders. In each case the affected individual was the product of a consanguineous marriage which increases the likelihood of expressing an autosomal recessive trait.

TABLE 2-2

CHARACTERISTICS OF AUTOSOMAL RECESSIVE INHERITANCE

1. Trait does not typically appear in every generation, may be sparsely scattered in a pedigree; when clustering of affecteds appears, it is in sibships.
2. When both parents carry the gene, there is a 25% chance for any one child to inherit the disease.
3. Sexes are equally affected.
4. Parents of affected child *may* be blood related.

When two carriers of an autosomal recessive trait mate, there is a 25% chance for each offspring to inherit two copies of the recessive gene and thereby exhibit the associated disease or trait; there is a 50% chance at each mating that the offspring will be a carrier, while there is a 25% chance that the offspring will not inherit the recessive gene. A summary of the criteria for autosomal recessive inheritance is presented in Table 2-2.

Occasionally, carriers of autosomal recessive disease will show mild abnormalities, such as in Usher's syndrome, Senior-Loken syndrome, cystinuria, sickle cell disease, and others.

X-LINKED RECESSIVE INHERITANCE

A trait or disease determined by a recessive gene carried on the X-chromosome is unique in its familial pattern. Males have only one X chromosome, so if they inherit the X-linked recessive gene from their mother they will be affected. If they are affected, they will give the X-linked gene to all daughters, who then have a 50% chance of passing the recessive gene to each offspring. Female carriers' daughters are, therefore, at a 50% risk of being carriers, and sons have a 50-50 chance of being affected (Table 2-3). A pedigree with X-linked recessive RP is presented in **Figure 2-11**.

The story is complicated further, since early in embryogenesis one X chromosome is inactivated in every cell of a female. This inactivation, called lyon-

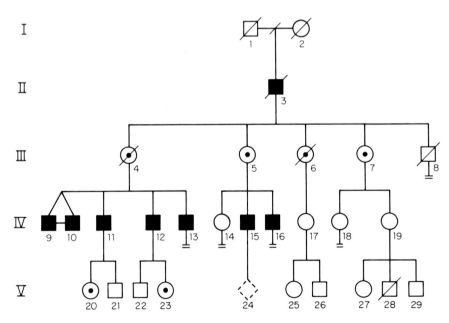

FIG. 2-11. X-linked recessive pedigree. Hemizygotes (female carriers) are denoted with a dot in the circle and are diagnosed by having affected male children, or they are the daughters of affected males and thus must inherit their fathers' X-chromosome. Some females at risk of carrying the gene for X-linked recessive RP or choroideremia, but who are not obligate carriers, such as IV-14, 17, 18, and 19, may be diagnosed by alterations seen on funduscopy.

TABLE 2-3

CHARACTERISTICS OF X-LINKED RECESSIVE INHERITANCE

1: Only males in pedigree are severely affected.
2. No history of male-to-male transmission.
3. Affected male gives the gene to all daughters, who give the trait to half their sons (on the average).
4. Incidence of trait in pedigree is almost all male (see discussion, lyonization).
5. Affected males in pedigree are related to each other through carrier female relatives.

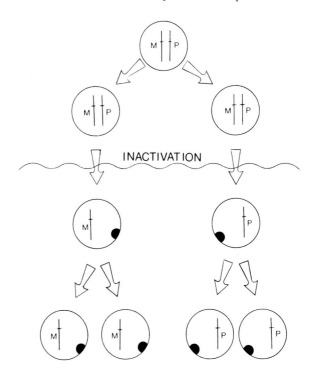

FIG. 2-12. Lyonization diagram. In females, early in embryogenesis one of the two X-chromosomes in every cell is randomly selected and is inactivated; therefore, in a heterozygote X-linked carrier of RP, on average, one-half of the X-chromosomes with the RP gene will be nonfunctional. But because the distribution of the inactivation fits a bell-shaped curve, a few carriers with a large percentage of inactivated normal X-chromosomes will be severely affected.

ization,[41] is random, so the X-linked recessive gene may be inactivated in some cells and the normal gene in the others (**Fig. 2-12**). This means that on the average about half of the cells of an X-linked recessive carrier female will have X-chromosomes containing the active abnormal gene. Since the distribution of affected cells is random, a bell-shaped curve would be representative of the number of cells affected or unaffected for a group of carriers. In practical terms this means that a few carriers will appear completely normal and some will appear to be affected to varying degrees with the disease or trait. X-linked dominant disease has never been demonstrated in the retinal dystrophies and will not be reviewed in this chapter. A summary of inheritance risk for offspring of the three Mendelian inheritance patterns is presented in Table 2-4.

SIMPLEX AND MULTIPLEX FAMILIES

A high percentage of RP patients present initially with no family history of RP; surveys in Europe and the USA have found that from 18% to 58% of patients have undefined or "sporadic" inheritance.[42] When there is only one affected member in a pedigree, the descriptive term *simplex* is used, while the term "sporadic" is generally avoided unless a mutational or environmental event is hypothesized. An example of a pedigree with simplex inheritance is presented in **Figure 2-13**. Simplex or isolated cases of RP may result from several mechanisms. First, since on the

TABLE 2-4

INHERITANCE RISK FOR OFFSPRING

GENE DISTRIBUTION IN PARENTS	NUMERICAL RISK*
One parent with autosomal dominant gene	50%
Both parents with one autosomal recessive gene	25%
One parent with autosomal dominant gene, history of nonpenetrance	Variable
Mother with X-linked recessive gene	
Sons	50%
Daughters (carriers)	50%
Father with X-linked disease	
Sons	0%
Daughters (carriers)	100%

* It is important to think of each pregnancy as an independent event, so the numerical risk remains the same for each, no matter what the prior occurrence has been.

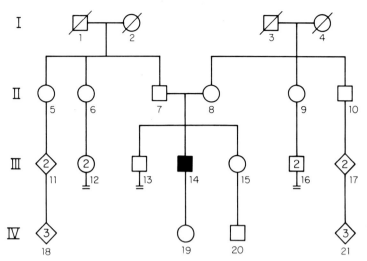

FIG. 2-13. Simplex RP pedigree. No other affected individuals are found even though a fairly extensive family history is obtained. While it might be assumed that this is an example of autosomal recessive inheritance, it could as likely be, for example, X-linked recessive in which prior RP members are unknown to the patient's mother, or a pigmentary retinopathy of nongenetic origin.

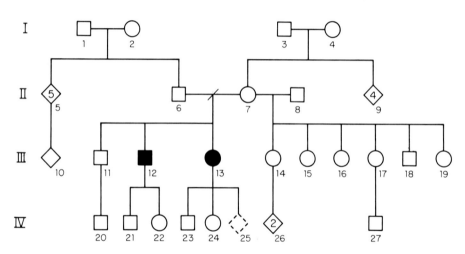

FIG. 2-14. Multiplex RP pedigree. Two affected individuals in the same sibship with no other affected members in the family. While this occurrence is stronger evidence for autosomal recessive inheritance, it still may not be conclusive evidence since nongenetic etiologies or unrecognized hereditary causes, such as autosomal dominant with incomplete penetrance in one of the parents, may be operating.

average only 25% of the offspring of carriers of autosomal recessive RP will be affected, many small families will by chance have only one affected individual. Genetic analyses have demonstrated, however, that there may be an excess of simplex families beyond probabilistic expectations.[43,44] The results of these analyses suggest that some additional factors, either genetic or environmental, may be important in the expression of RP in some cases.

Multiplex refers to families in whom more than one sibling is affected. A sample pedigree is presented in **Figure 2-14**; there are no other family members affected outside of the sibship. If other relatives are affected, other inheritance patterns must be considered. Although multiplex sibships do not all represent a single inheritance pattern, most are probably autosomal recessive. Several affected males and no affected females in a sibship, however, would be an indication to examine their mother, who may have carrier signs which would establish the diagnosis of X-linked recessive RP.

Authors commonly have assumed that simplex and multiplex RP patients always have autosomal recessive inheritance, but there is cumulative clinical evidence that these groups, particularly the multiplex patients, may not be expressing the disease in the same fashion as typical proven autosomal recessive RP patients. These differences are examined in Chapter 5. Another fascinating aspect of multiplex inheritance is that in a number of multiplex pedigrees the segregation ratio does not follow Mendelian rules in that frequently more than 25% of the siblings are affected. This higher percentage suggests that additional genetic factors may be operating.

Because RP represents a heterogeneous group of disorders, complications in clinical and research situations arise. Accurate recurrence risk data can be provided to families only if the mode of inheritance has been clearly delineated. For pedigrees meeting the criteria outlined above, Mendelian laws may be applied and resultant risk statistics for the inheritance of the gene provided (e.g., 50% for the offspring of an individual with autosomal dominant RP).

However, some pedigrees are incomplete where the family history may not be known, and in other cases the situation may be more complicated because variable expressivity or incomplete penetrance may be occurring. When the inheritance is unclear or complex, it frequently is necessary to examine other members of the family in order to obtain a reliable pedigree.

THE POPULATION PERSPECTIVE

RP may be an uncommon diagnosis among the patients in any one ophthalmologic practice, but in fact this group of disorders represents a relatively common form of genetic eye disease. Estimates of the frequency of RP in the general population vary among studies, with 0.25 per 1000 representing a conservative estimate. It is difficult to obtain accurate and comprehensive incidence figures, since many patients remain undiagnosed or are not ascertained in clinical studies.

Formal genetic studies take into account potential ascertainment biases, sex distribution, and family size. Application of genetic methods has permitted estimation of the proportion of the various genetic forms of RP. Some of these studies are summarized in Tables 2-5 and 2-6. Differences may in part be accounted for by selection procedures as well as methods of analysis. The distribution across studies is surprisingly similar, although the proportion of X-linked cases in the United Kingdom population is higher. The analytic methods used in the 1980 study were different, the proportion of "sporadic" being lower because it includes only the excess proportion of cases that could not be accounted for by recessive inheritance.

Some attempts have been made to characterize

TABLE 2-5

DISTRIBUTION (IN PERCENT) OF GENETIC TYPES OF RETINITIS PIGMENTOSA

INVESTIGATORS	YEAR	POPULATION	NO. PATIENTS	SIMPLEX "SPORADIC"	AUTOSOMAL RECESSIVE	AUTOSOMAL DOMINANT	X-LINKED
Pearlman[49]	1979	California	250	63	21	11	5
Boughman et al[50]	1980	USA	670	15*	69	10	6
Hu[51]	1982	China	151	48.3	33.1	11	7.7
Boughman & Fishman[52]	1981	Illinois	300	50	16.0	21.7	9.0
Jay M[53]	1982	England	426	42.1	15.5	24.4	18.0
Bunker et al[54]	1984	Maine	85	—	65	19	8
Heckenlively et al	1987	California	609	42.2	30.8	16.9	10.1

* Only that proportion of "simplex" not accounted for by probability alone

TABLE 2-6

DISTRIBUTION OF RP TYPES IN 609 PATIENTS, UCLA RP REGISTRY (1987)

PRIMARY DIAGNOSIS	FREQUENCY	PERCENT
Autosomal Dominant		
Rod-cone degeneration	47	7.7
Cone-rod degeneration	34	5.6
Nonspecific	6	1.0
Sector RP	11	1.8
Congenital onset	5	0.8
Autosomal Recessive		
Rod-cone degeneration	24	3.9
Cone-rod degeneration	12	2.0
Nonspecific	11	1.8
Usher I	35	5.7
Usher II	31	5.1
Preserved para-arteriolar RPE	6	1.0
Leber's amaurosis	15	2.5
Juvenile onset	4	0.6
Congenital RP with macular coloboma	8	1.3
Lawrence-Moon-Bardet-Biedl	19	3.1
Retinitis punctata albescens	4	0.6
Systemic RP types	18	3.0
Goldman-Favre	1	0.2
X-linked Recessive		
Rod-cone degeneration	23	3.8
Cone-rod degeneration	9	1.5
Nonspecific	1	0.2
Choroideremia	28	4.6
Simplex/Multiplex		
Rod-cone degeneration	73	12.0
Cone-rod degeneration	82	13.5
Nonspecific	52	8.5
Pigmented paravenous retinochoroidopathy	12	2.0
Pericentral RP	11	1.8
Unknown RP type	27	4.4
TOTAL	609	100.0

It should be noted that this is a biased sample, since data was inputed into the computer as patient's charts were available, and information on an additional 400 patients is currently not available.

the genetic types by studying clinical parameters or subclinical markers, but no procedure has been highly successful. Various forms of RP have been shown to have early onset of nyctalopia and specific refractive errors (see Chapter 5). Some specific ERG and ophthalmologic characteristics (as discussed earlier in this chapter and in Chapter 10) have been shown to occur in female carriers of X-linked RP. Some families with autosomal dominant RP have demonstrated specific ERG characteristics, such as delayed implicit times. Although the search continues for clinical correlates of specific genetic types of RP, the most characteristic aspect of all forms is the extreme variability in age of onset and progression of symptoms. Even within families, in which the same gene can be presumed to be operating, the clinical picture may vary considerably.

In the absence of clinical characteristics which differentiate RP types, new emphasis is being placed on the search for biochemical markers of specific forms of RP. Studies of marker loci linked to RP genes have shown promising results. Linkage studies first indicated in 1977 that one gene for autosomal dominant RP might be on chromosome 1.[45] More recently, the gene locus for X-linked RP[46 47] and for choroideremia[48] have been localized in the X chromosome using DNA markers. Recombinant DNA technology creates an essentially unlimited supply of markers by using different restriction enzymes and probes, making the possibility of mapping every single gene defect an eventual certainty.

In addition to determining inheritance patterns for accurate genetic counseling, the identification of homogeneous genetic entities is critical in research endeavors. The development and proper functioning of the retina are controlled by extremely complex biochemical and genetic processes. It is to be expected that several different defects might affect the photoreceptors and RPE, yet result in similar pathological deterioration (**Fig. 4-1**) (i.e., a retinal pigmentary degeneration is a common final pathway for a number of different diseases). The separation of RP types is a critical step in the process of determining the specific biochemical abnormalities responsible for the retinal degeneration and for the subsequent development of treatment protocols.

REFERENCES

1. Martin DA, Heckenlively JR: The normal electroretinogram. Doc Ophthalmol Proc Ser 31:135–144,1982
2. van Lith GHM: The macular function in the ERG. Doc Ophthalmol Proc Ser 10:405–415, 1976
3. Karpe G: The basis of clinical electroretinography. Acta Ophthal Kbh . 23(suppl):1–114, 1945
4. Björk A, Karpe G: The clinical electroretinogram. V. The electroretinogram in retinitis pigmentosa. Acta Ophthalmologica 29:361–371, 1951
5. Armington JC, Schwab GJ: Electroretinogram in nyctalopia. Arch Ophthalmol 52:725–733, 1954
6. Franceschetti A, Dieterle P: Die Differential diagnostische Bedeutung des Elektroretinogrammes bei tapeto-retinalen Degenerationen. Bibl Ophthalmol 48:161–182, 1957
7. Henkes HE, van der Tweel LH, Denier van der Gon JJ: Selective amplification of the electroretinogram. Ophthalmologica (Basel) 132:140, 1956
8. Armington JC, Gouras P, Tepas DI et al: Detection of the electroretinogram in retinitis pigmentosa. Exp Eye Res 1:74–80, 1961
9. Berson EL, Sandberg MA, Rosner B et al: Course of retinitis pigmentosa over a three-year interval. Am J Ophthalmol 99:240–251, 1985
10. Krill AE: Rod-cone dystrophies. In Krill AE, Archer DB (eds): Krill's Hereditary Retinal and Choroidal Diseases, pp 479–644. Harper & Row, Hagerstown, 1977
11. Berson EL, Gouras P, Gunkel RD. Progressive cone-rod degeneration. Arch Ophthalmol 80:68–76, 1968
12. Berson EL, Gouras P, Hoff M: Temporal aspects of the electroretinogram. Arch Ophthalmol 81:207–214, 1969
13. Berson EL, Gouras P, Gunkel RD et al: Dominant retinitis pigmentosa with reduced penetrance. Arch Ophthalmol 81:226–234, 1969
14. Berson EL, Simonoff EA: Dominant retinitis pigmentosa with reduced penetrance; further studies of the electroretinogram. Arch Ophthalmol 97:1286–1291, 1979
15. Berson EL: Hereditary retinal diseases: Classification with the full-field electroretinogram. Doc Ophthalmol Proc Ser 13:149–171, 1977
16. Berson EL, Gouras P, Gunkel RD et al: Rod and cone responses in sex-linked retinitis pigmentosa. Arch Ophthalmol 81:215–225, 1969
17. Berson EL, Rosen JB, Simonoff EA: Electroretinographic testing as an aid in detection of carriers of x-chromosome-linked retinitis pigmentosa. Am J Ophthalmol 87:460–468, 1979
18. Arden GB, Carter RM, Hogg CR et al: A modified ERG technique and the results obtained in x-linked retinitis pigmentosa. Br J Ophthalmol 67:419–430, 1983
19. Berson EL, Goldstein EB: The early receptor potential in sex-linked retinitis pigmentosa. Invest Ophthalmol 9:58–63, 1970
20. Steinberg RH: Interactions between the retinal pigment epithelium and neural retina. Doc Ophthalmologica 60:327–346, 1985
21. Arden GB, Barrada A, Kelsey JH: New clinical test of retinal

function based upon the standing potential of the eye. Br J Ophthalmol 46:449–467, 1962

22. Alexander KR, Fishman GA: Prolonged rod dark adaptation in retinitis pigmentosa. Br J Ophthalmol 68:561–569, 1984

23. Krill AE, Smith VC, Blough R et al: An absolute threshold defect in the inferior retina. Invest Ophthalmol Vis Sci 7:701–707, 1968

24. Weinstein GW, Maumenee AE, Hyvarinen L: On the pathogenesis of retinitis pigmentosa. Ophthalmologica 62:82–97, 1971

25. Weinstein GW, Lowell GG, Hobson RR: A comparison of electroretinographic and dark adaptation studies in retinitis pigmentosa. Doc Ophthal Proc Ser 10:291–302, 1976

26. Seiff SR, Heckenlively JR, Pearlman JT: Assessing the risk of retinitis pigmentosa with age-of-onset data. Am J Ophthalmol 94:38–43, 1982

27. Zeavin BH, Wald G: Rod and cone vision in retinitis pigmentosa. Am J Ophthalmol 42:253–269, 1956

28. Massof RW, Finkelstein D: Subclassifications of retinitis pigmentosa from two-color scotopic static perimetry. Doc Ophthalmol Proc Ser 26:219–225, 1981

29. Massof RW, Finkelstein D: Two forms of autosomal dominant primary retinitis pigmentosa. Doc Ophthalmol 51:289–346, 1981

30. Ernst W, Faulkner DJ, Hogg CR et al: An automated static perimetery/adaptometer using light emitting diodes. Br J Ophthalmol 67:431–442, 1983

31. Lyness AL, Ernst W, Quinlan MP et al: A clinical, psychophysical, and electroretinographic survey of patients with autosomal dominant retinitis pigmentosa. Br J Ophthalmol (in press)

32. Tyler CW, Ernst W, Lyness AL: Photopic flicker sensitivity losses in simplex and multiplex retinitis pigmentosa. Invest Ophthalmol 25:1035–1042, 1984

33. Ernst W, Tyler CW, Clover GC et al: X-linked retinitis pigmentosa: Reduced rod flicker sensitivity in heterozygous females. Invest Ophthalmol 20:812–816, 1981

34. Benson WE: An introduction to color vision. In Duane TD, Jaeger EA (eds): Clinical Ophthalmology, vol 3, chap 6. Philadelphia, Harper & Row, 1985

35. Retina and Vitreous, Section 4, Ophthalmology: Basic and Clinical Science Course, pp 84–93. San Francisco, American Academy of Ophthalmology, 1985

36. Franceschetti A, Francois J et al: Chorioretinal Heredodegenerations, pp 49–57. Springfield, IL, Charles C Thomas

37. Verriest G: Les deficiences acquises de la discrimination chromatiques. Mem Acad Roy Med Belg 2:35–327, 1964

38. Fishman GA, Young RSL, Vasquez V et al: Color vision defects in retinitis pigmentosa. Ann Ophthalmol 13:609–618, 1981

39. Heckenlively JR, Martin DA, Rosales TO: Telangiectasia and optic atrophy in cone-rod degenerations. Arch Ophthalmol 99:1983–1991, 1981

40. McKusick VM: Catalog of Mendelian Inheritance, 6th ed. Baltimore, Johns Hopkins University Press, 1983

41. Lyon MF: Gene action in the X-chromosome of the mouse (Mus musculus L.). Nature 190:372–373, 1961

42. Boughman JA, Caldwell RJ: Genetic and clinical characterization of a survey population with retinitis pigmentosa. In Cotlier E, Maumenee IH, Berman ER (eds): Clinical, Structural, and Biochemical Advances in Hereditary Eye Disorders, pp 147-166. Alan R Liss, 1982

43. Massoff RW, Finkelstein D, Boughman JA: Genetic analysis of subgroups within simplex and multiplex retinitis pigmentosa. In Berman E, Cotlier E, Maumenee I (eds): Birth Defects: Original Article Series, vol 18, pp 161–166, 1982

44. Jay M, Jay B: Families with retinitis pigmentosa: Problems in the analysis of sporadic, simplex and multiplex cases. Ophthalmologica Basel 185:61–64, 1982

45. Heckenlively JR, Pearlman JT, Sparkes RS et al: Possible assignment of a dominant retinitis pigmentosa (RP) gene to Chromosome 1. Ophthalmic Res 14:46–53, 1982

46. Bhattacharya SS, Wright AF, Clayton JF et al: Close genetic linkage between X-linked retinitis pigmentosa and a restriction fragment length polymorphism identified by recombinant DNA probe L1.28. Nature 309:253–255, 1984

47. Bhattacharya SS, Clayton JF, Harper PS et al: A genetic linkage study of a kindred with X-linked retinitis pigmentosa. Br J Ophthalmol 69:340–347, 1985

48. Lewis RA, Nussbaum RL, Farrell R: Mapping x-linked ophthalmic diseases. Provisional assignment of the locus for choroideremia to Xq13-q24. Ophthalmology 92:800–806, 1985

49. Pearlman JT: Mathematical models of retinitis pigmentosa: A study of the rate of progress in the different genetic forms. Trans Am Ophthalmol Soc 77:643–656, 1979

50. Boughman JA, Conneally PM, Nance WE: Population genetic studies of retinitis pigmentosa. Am J Hum Genet 32:223–235, 1980

51. Hu D: Genetic aspects of retinitis pigmentosa in China. Am J Med Genet 12:51–56, 1982

52. Boughman JA, Fishman GA: A genetic analysis of retinitis pigmentosa. Br J Ophthalmol 67:449–454, 1983

53. Jay M: On the heredity of retinitis pigmentosa. Br J Ophthalmol 66:405–416, 1982

54. Bunker CH, Berson EL, Bromley WC et al: Prevalence of retinitis pigmentosa in Maine. Am J Ophthalmol 97:347–365, 1984

3

Visual Fields in Retinitis Pigmentosa

JOHN R. HECKENLIVELY
HOWARD R. KRAUSS

Progressive visual field loss is one of the cardinal features of retinitis pigmentosa (RP) and a necessary finding in order to make the diagnosis. Because most RP patients initially present with a history and finding of visual field loss, serial visual field tests are not usually needed to confirm the diagnosis. However, if there is any doubt about whether a patient has RP, serial visual fields are requisite.

Examining the status of the visual field in patients with abnormal electroretinograms (ERGs) is an important step in detecting whether the patient has an RP-like process with constricted fields or signs of progressive visual field loss with ring scotomata, or stable peripheral fields as seen in patients with cone dystrophy.[1]

A few patients with pigmentary retinopathies from congenital rubella or toxic or inflammatory causes may have visual field loss (often asymmetrical), but a one-time retinal insult may be confirmed by relatively stable visual fields over time. Following patients from 5 to 10 years may be necessary to verify this stability.

In 1901 Gonin noted that visual field loss in RP began as a midperipheral annular scotoma with progression both outward and inward.[2] However, the findings on visual field testing depend on the stage of disease (Table 3-1); early findings typically include slight loss of vision in the superior peripheral field and scotomatous areas in the midequatorial field. In middle stages, multiple scotomatous areas become more confluent, so that partial to full-ring scotomata

TABLE 3-1

TYPICAL VISUAL FIELD FINDINGS IN RP

Constricted visual fields with or without peripheral islands

Superior field depression

Midequatorial scotomata (may be partial or advanced in which only central and peripheral islands remain)

Baring or enlargement of blind spot

Pseudoaltitudinal changes

Arcuate-like loss, usually representing paramacular loss connecting to blind spot (e.g., Fig. 3-5).

emerge. As the disease advances, the superior and nasal fields are lost, leaving a central island of field with elongated temporal islands. Obviously, in trying to summarize visual field findings in so many different diseases, there will be variability within patient populations and among diseases. Various examples of visual field changes in RP are presented in **Figures 3-1 to 3-10.**

In typical RP, the macular island of vision is quite resistant to the degenerative process. Whether this is due to the unique physiologic properties of the macula or redundancy of photoreceptors is not currently understood.

CONE-ROD VERSUS ROD-CONE DEGENERATION PATTERNS OF LOSS

Various features of visual field loss bear further discussion, particularly as they relate to rod-cone and cone-rod degenerative patterns. Distinctive visual field changes characteristic of cone-rod degeneration include ring scotomata nearer to fixation (5°–30°) than is typically seen in rod-cone degeneration

(30°–50°), pseudoaltitudinal loss, enlarged blind spots earlier in the disease process, and tight, concentric rings (similar to layers of an onion) with decreasing isopter size and intensity in later stages of the disease process (**Fig. 3-6A–E**).[3] The last finding is indicative of a demarcation line between normally and abnormally functioning retina.

Rod-cone degeneration patients more frequently show larger jumps in sensitivity on Goldmann kinetic perimetry between large and small isopters, although this finding is sometimes seen in patients with cone-rod patterns (**Fig. 3-7A and 3-10A**).

Both groups may show baring or enlargement of the blind spot, a feature that also is frequently found in patients with choroideremia.

Pigmented paravenous retinochoroidal atrophy (see Chapter 11) is a distinctive degenerative pattern wherein fundus changes are localized to areas adjacent to retinal veins.[4] Visual field disturbances include many changes seen in other RP subtypes, but these patients often uniquely demonstrate radial scotomata corresponding to the paravenous atrophic areas (**Fig. 3-11**).

(Text continues on p. 35)

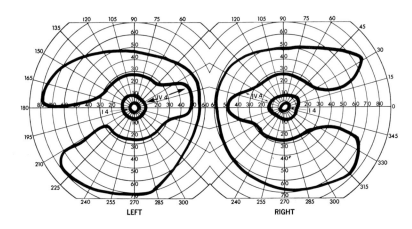

FIG. 3-1. Goldmann visual field of a 53-year-old woman with simplex cone-rod degeneration demonstrating contracted fields with a I-4-e isopter, ring scotoma, nasal extension, and temporal breakthrough with IV-4-e isopter.

FIG. 3-2. Goldmann visual field *(top)* and Octopus static perimetry *(bottom)* of a 33-year-old man with autosomal dominant rod-cone degeneration with retained central vision, superior depression, and mid-peripheral ring scotoma formation.

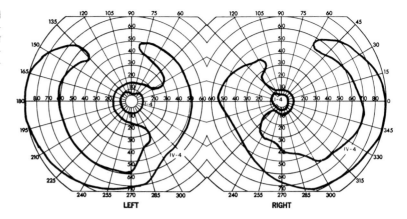

A

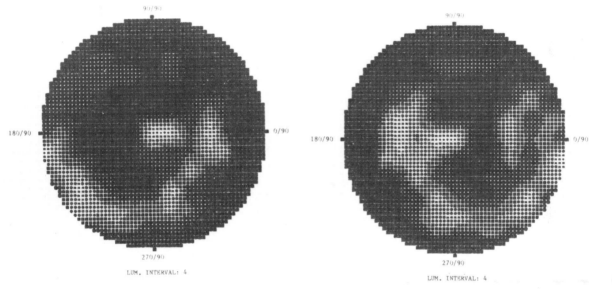

B

C

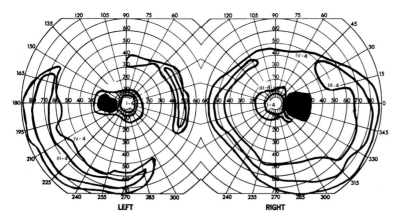

FIG. 3-3. Goldmann visual field *(top)* and Octopus static perimetry *(bottom)* of a 46-year-old man with choroideremia demonstrating enlargement of the blind spot, preserved central field, and large equatorial scotoma with superior depression.

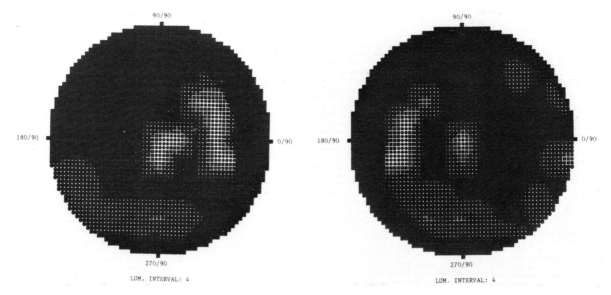

A

B

C

FIG. 3-4. Goldmann visual field studies in an 11-year-old boy with autosomal recessive cone-rod degeneration performed in 1976 *(top)* and 1980 *(bottom)* showing superior field depression (pseudoaltitudinal defect with small isopter) and progressive development of ring scotomata from 10° to 20°.

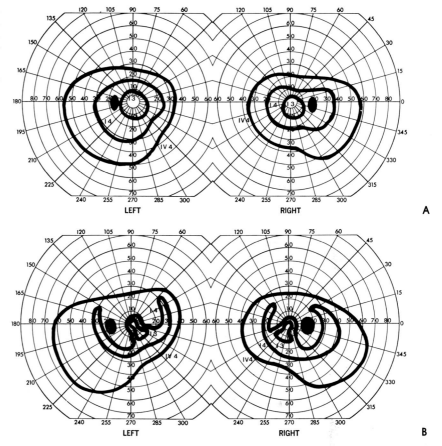

FIG. 3-5. Octopus visual field in a 30-year-old woman with early simplex cone-rod degeneration demonstrating "tight" partial ring scotomata near fixation and connecting to blind spots.

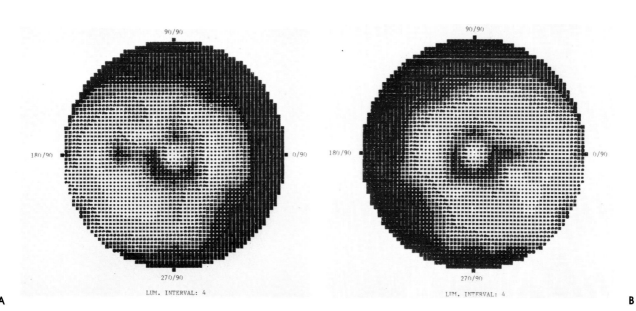

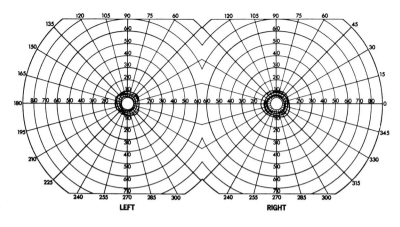

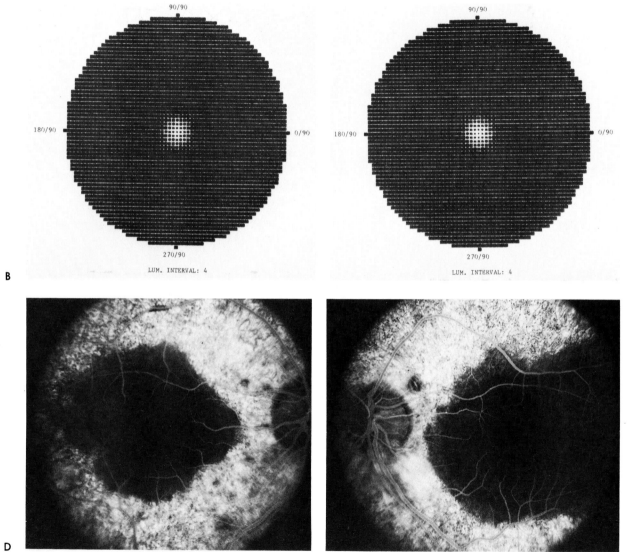

FIG. 3-6. A 27-year-old man with simplex cone-rod degeneration. *(A)* Goldmann visual fields demonstrate sharp (onion-like) layers to decreasing isopter size. *(B & C)* Octopus perimetry shows central preservation, and *(D & E)* fluorescein angiography shows only an intact macular island of RPE with a fairly sharp demarcation between normal- and abnormal-appearing retina. Concentric onion-like isopters, when present, are typically seen in patients with cone-rod degeneration.

FIG. 3-7. Goldmann visual fields of multiplex cone-rod degeneration of a 48-year-old man with an affected sister who demonstrates contracted visual field and enlarged blind spot in 1977 *(top)*, which progresses to ring scotomata with preserved central fields and several peripheral islands *(bottom)*, which are closer to fixation than seen in rod-cone degeneration.

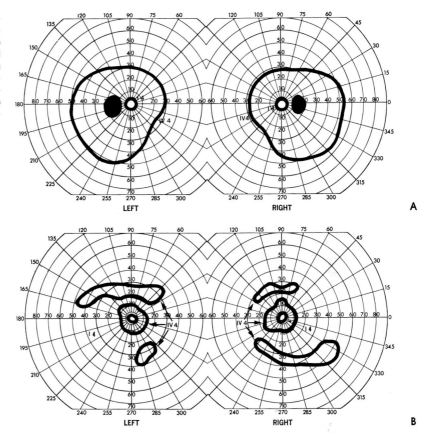

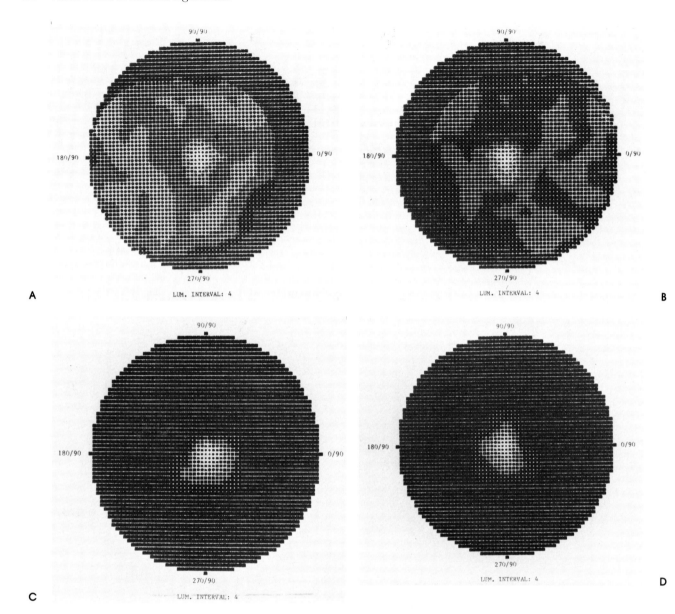

FIG. 3-8. Octopus visual fields of a 23-year-old man with Usher syndrome I with *(top)* midperipheral depression greater than far peripheral and *(bottom)* progression of visual field loss with only the central 10°-to-15° field remaining 4 years later.

FIG. 3-9. Goldmann visual field in simplex cone-rod degeneration performed in 1975 *(top)* and 1980 *(bottom)* demonstrating baring of blind spot, progression to superior field loss with the central field connected inferiorly to a peripheral island, with ring scotoma formation. This type of pattern *(bottom)* is commonly seen but is not limited to patients with X-linked RP.

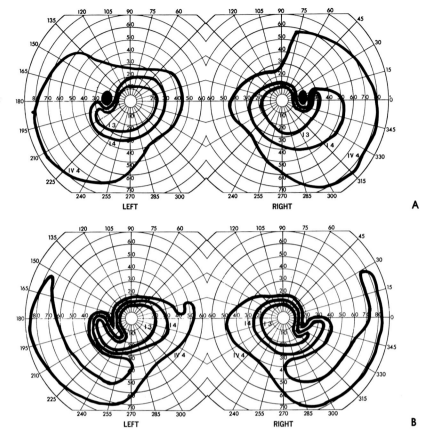

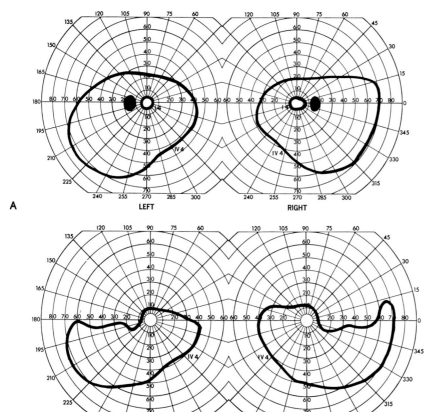

FIG. 3-10. Goldmann visual fields in autosomal recessive cone-rod degeneration in a 25-year-old woman in 1975 *(top)* and 1980 *(bottom)* showing contracted fields and later superior pseudoaltitudinal field loss.

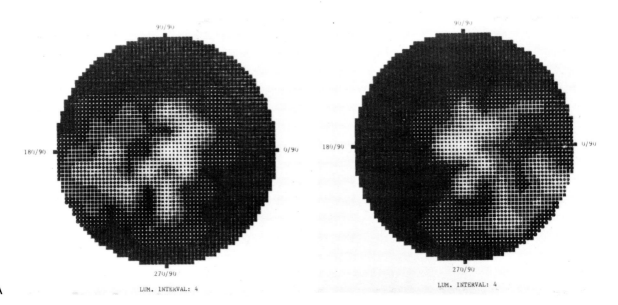

FIG. 3-11. Octopus visual fields in simplex-affected 26-year-old man with paravenous retinochoroidal atrophy showing nasal contraction and radial socotomata corresponding to paravenous areas seen on direct ophthalmoscopy.

SYMMETRY OF FIELDS

Patients with hereditary retinal disease normally have symmetrical findings between eyes, and when asymmetry is found on ERG, visual field, or fundus evaluation, nonhereditary causes for the pigmentary retinopathy must be considered (see Chapter 11). Massof found a high degree of interocular symmetry in 60 typical RP patients he examined,[5] and other authors have noted the importance of symmetrical findings to the diagnosis.[6,7]

FIELD SIZE AND NYCTALOPIA

In a number of RP patients, particularly those with cone-rod degeneration or "regional" loss, there is residual rod function; most of these patients do not describe difficulties with night vision until their visual field is less than 10°, after which they rapidly notice nyctalopia (see Table 5-3).

NATURAL HISTORY

Berson and colleagues examined visual field changes over a 3-year period in 92 RP patients; they found 21% worse and 16% better after 1 year, and 33% worse and 14% better at 3 years. Overall, they calculated about a 5° decline in field diameter over the 3-year interval with the V-4-e target. On average, their patients lost 4.6% of *remaining* visual field (not of total visual field) per year.[8] Occasionally, rapid progression is seen in an individual patient; such an example is seen in **Figure 3-8**, representing a 23-year-old patient with Usher syndrome who demonstrated a rapid loss of field over a 4-year period.

Sunga and Sloan evaluated 25 RP patients for periods up to 34 years. They concluded that the rate at which visual function is lost varies greatly even among affected members of the same family.[9]

VARIABILITY OF FIELD TESTING

Psychophysical testing, by its nature, is subjective and shows variability; factors that contribute to this inconstancy include patient and tester alertness and fatigue, variation in stimulus presentation, lack of calibration of equipment or between different pe-

rimeters, and changes in patient fixation. Parrish examined variability in normal subjects using static and kinetic perimetry, repeating the tests five times within a month.[10] Greater variability was seen with static perimetry in peripheral areas. With kinetic testing, higher standard deviations were found in temporal quadrants.

Ross performed variability studies in RP patients, examining interpatient visit and interexaminer variability.[11] RP patients of all genetic types were tested randomly by two examiners, with most of the patients completing their second visit within a 3-week period. A normal control group was used for comparison. Area and linear measurement of field size were obtained. Mean variability between visits was 4% to 6% in controls, compared with 10% to 16% in the RP population. The mean variability in the control subjects between two experienced field examiners was small, about 2% to 6%.

Many RP patients will announce on a particular visit that their visual field testing either went well or poorly depending on whether they are having a good or bad day (see "Good days, bad days" in Chapter 5). Some patients also demonstrate field loss during or immediately after a severe systemic illness or influenza, and vision usually recovers to pre-acute illness levels. Occasional histories of field loss in women undergoing pregnancy or child delivery appear to be uncommon, with only one of seven women evaluated during pregnancy at UCLA showing field loss after delivery (unpublished data).

METHODS OF PERIMETRY

Most recent reports of visual field studies of RP patients have used Goldmann kinetic perimetry or Octopus automated static perimetry with evaluation of the full field of vision. Tangent screen analysis may be useful for documentation of changes in the central field, but alone it is inadequate for evaluation of the RP patient because it ignores the 30°-to-40° region of field wherein lies much of the abnormality. Static perimetry is more accurate in determination of luminance sensitivity of specific points than is kinetic perimetry, but to map accurately the defects of an RP patient may be unreasonably time-consuming, since several programs may need to be run for each eye. The full-field quantitative Octopus program (#24) does not take long to run, but each test point is 15° away from the next adjacent point, allowing for serious gaps and misinterpretation of the true visual field based on interpolation, Therefore, we prefer to use the Goldmann kinetic perimetric technique in following RP patients with additional use of Octopus perimetry in selected cases, allowing a more accurate mapping of scotomata.

ISSUE OF LEGAL BLINDNESS

The definition of legal blindness in the U.S.A. was established by an act of Congress. As stated in the Social Security Act, blindness is defined as lens-corrected central visual acuity of 20/200 or less in the better eye, or limitation in the field of vision of the better eye such that the widest diameter of the visual field subtends an angle no greater than 20° (*i.e.,* a 10° field). This definition does not adequately cover RP patients who have tiny central fields, huge ring scotomata, and functioning anterior retina with temporal islands. On testing, an examiner may pick up the strip of functioning anterior retina and com-

pletely miss the huge ring scotomata surrounding the small central field (*e.g.,* Fig. 3-3 *top right*). These RP patients are functionally legally blind but might be excluded by an adverse interpretation of the law. Clearly these patients should be eligible for disability benefits. Weighted field loss determinations such as the Esterman technique[12] would appear to provide a fairer representation of visual disability than would a linear addition of arc of remaining field in the eight principal meridians.

STATIC PERIMETRY AS A RESEARCH TOOL

Two basic degenerative patterns have been delineated comparing perimetric measures of rod sensitivity to cone sensitivity. Massof and Finkelstein defined one group of RP patients with diffuse rod disease, and a second group with regionalized and combined loss of rod and cone sensitivity.[13-15] Similar findings have been found in RP patients by the Moorfield RP Research Group in a series of papers by Ernst, Arden, and Lyness.[16-19]

REFERENCES

1. Heckenlively JR, Martin DA, Rosales TO: Telangiectasia and optic atrophy in cone-rod degenerations. Arch Ophthalmol 99:1983–1991, 1981
2. Gonin J: Le scotome annulaire dan la degenerescence pigmentaire de la retina. Ann Oculist 125:101–130, 1901.
3. Krauss HR, Heckenlively JR: Visual field changes in cone-rod degenerations. Arch Ophthalmol 100:1784–1790, 1982
4. Heckenlively JR, Kokame GT: Pigmented paravenous retinochoroidal atrophy. Doc Ophthalmol Proc Ser 40:235–241, 1984
5. Massof FW, Finkelstein D, Starr SJ et al: Bilateral symmetry of vision disorders in typical retinitis pigmentosa. Br J Ophthalmol 63:90–96, 1979
6. Biro I: Symmetrical development of pigmentation as a specific feature of the fundus pattern in retinitis pigmentosa. Am J Ophthalmol 55:1176–1179, 1963
7. Pearlman JT: Retinitis pigmentosa: An improved clinical approach. Doc Ophthalmol Proc Ser 235–238, 1977
8. Berson EL, Sandberg MA, Rosner B et al: Course of retinitis pigmentosa over a three-year interval. Am J Ophthalmol 99:240–251, 1985
9. Sunga RN, Sloan LL: Pigmentary degeneration of the retina: Early diagnosis and natural history. Invest Ophthalmol 6:309–325, 1967
10. Parrish RK, Schiffman J, Anderson DR: Static and kinetic visual field testing. Arch Ophthalmol 102:1497–1502, 1984
11. Ross DF, Fishman GA, Gilbert LE et al: Variability of visual

field measurements in normal subjects and patients with retinitis pigmentosa. Arch Ophthalmol 102:1004–1010, 1984
12. Esterman B: Grids for scoring visual fields. Arch Ophthalmol 79:400–406, 1968
13. Massof RW, Finkelstein D: Two forms of autosomal dominant primary retinitis pigmentosa. Doc Ophthalmol 51:289–346, 1981
14. Massof RW, Finkelstein D: Subclassifications of retinitis pigmentosa from two-color scotopic static perimetry. Doc Ophthalmol Proc Ser 26:219–225, 1981
15. Massof RW, Finkelstein D: Vision threshold profiles in X-linked retinitis pigmentosa. Invest Ophthalmol 18:426–429, 1979
16. Ernst W, Faulkner DJ, Hogg CR et al: An automated static perimetry/adaptometer using light emitting diodes. Br J Ophthalmol 67:431–442, 1983
17. Lyness AL, Ernst W, Quinlan MP et al: A clinical, psychophysical, and electroretinographic survey of patients with autosomal dominant retinitis pigmentosa. Br J Ophthalmol 69:326–339, 1985
18. Arden GB, Carter RM, Hogg CR et al: Rod and cone activity inpatients with dominantly inherited retinitis pigmentosa: Comparisons between psychophysical and electroretinographic measurements. Br J Ophthalmol 67:405–418, 1983
19. Arden GB, Carter RM, Hogg CR et al: A modified ERG technique and results obtained in X-linked retinitis pigmentosa. Br J Ophthalmol 67:419–430, 1983

4

Pathologic Findings and Putative Mechanisms in Retinitis Pigmentosa

JOHN MARSHALL
JOHN R. HECKENLIVELY

The inherited pigmentary retinopathies comprise a disparate group of genetically determined conditions which differ from one to another in their modes of inheritance, their patterns of sensory loss, and occasionally their ophthalmoscopic appearance. Only a few distinct disease entities have been recognised within this group, and in no primary type is there comprehension of the underlying etiology.

One helpful subdivision in relation to these patients is made on the basis of their subjective symptoms. In those patients with early night blindness, a primary loss of rod function is implied, and on examination these patients are found to have loss of vision in the midzone of the visual field and morphological changes in the post-equatorial fundus. Electroretinographic testing in the earlier stages of these patients usually demonstrates a rod-cone degeneration, and psychophysical tests reveal diffuse rod dysfunction, with minimal cone dysfunction.

Some patients with inherited pigmentary retinopathy have a later onset of night blindness, and most though not all of these patients are found to have a cone-rod degeneration on the electroretinogram (ERG). Their psychophysical tests show loss of both cone and rod function.

In contrast to these two main divisions of retinitis pigmentosa (RP), in which rod dysfunction plays such an important role, patients with cone dystrophies have diffuse cone dysfunction, often with macular degeneration. The loss of visual function is noted in relation to cones, and the morphological changes are seen primarily in the central fundus. It can be assumed that the pathogenesis of conditions within the RP and cone dystrophy groups is through a spectrum of metabolic disorders that cause degeneration or dysfunction either primarily or secondarily of rods, cones, or a combination of both.

Recent knowledge concerning the involvement of the retinal pigment epithelium (RPE) in the maintenance of photoreceptor cell homeostasis has added a new set of factors to the putative causal agents in these diseases.

Table 4-1 summarizes histopathologic studies in RP.

(Text continues on p. 42.)

TABLE 4-1

SUMMARY OF HISTOPATHOLOGIC STUDIES IN RP

Autosomal Dominant

MEYER[124]

Clinical: Two brothers, aged 56 and 63, with advanced disease; correlation of histopathologic and clinical findings in living family members. Autopsy material.

Light: Underlying areas of bone spicules, RPE depigmented; partially degenerated areas show confluent drusen with overlying pigmented RPE. Glial hyperplasia optic nervehead, surface wrinkling of retina.

EM: Basal deposits in RPE.

KOLB[106]

Clinical: 68-year-old woman from 4-generation pedigree; 6 months before her death her visual acuity was OD 20/30, OS 20/25 with 8° visual fields. Fundus examination showed arteriolar narrowing and extensive peripheral pigmentation to retina.

Light: Remaining photoreceptors were in fovea contiguous with RPE. Outer nuclear layer nuclei reduced. Retina atrophic outside foveal area. Choriocapillaris appeared normal.

EM: Only photoreceptors found were cones. Outer segments were shorter with disorganized and disoriented discs. Inner segments distended. Foveal RPE cells were sliding over each other. RPE filled with lipofuscin, and melanin granules were rare. Peripheral RPE filled with dense, round melanin granules. Bone corpuscle-like pigmentation was composed of RPE devoid of lipofuscin and filled with dark, round melanin granules.

RODRIGUES[135]

Clinical: 66-year-old man whose father and two sisters had RP. Constricted fields, attenuated retinal vessels, posterior subcapsular cataract documented.

Light and EM: In areas of bone spicule pigmentation, RPE was found extending to level of inner limiting membrane. Choriocapillaris moderately occluded in severely affected areas. Foveal 20% reduction in cones. RPE in preserved areas stated to have changes consistent with the patient's age.

Biochemistry: Cyclic GMP was lower and cyclic AMP higher than controls. Interphotoreceptor retinoid-binding protein was low.

DUVALL[127]

Clinical: Two brothers with pigmentary retinopathy in which nyctalopia presented late (fifties). Central vision was reduced in both patients. The EOG was reported flat and ERG reduced in one patient. Areas of circular RPE loss seen in transition area between severely and mildly involved areas. Atypical RP, pericentral form.

Light: Photoreceptor layer atrophied except macula, where photoreceptors with stunted outer segments were occasionally seen in one brother, while the other had some peripheral rods and cones which were shorter and disorganized. In the RPE, melanin and lipofuscin granules confined to apical aspect. A thick basal deposit was present on the retinal surface of Bruch's membrane in both brothers with irregularly occurring nodules protruding towards the retina. The choriocapillaris was patent in most areas.

EM: Bruch's basement membrane missing. Filamentous structure seen to deposit external to RPE. Scanning EM showed frond-like appearance to subretinal deposit.

RAYBORN/HOLLYFIELD[111,136]

Clinical: 79-year-old woman who noted visual loss at age 57 and who was diagnosed as having RP and "bilateral papilledema." At age 72, the patient's vision was HM OU. Both optic discs were gray-white and atrophic. Severe chorio-retinal atrophy was noted with bone spicule pigment noted nasally.

Light: Foveal cones were present but reduced in number. Abrupt transition from nearly normal to retinal atrophy and gliosis. Choriocapillaris was present in macula and greatly reduced to absent in other areas.

EM: In central areas with photoreceptors, the RPE had normal thickness and no drusen below the basal surface. Bruch's membrane filled with fine vesiculated electron-lucent profiles. In abnormal retinal areas, the RPE had reduced apical to basal height, loss of melanosomes, and presence of drusen. Choriocapillaris under the fovea had normal fenestrations, but the endothelium was thick with·no fenestrae in other areas.

TABLE 4-1 *(continued)*

SUMMARY OF HISTOPATHOLOGIC STUDIES IN RP

Biochemical: In nondegenerate regions, marked accumulation of ³H-GABA by Müller cells was seen. Uptake of ³H-muscimol, a GABA analog, was decreased, indicating few GABAergic neurons remained. ³H-dopamine cell terminal sites were decreased. Tritiated Mannose labeling was more pronounced in cone photoreceptors than rods, the reverse of the normal control.

Autosomal Recessive

LAHAV[107]

Clinical: 46-year-old man, product of consanguineous marriage; two affected brothers. Visual problems from childhood. Exact inheritance not known.

LM: Retinal architecture disorganized. RPE atrophy, hypertrophy, intraretinal migration. Focal areas of RPE proliferation often continuous with intraretinal perivascular pigmented cells.

EM: Variable melanin content RPE. Electron-dense globular bodies in RPE apical region. Amorphous deposits outside basement membrane. Scanning EM showed sieve-like appearance of retinal architecture.

X-Linked Recessive

SZAMIER[110]

Clinical: 24-year-old man (hemizygote) with affected brother and maternal uncle, and mother with carrier signs. He reported night blindness at age 10, and by age 24 his visual acuity was OD 20/80 and OS 20/50. Visual fields were constricted, and dark adaptometry showed no evidence of rod-cone break and a 4.0 log unit elevation of the final rod threshold at 11° but near normal thresholds in the far periphery.

EM: Foveal cones reduced by 50% and had shortened and distorted outer segments. Foveal inner segments twice normal diameter with swollen mitochondria. Peripheral retina had both rods and cones with shortened outer segments with RPE villi which were distended. The RPE in the most affected areas had basally placed nuclei and large numbers of melanolysosomes and lysosomes. The choriocapillaris was normal.

SZAMIER[137]

Clinical: 79-year-old asymptomatic heterozygote (carrier) who had a 35-year-old son with advanced RP. On fundus examination, she had retinal vascular attenuation, equatorial and peripheral areas of bone spicule pigmentation, and retinal atrophy.

Light and EM: Patchy involvement of the mid- and far peripheral retina; inner retina was intact except over severe areas of photoreceptor degeneration. In transition zones, rod outer segments were truncated with pyknotic nuclei while cone pedicles were normal. A few RPE cells extended between photoreceptor cells to the external limiting membranes, and photoreceptors in these areas were abnormal. The choriocapillaris was normal in all areas.

Choroideremia

RODRIGUES[138]

Clinical: 19-year-old asymptomatic man (hemizygote) with typical fundus findings of choroideremia who died of injuries received in a diving accident. Mother had typical pigmentary stippling of midperipheral retina.

Light: In affected area, marked degeneration of outer and midportions of retina with loss of RPE and Bruch's membrane, and absence of choriocapillaris. RPE and choriocapillaris were present in areas where photoreceptors were retained.

EM: Macrophage-like cells with trilaminar structures; remnants of photoreceptors were adherent to these cells.

Biochemistry: Interphotoreceptor retinoid-binding protein reduced, cyclic AMP higher in RPE-choroid complex tested.

McCULLOCH[139]

Clinical: Five eyes are reported, four from elderly and one from a 43-year-old man whose left eye was enucleated for a tumor.

Light: Extensive atrophy of choroidal vascular, RPE and Bruch's membrane. Middle and inner retina relatively uninvolved. Optic nerve was abnormal with increased glial tissue within septa and mild cystoid degeneration among axons in neural channels.

(continued)

TABLE 4-1 *(continued)*

SUMMARY OF HISTOPATHOLOGIC STUDIES IN RP

KRILL[140]

Clinical: 84-year-old woman from known pedigree with choroideremia. Her visual acuity was 20/50 OU. There were granular peppery areas in the mid- and far periphery. She was asymptomatic.

Light: RPE had alternating areas of atrophy and pigment clumping. Retinal structures were normal.

Simplex

BUNT-MILAM[113]

Clinical: 31-year-old man found to have choroidal melanoma in one eye. The patient has an identical twin, who also has RP. The family history was negative for RP.

Light: Photoreceptors were reduced and outer segments absent in region of poorest vision. In area of best vision, outer segments were shortened and disorganized. RPE in some areas were reduplicated, depigmented, while pigmented RPE cells or macrophages appeared to be invading retina.

EM: Apical pyramid-shaped villi of RPE were filled with melanin granules and enclosed short cone but not rod outer segments. Inner segments had swollen mitrochondria.

MIZUNO[120]

Clinical: Case 1 was a 74-year-old man with reduced vision and night blindness from youth. There was no family history, and serum tests for syphilis were negative. He had a sudden attack of glaucoma OD. The visual field in the left eye was 10° and visual acuity 0.3.

Case 2 was a 51-year-old man with a 25-year history of night blindness with a visual acuity of OD 0.06, OS 0.05. Visual fields were constricted to 2°–3° in both eyes. Marked retinochoroidal atrophy was noted. Family history is not mentioned. When the patient's left eye was being repaired for a stab wound, prolapsed retina and choroid were excised and examined.

Light: In case 1 some cones were seen, blood vessels had hyaline degeneration. Choroidal changes not seen. Case 2 had no retinal visual cells, and the RPE was atrophied.

EM: Case 1 had irregularly thickened RPE basement membrane, and the various layers were hard to discern. Basal infoldings less frequent. Melanin granules greater than usual in apex of RPE. Variable findings seen with cones. Degeneration of the photoreceptors coincided with attenuation of basal infoldings and thinning of basement membrane of RPE.

Case 2 had a thin Bruch's membrane though the collagenous fibers were denser. Parts of RPE had balloon-like appearance, other areas were atrophied with scanty mitochondria.

Syndromes

Bardet Biedl (Laurence-Moon-Bardet-Biedl)

STANESCU[142]

Clinical: A 28-year-old man with mental deficiency, obesity, hypogonadism, polydactyly, RP. Foveal and parafoveal yellowish patches.

Light: Retinal atrophy, external limiting membrane intact, ganglion cells reduced in number, RPE "massively proliferated" with pigmentary isles migrated in the superficial layers.

EM: None

Laurence-Moon-Biedl

RUNGE[112]

Clinical: A 4-year-old boy, born full-term from an unremarkable pregnancy. He was normal at birth except for polydactyly consisting of one complete extra toe on each foot. Failure to thrive developed by 4 months. By 6 months, he was admitted for evaluation and found to have renal failure, although the IVP and cystogram were normal. At 10 months, photophobia was noted, and by 13 months, occasional nystagmus was present, which was continuous by 14 months, at which time the fundus examination was normal. Evaluation under anesthesia showed +5.00 refractive errors O.U. Rod ERG was reported markedly subnormal, and flicker response reduced. By age 2 years, 3 months, optic nervehead pallor, attenuated vessels, and RPE alterations were noted. By 3 years, 10 months, peritoneal dialysis was started, and renal transplantation performed. By 4 years, posterior subcapsular cataracts were present. He had several episodes of graft rejection and died of associated complications.

TABLE 4-1 *(continued)*
SUMMARY OF HISTOPATHOLOGIC STUDIES IN RP

Light: The most severe changes were seen in the macula. The outer segments were lost, and the inner segments were swollen. The RPE was filled with lipofuscin in a concentration that would be found in eyes 20 years older. In the midperiphery, outer segments were shortened and disoriented in relation to the surface of the RPE.

EM: Central RPE were packed with lipofuscin granules, melanolysosome, and melanolipofuscin. Apical and basal membranes had reduced microvilli and convolutions, respectively. More peripheral areas had whorls or sheets of membranous outer segments which covered the apical surface of the RPE and extended into the extracellular space between adjacent cells. In the cone inner segments, outophagic vacuoles, reduced mitochondria, and dissolution of the myoid region were seen, while in the outer cone segments, discs were misaligned and disoriented. An inadequate phagocytic process is hypothesized.

Cockaynes

LEVIN[143]

Clinical: A 44-month-old black male who died of bronchopneumonia, with two affected sisters. One died of sudden infant death syndrome at the age of 8 months, and at autopsy the brain was small with diffuse cerebral demyelination. The other sister developed regressive mental changes, bird-like facies, salt-and-pepper fundi, optic atrophy, cataracts, peripheral neuropathy; she died at age 55 months of pneumonia, and autopsy revealed a small brain with diffuse demyelination. The male patient showed motor developmental delay. While he would follow objects with each eye, he had nystagmus, unreactive pupils to light, salt-and-pepper pigmentary retinopathy with vessel attenuation. Urine metabolic screening tests were normal in patient and his older sister. Autopsy revealed atrophic cortical white matter, diffuse calcification of cortex, globus pallidus, putamen, and cerebellum.

Light: Ganglion cell layer and other nuclear layer reduced, outer segments absent, inner segments reduced. Rods and cones equally affected. RPE intact, with loss of pigment granules. Choroid and choriocapillaris normal. Optic nerve fiber bundles reduced.

EM: No abnormal inclusions in retinal neurons or RPE. Excessive lipofuscin present in RPE.

Kearns-Sayre

McKECHNIE[143]

Clinical: Atypical case. Simplex case with psychomotor delay, admitted to hospital with pancytopenia, age 13 months; recovered after blood transfusion. At 7 years, he had short stature, mental retardation, cerebellar ataxia, dysarthria, bilateral ptosis, progressive external ophthalmoplegia, macular atrophy, sensorineural deafness, and generalized muscle weakness. Metabolic studies showed partial growth hormone deficiency and primary hypoparathyroidism. Muscle biopsy showed ragged red fibers. At age 12, he had a cardiac pacemaker for heart block. Patient died at age 14 of heart failure.

Light: Photoreceptors absent except posterior pole. RPE cells present. Peripheral retina showed complete atrophy. Patchy preservation of RPE–photoreceptor complexes.

EM: RPE had loss of apical microvilli and basal infoldings, was devoid of melanosomes, and had no evidence of phagocytosis of photoreceptor debris. The RPE cytoplasm had numerous enlarged mitochondria. There were numerous macrophages in subretinal space.

RUNGE[112]

Clinical: The patient was normal until 8 months, when she was noted to be pale, and bone marrow red cell hypoplasia was found. Failure to thrive with height and weight below 10th percentile. Renal failure was diagnosed at age 9 years, and a renal transplant was performed at age 11. Visual acuity at age 9 was 6/9 OU, extraocular movements normal, and ERG reported normal. By 12 years, visual acuity was 6/36. Cerebellar and cerebral atrophy with ataxia were noted by age 12, and seizures began at age 9 years. Hearing loss was severe by age 12. Neurological examination at age 12 years revealed marked ptosis, muscle wasting, hyeflexia. Muscle biopsy showed ragged red fibers. EKG showed left bundle branch block and left anterior hemiblock.

Light: RPE contained sparse melanin. Midperiphery showed most degeneration with focal areas of denuded Bruch's membrane exposed to remnants of interphotoreceptor matrix or recolonized by amelanotic cells. Beneath areas of RPE loss, the choriocapillaris was correspondingly lost. Throughout the retina, outer segments were in poor condition; where inner and outer segments survived, they were juxtaposed to RPE.

EM: RPE and inner segments were missing many of their organelles including melanin granules and lipofuscin in the RPE, and mitochondria in both. Atypical mitochondria cristae seen in inner segments. Globular lipid-like inclusions seen in rod outer segments.

(continued)

TABLE 4-1 *(continued)*

SUMMARY OF HISTOPATHOLOGIC STUDIES IN RP

Refsum

    TOUSSAINT[145]

Clinical: 44-year-old woman with profound weakness, ataxia, muscle wasting, loss of deep tendon reflexes. She had generalized icthyosis, intentional tremor, and was blind and deaf.

Light: Receptor layer missing, outer nuclear and outer plexiform layers atrophic. Inner nuclear layer thinned and ganglion cells reduced in number. Nerve fiber layer thickend by gliosis. RPE was uniformly loaded with lipid material, as were the sclera, trabecular meshwork, and iris.

EM: None

CONCEPTS OF PATHOGENESIS IN INHERITED RETINAL DYSTROPHIES

In general, hereditary disorders are caused by defects in the genetic code, which, in turn, result in an abnormal amino acid composition of specific proteins. If a defective protein is coded by a gene whose activity is confined to a single cell type, the primary effect will be localized in that cell type, even though secondary effects may occur in other cells. Thus, the effects of defective coding for a visual cell protein will be restricted primarily to the type of visual cell containing that protein. Alternatively, a systemic metabolic abnormality may result in the degeneration of a specific cell type, such as visual cells, by depriving them of vital metabolites or causing disruption of some metabolic process.

During the past 20 years, knowledge of the micrometabolism of retinal cells has increased immensely, particularly with regard to the interactions between the photoreceptor cells and the RPE.[1] One of the most significant findings pertinent to the etiology of the receptor dystrophies is that the light-sensitive disk membranes in the outer segments of the photoreceptor cells are being renewed throughout life.[2-4] This process involves multiple steps, each of which may require specific proteins and enzyme systems for fulfillment. Since each of these processes has to be integrated with the next, there are abundant opportunities for defects in the genetic codes to disturb renewal mechanisms and lead to cell abnormalities or death.

That a defect in cell support systems may cause retinal dystrophies is not a new concept, but recent work has served to identify some of the specific metabolic attributes of receptor cells that may be involved in the pathogenesis of these disorders.

THE NORMAL SYSTEM

METABOLIC INPUT

The main stages in the process of photoreceptor maintenance are illustrated in **Figure 4-1**. Blood-borne metabolites within the choriocapillaris are free to diffuse out of the vessel lumen through fenestrations in the endothelial lining. They pass through Bruch's membrane and into the extracellular spaces both beneath and between the RPE cells. Free diffusion into the neural retina is prevented by junctional complexes, zonulae occludens, which occur between the apical portion of the lateral membranes of adjacent epithelial cells. These junctions constitute a blood–retinal barrier.[5] In contrast, the basal membrane of the RPE is highly convoluted and contains specific receptor sites,[6] which enable metabolites to be actively accumulated within the RPE.[7] Inside the epithelial cells, those molecules required by the photoreceptor cells are transported by special intracellular carrier proteins[8-10] to the apical surfaces of the underlying RPE cells. This surface is specialized in two ways: first, it possesses microvilli, and, second, special sheaths of RPE surface membrane envelope the tips of the photoreceptor cells. It would seem that rapid transport could be achieved by transfer from these sheaths directly into the outer segments, but autoradiographic evidence from animals shows that metabolites are actively accumulated in the inner segments of the photoreceptor cells and that, in some cases, this may involve extracellular diffusion[11] via the inter-receptor matrix.[12] Whatever the route, uptake into the photoreceptor cells requires the existence of specific receptor sites within their cell membranes. The necessary molecular moieties, having accumulated within the inner segments of the photoreceptor cells, are then utilized

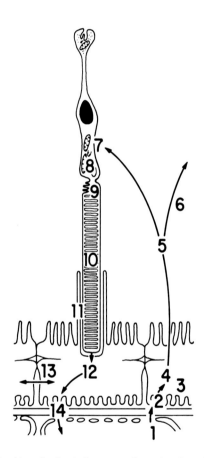

FIG. 4-1. Hypothetical diagram of mechanisms that may be involved in the degeneration of photoreceptor cells: *(1)* uptake or transport defect, *(2)* abnormal membrane receptor sites in RPE, *(3)* intracellular RPE metabolic defects, *(4)* transepithelial transport defect, *(5)* RPE to photoreceptor donor defect, *(6)* RPE to other retinal cells (e.g. Müller cells) defect, *(7)* abnormal sites in photoreceptor cell, *(8)* micrometabolism malfunctions, *(9)* faulty membranogenesis, *(10)* inability to stabilize membranes, *(11)* malfunction in phagocytosis, *(12)* malfunction in lysis, *(13)* defective RPE lateral transport and communication, *(14)* inability to void lytic products.

in the metabolic processes essential for both cellular renewal and integrity.[13] After synthesis, the proteins, glycoproteins, and phospholipids begin to move to various cellular locations. A considerable portion of the protein, much of it now complexed with carbohydrate and possibly lipid, moves through the cilium to reach the photoreceptor outer segment.[14]

PHOTORECEPTOR RENEWAL

There is a striking difference between the renewal systems in rods and cones. In rods the newly formed proteins are incorporated into small membranous outgrowths in the outer segment portion of the cilium (**Fig. 4-2A**). By a complex mechanism of membrane fusion and migration, these outgrowths are eventually embodied into the rod outer segments and form the hollow, coin-like disk membranes. Each disk is a discrete structure isolated from both its neighbors and the boundary membrane of the rod. With successive disk production, units are progressively displaced down the outer segment toward the RPE. In monkeys the outer segment transit time for a disk is 9 to 13 days,[15] and since each rod contains approximately 1000 disks, between 30 and 100 new disks are made each day. In normal eyes there is a high degree of membrane stability in the disks, and no structural differences can be detected between new and old structures. To prevent large fluctuations in rod length, old disks are removed from the tips of the outer segments by phagocytic action of the pigment epithelium.[16] This process seems to be initiated by the onset of light[17,18] but may also be mediated by hormones, since a diurnal rhythm of disk shedding is exhibited even in prolonged periods of darkness.[18,19] The exact mechanism whereby rod disks are shed is also a subject of debate, with some workers having opined that there is active ingression of the retinal pigment epithelial sheath into the tips of the rod cells,[20] and others having suggested a passive role for the pigment epithelium in response to an active shedding of spent disks by the rods.[3] But whatever the mechanism, the phagocytosis of the disks depends upon the triggering of membrane recognition sites within the apical membrane of the RPE.[21–24]

Experimental studies on cones are more difficult

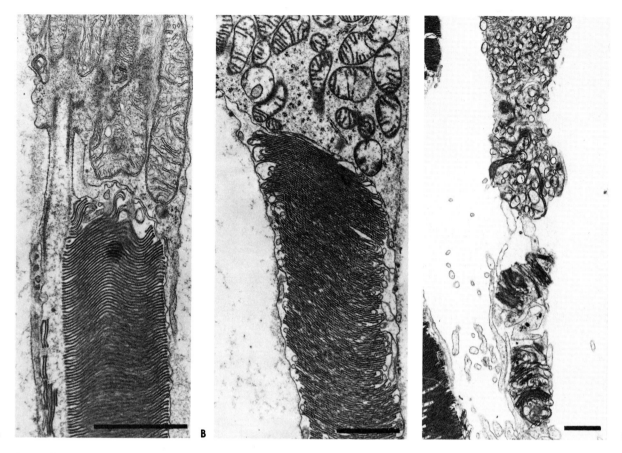

FIG. 4-2. Electron micrographs of normal human photoreceptor cells; *(A)* a 30-year-old rod, *(B)* a 28-year-old cone, and *(C)* a 78-year-old cone showing age-related membrane changes. (The bar markers are I μm.)

to interpret. This is because the light-sensitive membranes in the cone outer segments do not form discrete disks but are a continuum (**Fig. 4-2B**).[25] Thus, since newly formed proteins are free to diffuse to any part of the cone outer segment membrane, radioactive tracer studies on cones always show a random and diffuse distribution of the label.[4] Nevertheless, there is morphological evidence of cone renewal[13,16,26] with cone shedding at night. It would seem, however, from studies of cone function after detachment surgery[27] and of cone morphology during aging[28] that the capacity for membrane replacement in cones is less well developed than that of rods (**Fig. 4-2C**).

RETINAL PIGMENT EPITHELIUM PHAGOCYTOSIS AND DIGESTION

Once inside the RPE, the group of disks, engulfed in a phagosome, undergo lysis, which results in their progressive degradation.[29–31] Some of the breakdown products of this process may be recycled back to the photoreceptor cells, but others are voided into the choriocapillaris via Bruch's membrane. The RPE is a system of normally nondividing cells, and with increasing age there is a net loss of cells from this layer with a resulting increase in size of those remaining. Coupled with this reduction in available cells, both the lytic and voiding capabilities of those remaining seem to decline, resulting in the accumulation of incompletely degraded phagosomal particles called lipofuscin granules (**Fig. 4-3A**).[32] In the absence of disease, lipofuscin becomes apparent within the RPE by the age of 10 years, and by the age of 40 years occupies some 8% of the cytoplasmic volume of the cells.[33] By 80 years of age, this figure has risen to more than 20%.

The lipofuscin granules seen within the RPE cells of the elderly[34–36] have been attributed to the retention of incompletely degraded remnants of phago-

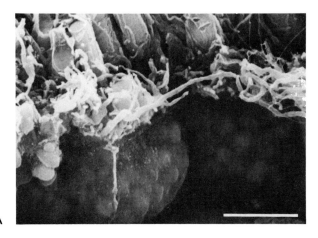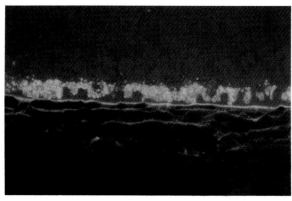

A

B

FIG. 4-3. *(A)* Scanning electron micrograph of the junctional zones between the photoreceptor cells and the RPE, and the RPE and Bruch's membrane of a 30-year-old man. The lateral margins of the RPE cells are displaced by the numerous underlying granules of lipofuscin. (The bar marker is 5 μm.) *(B)* Fluorescent light micrograph to demonstrate the brilliant yellow autofluoresence of lipofuscin within the RPE of a 43-year-old.

cytosed photoreceptor outer segments.[29,37] They are comparable to the lipofuscin granules described in many other parts of the body, such as the central nervous system and the myocardium, which are considered to be the oxidized and polymerized residues of inadequate lysosomal hydrolysis.[38] In nonocular tissues the evidence suggests that they originate from the catabolism of mitochondria and various forms of intracellular lipid.[39] Since lipofuscin is not extruded from the cell but slowly accumulates with the passing years, it is particularly obvious in the tissues of older individuals. In the context of the RPE, the heavy demands on lysosomal activity caused by the need to dispose of engulfed photoreceptor material may increase the predisposition to lipofuscin formation. The situation is complicated by the presence of melanin, which although apparently exposed to lysosomal enzymes,[40] appears to be little affected by them.[41] In some instances, particles of melanin pigment and lipofuscin granules occur in the same organelle.[34] There are, consequently, several terms describing the various types of residual body seen in the retinal pigment epithelium[34]:

1. Lipofuscin granules. These are golden brown, autofluorescent residues of incomplete lysosomal hydrolysis of phagocytosed and endogenous lipid (Fig. 4-3*B*).

2. Melanolysosomes. These are formed by the fusion of melanosomes with primary lysosomes.

3. Melanolipofuscin. This presents as melanin with a surrounding rim of lipofuscin and represents a residual body formed by the fusion of the partially degraded products of a melanlysosome with one or more lipofuscin granules.

Recently some interesting observations have been obtained from studies on human RPE cells grown in culture. First, it is well established that the rate of cell division in culture depends upon the age of the donor from whom the cells were obtained, with fastest growth curves being displayed by cells from the young.[42,43] This finding relates to the decline in rates of cell division in open or dividing systems observed in vivo. The new observation is that in any given individual, cells derived from the macula grow less well than those from the retinal periphery, and that this differential increases with age.[44] A major difference between cells obtained from these two locations is that those from the macula contain more lipofuscin than those from the periphery.[36]

There are potential specific implications for the degeneration pattern seen in RP from the differential growth pattern seen in equatorial versus macular RPE. Since a higher potential for division is found in equatorial RPE, any process which causes dysfunction in the RPE with subsequent visual loss will result in a scotoma, and the location being such, this will produce a ring scotoma in many patients. Conversely, it is possible that the low potential for division found in macular RPE may be in some fashion related to the preservation of central vision in typical RP. While this explanation is currently speculative, until the growth differences between macular and peripheral RPE was noted, there had been no good explanation for the ring scotomata so commonly seen in RP.

In a further series of experiments, Boulton and Marshall have shown that if retinal pigment epithelial cells of any age are artificially fed lipofuscin granules in their culture media, cell division and metabolic activities are reduced as lipofuscin content increase, and beyond a certain critical level the cells die.[45] From these studies it would appear that the onset of senescence in the RPE is at least in part due to the accumulation of lipofuscin, which in turn reflects the demands made upon it by the constant phagocytic load of photoreceptor cell membranes.

It may well be that this age-related decrement in performance of the RPE acts synergistically with the gene defect in those diseases in which the gene expression is within the RPE, and the combined effects of inheritance and aging eventually result in cell death. This would to some extent explain the long time course seen in many of the retinal dystrophies and also the acceleration in disease processes in later years.

THE ABNORMAL SYSTEM

In a number of conditions involving degeneration of visual cells, it is now possible to identify specific malfunctions in their maintenance cycle (**Fig. 4-1**). Much of this knowledge is derived from experimental studies, particularly in animals with inherited retinal dystrophies. Although the relevance of such animal homologues to human disease is tentative, they remain our best opportunity to comprehensively study diseased retinal tissue of genetically induced origin other than tissue culture.

SYSTEMIC DISORDERS

Systemic disorders may result in a secondary degeneration of visual cells (**Fig. 4-1**). A recent example

of this is the finding that cats fed on a taurine-free casein diet developed both plasma and retinal taurine deficiency followed by a central degeneration of rods and cones.[46-48] In humans the visual problems associated with an absence of vitamin A (retinol) from the diet have been known for some time[49-51] and arise through an inability to replenish the rod retinal pigment rhodopsin (retinol plus a protein, opsin). The initial symptoms are highly variable and presumably relate to storage levels of the vitamin in the liver and RPE, but eventually a rise in both rod and cone dark adaptation thresholds is noticed and in extreme cases "night blindness" results. In protracted studies on animals, the visual cells are seen eventually to degenerate.[52,53] The similarities in symptoms between this deficiency and the RP group of diseases had led to extensive investigations of vitamin A levels in the blood of the latter, with a profusion of claims and counterclaims in the literature. However, no convincing relationships have been discovered,[54,55] and no beneficial results have been obtained by administering this vitamin to RP sufferers.[56-58]

Other workers have suggested that the RP group of disorders may be the result of a problem of retinol availability, and that they may arise through a malfunction in the serum carrier lipoprotein for this vitamin. They hypothesize that the retinol-binding protein may be present in too low a concentration to be effective or that its binding properties are altered in some way to make it either inefficient in carrying retinol or hyperefficient and therefore unable to release bound retinol. There is no evidence concerning the second of these hypotheses, and that relating to the first is confusing. In a group of RP patients with a variety of modes of inheritance, Rahi[59] reported a low serum retinol-binding protein level, but a more recent study found no significant variation between affected individuals and those from control groups.[60]

The most persuasive evidence against vitamin A deficiency as a cause of RP is derived from the work of Ripps and colleagues,[61] in which it was demonstrated that the rhodopsin concentration of the rods differed markedly between a limited number of patients with RP and one patient with vitamin A deficiency. These findings have been confirmed[62] and imply that investigation of vitamin A metabolism is unlikely to reveal abnormalities in RP patients unless it can be demonstrated in some patients that rod sensitivity is reduced to below that of cones with a small reduction of rhodopsin concentration only.

A similar systemic defect resulting in degeneration of visual cells is seen in the Bassen-Kornzweig syndrome, a condition in which the primary defect seems to interfere with synthesis of the protein component of serum β-lipoproteins in the liver. Because these serum lipoproteins normally transport lipids through the blood, plasma lipid fractions, including vitamin A, are markedly reduced in this disease. Visual cell degeneration probably ensues as a result of a derangement in the renewal of lipids in the disk membranes.[63]

TRANSPORT AND METABOLIC PATTERNS

There is little experimental evidence for a deficit in the supply of metabolites (stages 2–5, **Fig. 4-1**) being responsible for visual cell loss, although the isolation of the photoreceptor cells from their metabolic input is presumed to be fundamental to the degenerative changes seen in retinal detachment.[64] Investigations of receptor sites in the basal membranes of RPE cells in animals with inherited retinal dystrophies indicate that such sites are similar to those of unaffected animals.[6] Little is known about the mechanism of transepithelial transport, but a failure of this system may give rise in part to the receptor degeneration seen in Refsum's syndrome. This latter is an autosomal recessive disease in which the defect is an absence or deficiency of the enzyme that oxidizes phytanic acid, so that abnormally high levels of this substrate build up in the blood.[65] Phytanic acid is a fatty acid similar to palmitic acid (branched); furthermore, experimental studies have shown that rod outer segment renewal systems become disorganized if fatty acids (polyunsaturated) are withheld from the diet,[66] but subsequent investigation has shown this issue to be unclear.[67] In Refsum's syndrome the earliest symptom is night blindness, and this is followed by a pigmentary retinopathy, progressive visual field loss, partial deafness, as well as other systemic manifestations (see Usher section,

chapter 12). Receptor degeneration is associated with huge lipid deposits rich in phytanic acid within the RPE.[68,69] Such findings may be interpreted as indicating either a failure in the transepithelial transport of fatty acids, or a limited ability to degrade phagocytosed particles of rod outer segments containing abnormal lipid components. A number of carrier proteins have been isolated from the interreceptor matrix, but as yet no fault associated with these systems has been implicated in any receptor dystrophies.

In recent years, increasing attention has been given to the micrometabolism of the photoreceptor cells and in particular to those systems concerned with the manufacture and functional stability of the outer segment membranes. A common biochemical defect has been identified in early-onset retinal dystrophies in three different species of animals: rats,[70] mice,[71] and dogs.[72] In each of these animals there is evidence of an abnormality in the cyclic nucleotide metabolism, leading to the death of photoreceptor cells. In the early 1970s it was suggested that cyclic nucleotides may be involved in transduction.[73] Subsequently, a light-activated phosphodiesterase was discovered in rod outer segments,[74] which catalyzes the hydrolysis of guanosine 3'5'-monophosphate (cGMP). In neurons of other tissues, the cyclic nucleotides are cofactors for a kinase able to catalyze the phosphorylation of a membrane protein which is believed to control membrane permeability to ions. The discovery that under certain conditions there is a correlation between the permeability of the rod outer segment membrane and the level of cGMP confirmed the suggestion that cyclic nucleotides are involved in transduction. In both the C3H mouse and the dystrophic Irish setter dog, photoreceptor cells do not become fully developed and subsequently degenerate, owing to an accumulation of cGMP arising from deficiency in cGMP-phosphodiesterase activity. The causal relationship between the elevation of cGMP and photoreceptor cell degeneration has been confirmed in vitro using normal eye rudiments of *Xenopus laevis* cultured in the presence or absence of phosphodiesterase inhibitors.[70] In the latter studies the addition of cGMP-phosphodiesterase inhibitor (isobutylmethylanthine) to the culture always resulted in an elevation of cGMP, followed by disorganization and death of the visual cells. The authors postulated that since cGMP is fundamental to the basic function of rod photoreceptors, inherited dystrophies affecting visual cells may arise from errors in cGMP metabolism. Their conclusions are supported by the findings that cGMP metabolism is also disturbed by a feedback mechanism emanating from the extracellular outer-segment debris in the Royal College of Surgeons (RCS) dystrophic rat.[75]

PHOTORECEPTOR MEMBRANE REPLACEMENTS AND STABILITY

Even in cells with a normal metabolic support mechanism, the light-sensitive membranes contained within the visual cell outer segments may be induced to undergo degenerative changes by relatively mild changes in their environment. Perhaps the most surprising finding concerning the response of visual cells to environmental change was that described by Noell[76]; in a series of experiments laboratory rats were exposed to fluorescent lamps which produced a maximum cage illumination of 2500 lux. Exposure varied for periods up to 24 hours, and animals were examined subsequently using electrophysiologic and histologic techniques. It was found that the visual cells in these animals degenerated and that the rate of degeneration could be altered by changing either the duration of the light exposure or the illuminance. Noell considered that this damage was photochemical and resulted from the build up of some toxic photoproduct, although attempts to identify such products were unsuccessful. Strangely, however, it was found that a dietary deficiency of vitamin A reduced the damaging effects of light exposure.[77,78] Subsequent work has supported Noell's findings and extended them to diurnal species.[79-84] Further, it has been demonstrated that if RCS rats are deprived of light, the rate of degeneration is retarded[4,85] and that a similar decrease in degeneration occurs if the animals are deprived of vitamin A.[86,87] These findings resulted in some workers suggesting that RP sufferers should occlude one eye in hope that such light deprivation would extend their visual life.[88] However, there is increasing evidence that cones are more sensitive to light-induced damage than rods[82,89-91] and that this sensitivity may not represent a different threshold for damage, but may be related to differences in membrane replacement mechanisms.[92] Rods have an incremental repair system, making 10 to 100 disks per day, so that if some of their outer segments are damaged by phototoxic substances, they can rapidly resynthesize and replace damaged membranes by disk displacement. The confluent nature of cone membranes means that the whole unit must be replaced if it is damaged. This difference may also explain the differences in aging of the two types of photoreceptor cells, since it has been observed that after the fifth decade, degenerative changes are increasingly apparent in the outer segments of cone cells (**Fig. 4-2**).[28,93] Perhaps there is a synergistic relationship between the light history of an eye and aging processes; if so, limiting light input may theoretically be of benefit. In experimental studies in monkeys, the stabilized image of the indirect ophthalmoscope has been shown to result in focal degeneration of photoreceptor cells,[94-96] and RP patients always complain about the persistent decrement in their visual performance after ophthalmic examinations. There is no direct evidence, however, that any particular type of RP is made worse by extensive light exposure, though the question of light toxicity in RP needs futher evaluation.

RETINAL PIGMENT EPITHELIUM PHAGOCYTOSIS AND LYSIS

A failure of the phagocytic relationship between the photoreceptor cells and the RPE will lead to degenerative changes in the photoreceptor. Such a situation arises in the RCS strain of rat, in which the RPE shows an absolute inability to phagocytose the disks shed from overlying rod cells. The spent disks progressively accumulate between the tips of the visual cells and the apical surface of the RPE.[85,97-99] There are four primary mechanisms by which such a development could occur[100]:

1. The RPE lacks some component necessary for phagocytosis.

2. The rod outer segment either lacks an essential

inducing agent, or possesses an inhibiting agent that precludes phagocytosis.

3. Both mechanisms above are present in some combination and contribute collectively.

4. Complementary defects are present in the rod outer segment and the RPE such that disease manifestations are expressed only when both defects are combined.

Until recently, most of the experimental evidence seemed to indicate that the primary abnormality was in the outer segments of the receptor cell.[24,100,101] However, that the fault occurs solely within the RPE was elegantly demonstrated in a series of experiments by Mullen and LaVail.[102] These workers created chimeric rats by first flushing out eight-cell embryos from the oviducts of both normal and dystrophic animals, then aggregating them in culture overnight before implanting the fused blastocysts into the uteri of pregnant or pseudopregnant females. By using albino dystrophic animals and combining them with pigmented normal individuals, the distribution of the RPE in the resultant chimera represented a mosaic of both genotypes. In such animals, degeneration of the photoreceptor cells occurred only in relation to areas of nonpigmented epithelium. Clearly, given the complex and separate sequences of invagination and differentiation undertaken by the RPE and neural retina during their embryonic development, it is unlikely that areas of dystrophic retina would always come to lie adjacent to dystrophic RPE.[103] This led the authors to conclude that in RCS rats, the genetic defect is expressed soley within the RPE. Recent work has both confirmed and refined these conclusions, and demonstrated that the defect is not in the initial part of the phagocytic mechanism (i.e., binding and recognition), but occurs in the middle stages of ingestion or engulfment.[104] It appears that in the RCS rat there is a massive reduction of ingestion of outer segment particles. Although there is no direct evidence of failure of the phagocytic mechanism in any of the human dystrophies, subretinal membranous deposits could account for both the small white dots in the fundus of many RP patients and for the hypofluorescent or dark choroid effect seen in some types of RP, bull's-eye dystrophies, as well as fundus flavimaculatus (although in this latter condition, an RPE intracellular buildup of lipofuscin-like products has been well demonstrated).[105] In the limited number of RP cell tissues studied to date no failure in phagocytosis has been identified.[42]

Secondary problems caused by a defective RPE are also present in the RCS rat early in the development of the disease process at the same time as spent disks are beginning to accumulate beneath the retina; abnormal biochemistry has been recorded in the interphotoreceptor cell matrix.

It is difficult to determine the boundaries between physiological and pathological process in the age-related changes associated with phagosome degradation and voiding mechanisms of the RPE. In all human eyes there is progressive accumulation of intracellular lipofuscin with increasing age.[34,36] Unlike any other macrophage which has a transient existence and having fulfilled its role by ingesting its target material dies to be replaced by a new cell, the same RPE cell must continuously engulf some 300 million million discs during a 70-year life span. At about the age of 40 years, RPE cells become too full with waste products; they remedy this by pushing the waste products out through Bruch's membrane (see below). Over the age of 40 years in normal individuals, focal aggregations of such subpigment epithelial debris are observed, and these excrescences on Bruch's membrane are called drusen. Many RP patients well under the age of 40 have multiple areas of drusen throughout the posterior pole, and presumably are demonstrating an acceleration of debris accumulation beneath the basal layers of the RPE.

The observations of both lipofuscin and debris within Bruch's membrane in several dystrophic human retinas suggest that phagocytic processes are occurring within these eyes, but do not exclude some quantitative fault in the process.[35,106 – 108]

For example, the lipofuscin content within some of the RPE cells of a 24-year old X-linked RP patient was comparable to that of a 70- or 80-year-old normal individual (**Fig. 4-4**).[108] However, at present we cannot determine whether this represents an inundation of the degradative capacity of the RPE by

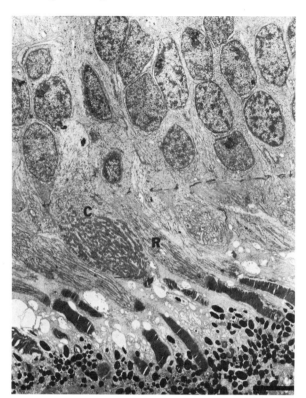 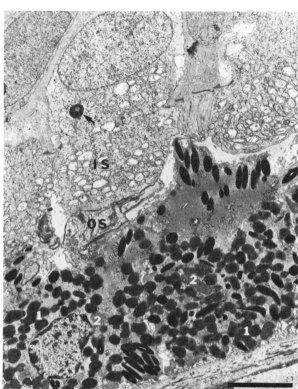

FIG. 4-4. *(A)* Representative cone *(C)* and rod *(R)* in the far periphery of donor eye with sex-linked RP; outer segments are shortened in length. Inner segments of photoreceptors cells appear normal. Swollen microvillous processes of the RPE extend up to the inner segments. Free melanin granules are prominent in the apical portion of the RPE. *(B)* Cones in the central fovea have enlarged inner segments *(IS)* and distorted remnants of outer segments *(OS)*. Autophagic vacuoles *(arrows)* are seen in the perinuclear cytoplasm. RPE cells contain large numbers of melanolysosomes *(1)*, lysosomes *(2)*, and few free melanin granules. Apical protrusions of these cells extend between cone inner segments. (The bar markers are [A] 6 μm and [B] 3 μm.) (Photographs courtesy of Professor Eliot Berson; Invest Ophthalmol 18:156, 148, 1979)

prematurely degenerating receptor cells or whether the receptor cell degeneration is secondary to reduced metabolic exchange by prematurely aged RPE cells.

BRUCH'S MEMBRANE AND CHOROID

Bruch's membrane is an acellular structure that can be subdivided into five substrata; two are basement membranes, two are collagenous, and the remaining one is composed of elastin. A useful analogy is to consider the fibrous layers as the wires in a garden sieve. With age the fibrous components increase in number, and presumably there is progressive resistance to the passage of particles. This increased resistance, coupled with an increased outflow of cel-

lular detritus, results in an accumulation of debris, which in turns tends to displace the overlying RPE cells.

In addition to the alteration induced in Bruch's membrane by phagocytic problems of the RPE, other aging changes occur which are also thought to have functional significance, and of these the most prominent are the accumulation of fine granular deposits on its innermost margin, termed by Sarks the "basal linear deposit."[109] This deposit is a thickened and chemically modified basement membrane of the RPE. In association with these basement membrane changes the basal border of the epithelial cells undergoes a reduction in the complexity of its convolutions, a finding that would suggest a progressive decline in active transport with age.

LABORATORY STUDIES IN MAN

Laboratory studies of inherited retinal dystrophies in man have been severely handicapped by two major constraints:

1. A general lack of availability of tissue for study
2. The little tissue that has been obtained has been with a few exceptions from elderly blind eyes with advanced stages of the diseases.

One notable exception to this generalization has been the eyes of elderly female hemizygotes with X-linked disease, where the disease process may still be active and mild, but the pathology is complicated by the presence of natural aging processes (**Figs. 4-5 and 4-6**). The laboratory investigation of R.P. material 20 years or more after the onset of severe visual handicap or total blindness in most cases gives little information about the subtle causal mechanisms or conditions that prevailed 60 or more years previously. These problems are now being overcome.

First, in several countries emergent patient organizations are establishing eye donor schemes for RP sufferers to donate their eyes after death for laboratory research. Since the inception of the Eye Donor Scheme of the British Retinitis Pigmentosa Society in 1980, 22 pairs of eyes have reached research laboratories, and a similar response has occurred in the USA to the Eye Donor Program of the RP Foundation Fighting Blindness. The importance of these eye donation programs can not be overemphasized.

Second, several centers have been experimenting with retinal biopsy procedures in animals. It may well be that as laboratory techniques develop it will be possible to use increasingly smaller tissue samples. At such time, some patients may wish to volunteer to provide samples of their retina which show early or active disease processes. The medical ethics of retinal biopsy in such a situation are as yet unclear, though there is clear historical precedence for this approach. If laboratory concepts develop theories that need testing in relation to specific disease processes, it may well be that such objections that exist

FIG. 4-5. *(A,B)* Representative sections from a patch of photoreceptor degeneration in the midperipheral retina of a carrier of a X-linked RP. Small abnormal foci may involve only a few receptors and one or two RPE cells. *(A,B,C)* In these patches, RPE cells extend between receptors to the level of the external limiting membrane. *(B,C)* Rod and cone outer segments overlying and adjacent to these extended RPE cells are distorted, and the outer segments are short. Cone nuclei are occasionally observed in the inner segments. *(C)* The RPE contains few melanin granules, some melanolysosomes, and large numbers of lipofuscin bodies. (The bar markers are *[A]* 40 μm, *[B]* 20 μm, and *[C]* 10 μm.) (Photomicrograph courtesy of Professor Eliot Berson. Ophthalmology 92:275, 1985)

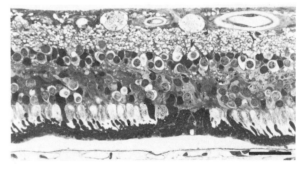

A

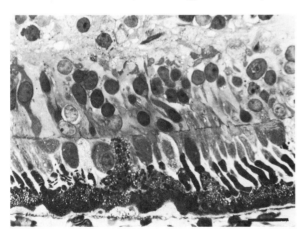

B

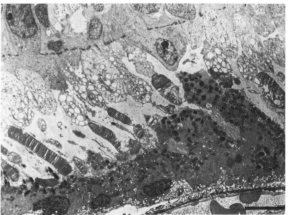

C

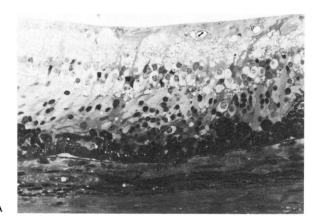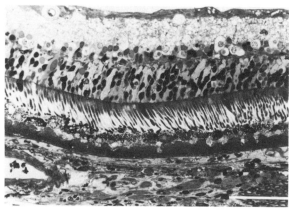

A

B

FIG. 4-6. Light micrographs of *(A)* peripheral and *(B)* paracentral areas of the retina of a 74-year-old man with autosomal dominant RP. The inner retinal layers are relatively well preserved in all areas examined. (The bar marker is 50 μm.)

will be withdrawn. It is hard to see how any cures can be derived without examining diseased tissue.

Major advances in tissue culture procedures over the past decade offer the opportunity for preservation and propagation of rare samples, such that cells derived from a specific donor eye may be amplified and ultimately stored for study by several laboratories. This concept was realized in 1983 when cultures of RPE cells from donors in the United Kingdom were shipped to the Wilmer Institute in Baltimore, Maryland, and has since been reciprocated in 1984 when cells from donors in the USA traveled to the UK.

HISTOPATHOLOGY OF INHERITED RETINAL DYSTROPHIES

For the reasons previously stated, with few exceptions, histopathological reports are based on inadequately preserved material and describe structural changes in advanced stages of retinal degeneration. However, there are reports where postmortem times are minimal, 1 hour or less between death and enucleation[108,110–112] or where a single eye was surgically enucleated for a choroidal tumor.[113] Reports on young RP eyes, less than 32 years of age, are themselves limited and do not necessarily describe early disease (31 years: Bunt-Milam, Kalina, Pagon[113]; 23 years: Szamier, Berson Klien and Myers[110]; 19

years: Rodrigues, Ballintine, Wiggert, Fletcher and Chader[138]; 14 years: McKechnie, King, and Lee[143]; 13 and 14 years: Runge, Culver, Marshall and Taylor[112]; see Table 4-1).

Even when eyes reach the histopathologist in optimal condition, interpretation of disease processes is complicated by a somewhat limited spectrum of responses exhibited by the retina when confronted with injurious agents. It is therefore not surprising that the histological appearances of advanced cases of RP are remarkably similar regardless of the genotype of the disease.[69,106,108,114–121] With the exception of Best's disease and some of the lipidoses[122] where specific cytoplasmic inclusions are seen, the general picture of retinal degeneration holds true for all the inherited pigmented retinal dystrophies.

In RP the primary abnormality, with virtually 100% incidence in pathologic specimens, is the focal disappearance or loss of both rods and cones. The next most common finding are anomalies within the RPE; these may be depigmentation, atrophy, degeneration, or proliferation, and generally when present are more pronounced in the midperipheral retina (**Fig. 4-7**). In the inner retina the histological appearance in any given eye may vary widely between the two extremes of total loss of all retinal neurons and their replacement with glia (**Fig. 4-8**) to an apparently normal substructure (**Fig. 4-9**). Both extremes may also present in different locations within a single

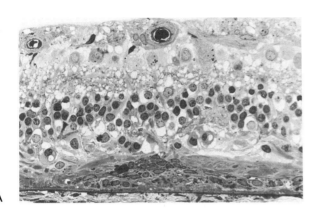
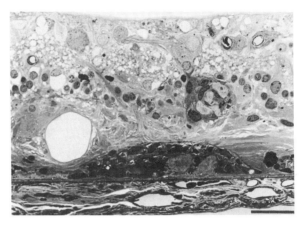

A

B

FIG. 4-7. Light micrographs of areas of the retina of a 74-year-old woman with RP of unknown genetic type. Note hypoplasia of the RPE in both *A* and *B*, but in *A* the inner retinal layers are relatively well preserved while in *B* they are almost lost. (The bar marker is 50 μm.)

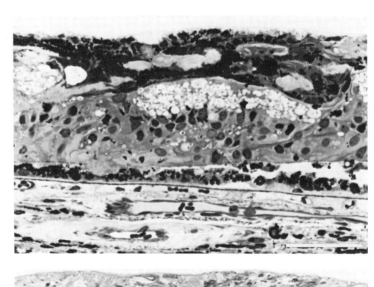

A

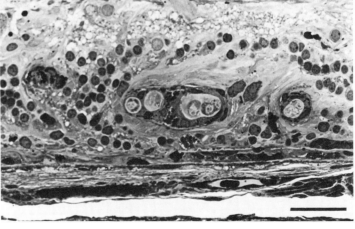

B

FIG. 4-8. Light micrographs of areas of the bone spicule zone of the retina of a 67-year-old man with RP of unknown genetic type. The inner retinal layers are disorganized, and pigment cells are located *(A)* beneath the inner limiting membrane and *(B)* around highly attenuated or occluded vessels. (The bar markers are 50 μm.)

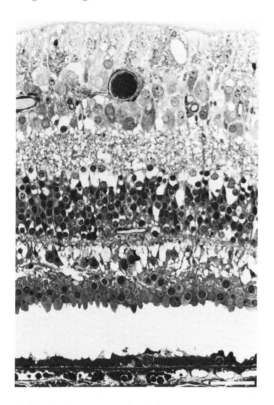

FIG. 4-9. Light micrograph of the macular area of the retina of a 74-year-old woman with RP of unknown genetic type. The inner retinal layers are virtually normal apart from post mortem artifacts. Macular cones remain in a simplified form having lost their outer segments. (The bar marker is 50 μm.)

eye. In all RP eyes showing a classical bone spicule region, the underlying cause is seen in the inner retinal layers with displaced pigment cells usually concentrated around extensively hyalinurized and often sclerotic retinal vessels. One further common finding in the pathology of these eyes is the development of cellular epiretinal membranes in advanced disease (**Fig. 4-10**). These appear to be glial in origin[123] and are often associated with a marked gliosis at the optic nervehead,[124] a finding which may account for the pallor and small cup-to-disc ratio seen clinically.

Given the limited data base in the pathology of RP, with relatively few eyes studied and the progressive convergence to a common endpoint morphology in advanced disease, it is perhaps not useful to describe findings in relation to modes of inheritance. For this reason we have elected to describe the spectrum of change seen in each cell layer and highlight the genetic type only where a specific observation seems to be apparent. It is also a useful generalization to divide these eyes into four morphological zones: macula, preequatorial, bone spicule, and far peripheral retina. The zones will vary dramatically in exact dimension and geographical extent between individual eyes, but they are always apparent in some configuration.

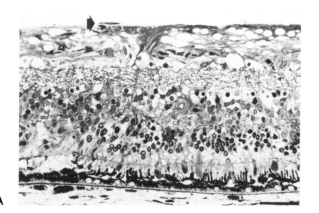

A

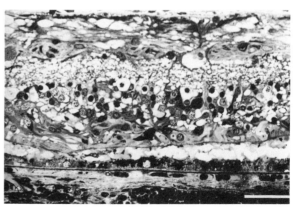

B

FIG. 4-10. Light micrographs of areas of the retina *(A)* with and *(B)* without presence of photoreceptors, from the eye of a 67-year-old man with RP of unknown genetic type. In both regions epiretinal membranes can be seen *(arrows).* (The bar markers are 50 μm.)

PHOTORECEPTOR CELLS

Electron microscopical studies have revealed that in advanced autosomal dominant (presumably rod-cone) disease[106,108] and possibly in others,[120,126] the only remaining photoreceptor cells in the retina are cones. The surviving cones are located in the posterior pole, are few in number, and have an atypical appearance (**Fig. 4-11**). Clearly, with any insidious disease process, the degree of cellular change is unique to a given individual at a particular time, and therefore care must be exercised in interpreting the cytopathology of a limited number of specimens. However, in each of the eyes described immediately above, only the foveal cones had outer segments, and these were truncated and composed of small groups of disoriented disk membranes, many of which had degenerated into a vesicular form. The outer segments were connected to abnormally wide and short inner segments via an apparently normal cilium. Many of the cells contained autophagic vacuoles.[125] The cone nuclei were also swollen to a diameter 30% larger than normal.[108] In the macula, cone remnants became progressively more degenerate with increasing distance from the fovea (**Fig. 4-12**). These changes occurred first as a loss of the outer segment, with subsequent swelling of the inner segment, and finally as a loss of both inner and outer segments to leave a residual photoreceptor cell of spherical shape with little cytoplasm (**Figs. 4-13 to 4-15**). These changes are morphologically identical to those exhibited by cones in areas of retinal detachment[126] or those exposed to mild light damage.[82] In most eyes in the advanced stages of RP, photoreceptor cells have not been observed beyond 5 mm from the macula. In the peripheral regions, proliferated glial tissue is in direct contact with the RPE.

In less advanced disease[113,127,135] elements of both rods and cones may be present in the peripheral or

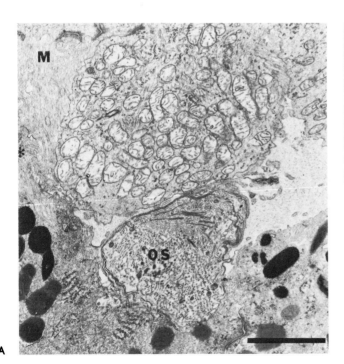
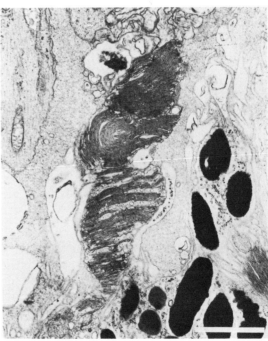

A   B

FIG. 4-11. Electron micrographs of cones from the retina of a 24-year-old man with X-linked RP. *(A)* Central foveal cones have outer segment discs *(OS)* that are vesiculated and disrupted. Rough endoplasmic reticulum is prominent in apical portions of RPE cells. Apical microvillous processes *(asterisk)* of RPE cells abut on Müller cell microvillous processes *(M)*. *(B)* Cone outer segment discs are vesiculated and disoriented. Outer segments are surrounded by distended microvillous processes of the RPE. (The bar markers are 2 μm.) (Photographs courtesy of Professor Eliot Berson; Invest Ophthalmol 18:149, 159, 1979)

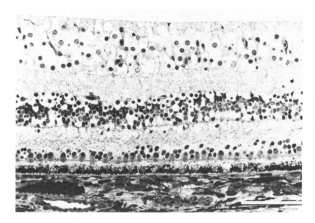
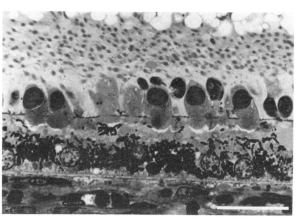

A

B

FIG. 4-12. Light micrographs of the macular retina of a 4-year-old boy with Laurence-Moon-Bardet-Biedl syndrome. The inner retinal layers are well preserved but there is a loss of outer cone segments and rods. The "rounded-up" inner segments and nuclei of cones make them particularly prominent. (The bar markers are [A] 100 μm and [B] 20 μm.)

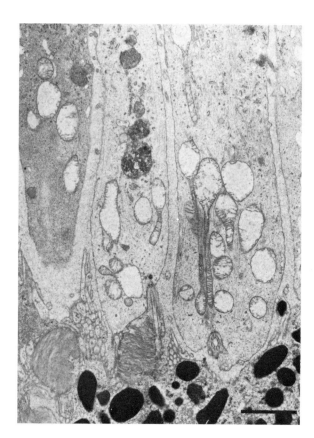

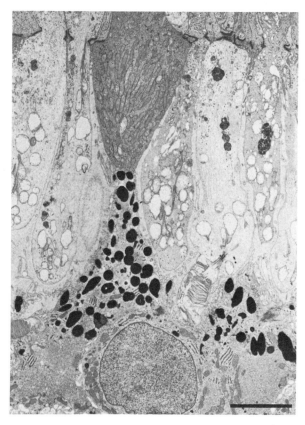

FIG. 4-13. Electron micrograph of a rod cell remnant from the retina of a 31-year-old man with autosomal recessive disease. The inner segments of the rods have swollen mitochondria and electron-dense granular inclusions. (The bar marker is 2 μm.) (Photographs courtesy of Professor Ann Bunt-Milam; Invest Ophthalmol 24:464, 1983)

FIG. 4-14. Electron micrograph of the interface between photoreceptor cells and RPE in the retina of a 31-year-old man with autosomal recessive RP. The sample of cones is from an area 50° eccentric from the macula and shows apical protuberances which contain melanin and enclose cone but not rod outer segments. (The bar marker is 5 μm.) (Photograph courtesy of Professor Ann Bunt-Milam; Invest Ophthalmol 24:463, 1983)

equatorial retina outside the bone spicule zone. In this location they usually exhibit atypically short outer segments with disorganized disk membranes (Fig. 4-16). Many cells have a further indication of compromised function in that their nuclei are displaced towards the RPE, having passed through the outer limiting membrane.[128] Towards the central margins of this peripheral zone of photoreceptors, the outer segments become progressively shorter and increasingly deranged especially at their outer ends (Figs. 4-17 and 4-18). It is perhaps surprising that there is often an abrupt transition between this zone of photoreceptor cells with inner and outer segments, and the peripheral edge of the bone spicule zone where glial cells may be in contact with the RPE (Figs. 4-6, 4-10, and 4-15). Abrupt transitional zones may well be instructive in terms of underlying mechanism. Focal degeneration in the outer retina which corresponds to the size of choriocapillaris lobules is a relatively common finding in the inherited retinal dystrophies (Fig. 4-19). Even in the bone spicule zone, small cave-like regions may be observed, occasionally containing remnants of both inner and outer segments. In such regions the roofs of the cave are delineated by the outer limiting membrane which describes an arc curving away from the RPE but in apposition to it at the cave margins. Photoreceptor cell remnants have not been found in the absence of RPE.

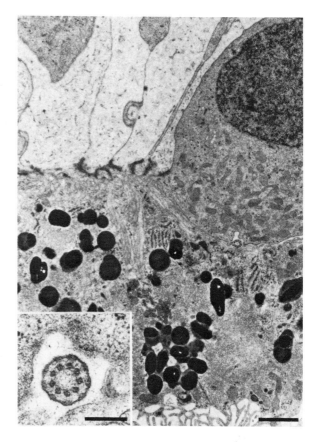

FIG. 4-15. Electron micrographs of the peripheral retina of a 31-year-old man with autosomal recessive disease showing the RPE and a cone inner segment and nucleus that appear normal morphologically. Note hypertrophy of Müller cell processes at the level of the external limiting membrane that abuts the RPE. *(Inset)* Cross section of cone connecting cilium that shows normal fine structure. (The bar markers are 2 μm and [*inset*] 0.25 μm.) (Courtesy of Professor Ann Bunt-Milam; Invest Ophthalmol 24:465, 1983)

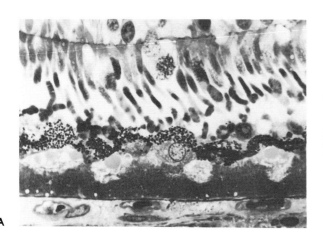

A

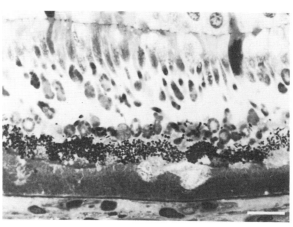

B

FIG. 4-16. Light micrographs of the midperipheral retina of a 74-year-old man with autosomal dominant RP. The outer segments of the photoreceptor cells are reduced in length and contain disorientated discs. Beneath the RPE is a massive accumulation of extracellular deposit which stains as a multilayered system. (The bar marker is 10 μm.)

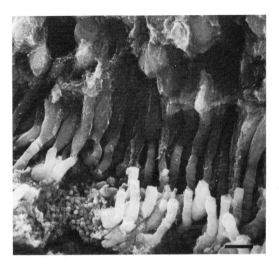
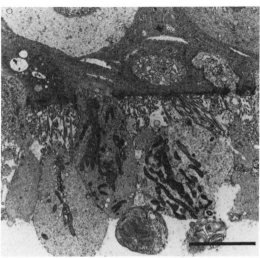

FIG. 4-17. *(A)* Scanning and *(B)* transmission electron micrographs of the photoreceptor cell remnants in the midperipheral retina of a 74-year-old man with autosomal dominant RP. Note the disorientated outer segments. (The bar markers are 5 μm.)

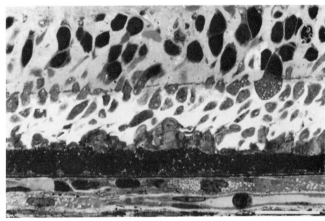

FIG. 4-18. *(A)* Light and *(B,C)* electron micrographs of the interface between the photoreceptor cells and RPE in the midperipheral retina of a 4-year-old boy with Laurence-Moon-Bardet-Biedl syndrome. The RPE contains an abnormally high concentration of lipofuscin for the individual's age; there is an accumulation of outer segment debris on the apical surface of these cells. (The bar markers are *[A]* 30 μm, *[B]* 5 μm, and *[C]* 2 μm.)

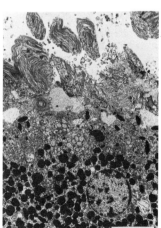
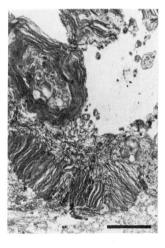

FIG. 4-19. *(A,B)* Light and *(C)* electron micrographs of the midperipheral areas of the retina of a 12-year-old girl with mitochondrial cytopathy (Kearns-Sayre syndrome). *A* shows a "cone" of partially preserved photoreceptor cells but all demonstrate the presence of lipid droplets seen at higher power in *C*. In areas of more advanced disease, the photoreceptor remnants are lost and large aggregations of lipids are seen. (The bar markers are *[A]* 100 μm, *[B]* 25 μm, and *[C]* 1 μm.)

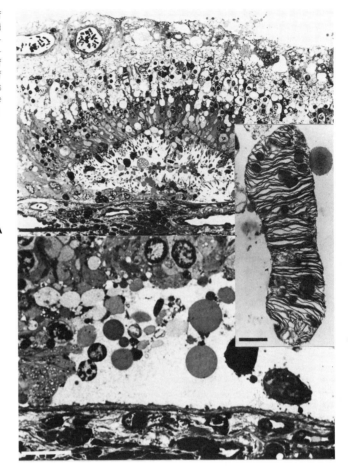

Perhaps the best example of the ultrastructural changes in photoreceptor cells in early disease is that of a 23-year-old man who had X-linked RP.[108] This patient had a typical annular zone of pigment distributed in a bone-spicule pattern between about 45° and 60° from the fovea. Although all the remaining photoreceptor cells in this patient exhibited abnormalities, there were marked differences beween the center and the periphery. Central foveal cones were reduced in number by about 50% and had shortened and severely distorted outer segments containing vesiculated and disrupted disk membranes similar to the remnants seen in advanced disease. A further similarity was noted in the parafovea, where cones first lost their outer segments and then became progressively more disorganized as the distance from the fovea increased. In the major portion of the zone showing bone-spicule formation,

only occasional vestiges of cones were noted, these being identified by their swollen tigroid nuclei and in some cases tiny ellipsoids protruding through the outer limiting membrane. On the outermost border of this zone, inner and outer segments of both rods and cones were apparent, and these became progressively more organized toward the periphery. Both rods and cones had outer segments at least 25% shorter than those in a comparable location in a normal control eye, but whereas the disk membranes of the rods were well ordered and nearly normal in appearance, those of the cones were both disoriented and vesiculated. Thus, the cones in this young patient were similar to those of the very elderly.[28] Similar photoreceptor changes have been observed in the eyes of an 80-year-old female carrier of X-linked disease.[129] Athough all the foveal cones were lost in these eyes, cone nuclei and their fiber components in the layer of Henle could be seen in the macula. A small island of both rods and cones with shortened outer segments was observed in each eye on the nasal side of the disk central to the bone spicule zone. As in the young X-linked specimen reported by Szamier, the rods had well-ordered disks in their outer segments, whereas those of the cones were extremely degenerate.

RETINAL PIGMENT EPITHELIUM

Changes in the RPE in RP may be divided into three main classes, which roughly correspond to the degree of retinal eccentricity:

1. Cells from the central region are typically tall cells with apically displaced nuclei and a cytoplasm crammed with electron-dense inclusions interpreted as lipofuscin[106] or melanolysosomes.[108,110] They contain few melanin granules and occasional phagosomes,[113] the latter having been found only in cells associated with cones possessing vestigial outer segments. Where extensive photoreceptor degeneration has occurred, the cells of the RPE have been identified in various stages of budding or migration from Bruch's membrane.

2. Cells from the central region or bone spicule area may be flattened and devoid of either melanin granules or lipofuscin. These cells may occur in more than one layer and are often found with macrophage-like cells whose processes often penetrate to the midlayers of Bruch's membrane.

3. In the periphery, in contrast to the center, the RPE cells contain little lipofuscin but many pigment granules. In some specimens, particularly on the peripheral edge of the bone spicule zone, localized circular regions of epithelial loss with sharply demarcated borders are found, although it is to be noted that similar findings have also been reported in the eyes of the elderly.[130]

The geographic differences in RPE, and the variations in different regions with increasing age[36] make the analysis of ultrastructural studies in this region in RP even more difficult. In essence there are no unique findings in this layer in RP, but there

are differences in both spatial and temporal distributions of inclusions and organelles. The most striking feature is the distribution of subpigment epithelial deposits on Bruch's membrane. These are particularly apparent when the abrupt transition zones between areas of residual photoreceptor cells and glial scars are examined. In such regions it can be seen that beneath the RPE overlaid with photoreceptor cells Bruch's membrane may show a relatively normal content of debris or basement membrane material. In contrasting the region of glial contact with attenuated RPE cells, the underlying membrane may be distorted with a high concentration of lipid globules or predrusen deposits. Deposits on Bruch's membrane may be related to the increased phagocytic load of the RPE cells in these areas of retina where disease has resulted in total loss of photoreceptor cells. Equally, it could result from some disturbance in the metabolism of the RPE cells or choroid. In some RP eyes extensive deposits of amorphous material are present on Bruch's membrane, and observations have been made in at least two genetic varieties, X-linked (Santos-Anderson et al, 1982) and autosomal dominant.[126,129] These deposits are thicker than the basal laminar defects seen in aging,[109] and the geographic distribution is different in that it is fairly uniformly distributed from the ora to the optic nerve rather than centered at the posterior pole as in senile eyes (**Figs. 4-20 and 4-21**).

Recently, biochemical analysis of Bruch's membrane from eyes of two different subjects with autosomal dominant diseases showed differences from the age-matched norms in both composition and ratios of proteglyceon components. As these molecular moieties contribute to the structural and filtration properties of Bruch's membrane, the abnormal configurations and concentrations in RP eyes may well further exacerbate the disease process.

Deposition of amorphous material under the RPE and in the inner collagenous layer of Bruch's membrane has been described in Doyne's choroiditis[131,132] and has been presumed to be secondary to disease in the choroid. This view was also taken in describing a similar deposit in an inherited retinal dystrophy by Ashton and Sorsby.[133] It is difficult to sustain this concept, since the deposit is not

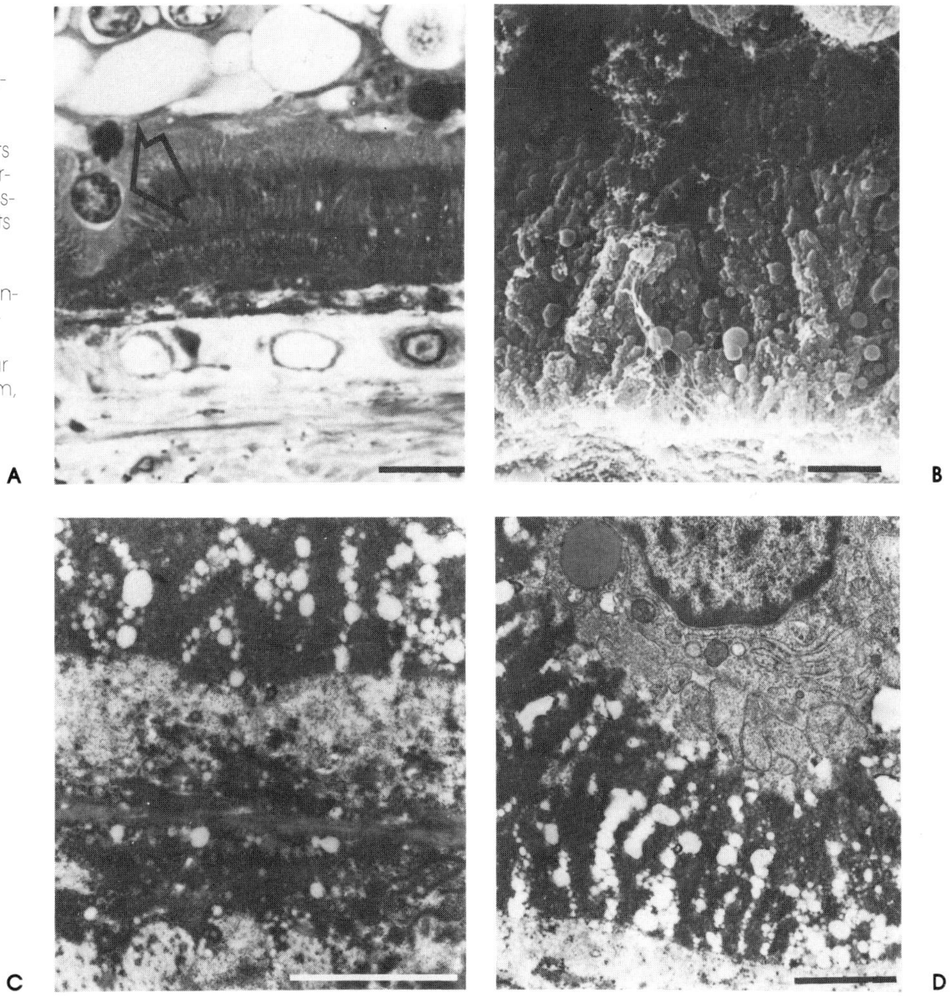

FIG. 4-20. *(A)* Light, *(B)* scanning, and *(C,D)* transmission electron micrographs of the subpigment epithelial deposits seen in the retina of a 74-year-old man with autosomal recessive disease. Identical deposits were seen in this patient's 62-year-old brother. The deposits often show a dichromatic staining pattern. Occasional mononucleate cells *(arrows)* are seen in such deposits. (The bar markers are *[A]* 5 μm, *[B]* 2 μm, and *[C,D]* 1 μm.)

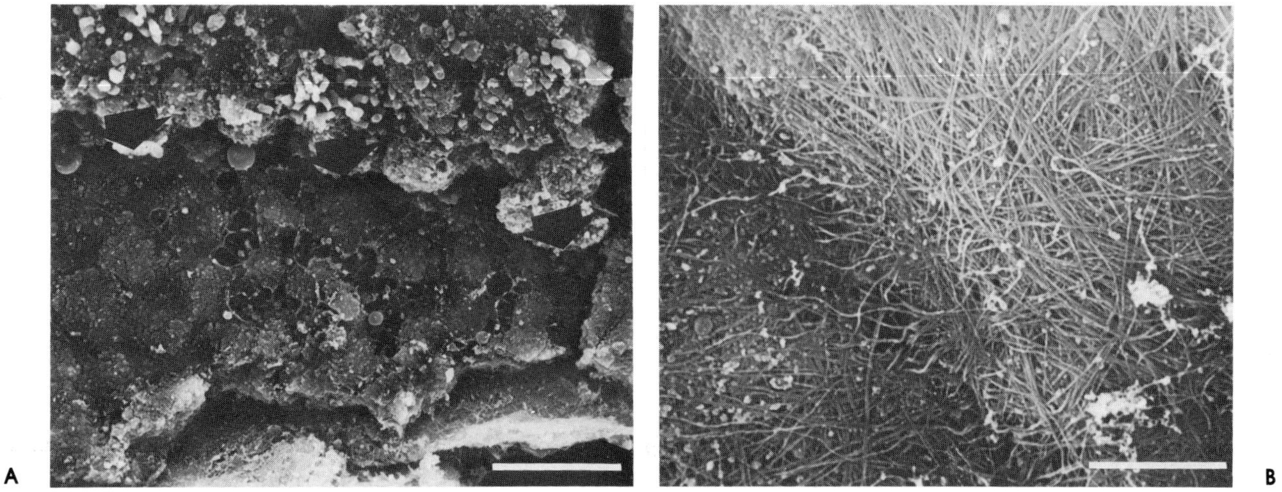

FIG. 4-21. Scanning electron micrographs of *(A)* the RPE and *(B)* Bruch's membrane from the eye of a 74-year-old man with autosomal dominant RP. The subepithelial deposits can be seen in *A* in an area where the RPE cells have been artificially detached *(arrows)*. The coarse, high-resistance structure of the inner collagenous layer of Bruch's membrane is demonstrated in *B*. (The bar markers are *[A]* 20 μm and *[B]* 5 μm.)

61

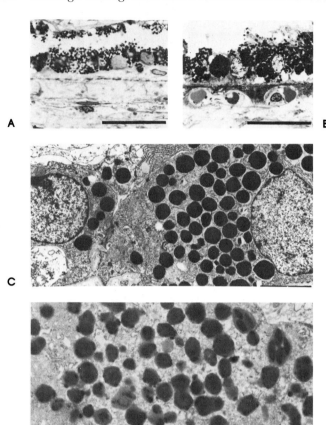

A

B

C

D

FIG. 4-22. *(A,B)* Light and *(C,D)* electron micrographs of the RPE, of a 68-year-old woman with autosomal dominant RP. *A* and *C* show the peripheral epithelium and *B* and *D* the foveal epithelium. Note the preponderance of lipofuscin granules in the central epithelium. (The bar markers are *[A,B]* 30 μm, *[C]* 3 μm, and [D] 2 μm. (Photographs courtesy of Professor Peter Gouras; Invest Ophthalmol 13:490–491, 1974)

patchy or lobular as is the choriocapillaris nor is there a high concentration at the posterior pole where the choroidal vascular bed is richest.

The presence of lipofuscin in RPE cells in RP eyes[106] suggest that in most of these patients the phagocytosis cycle involving photoreceptor cells and RPE is functional at some level although not necessarily normal (**Figs. 4-22 and 4-23**). Attempts to demonstrate a phagocytic problem in human disease using tissue culture of RPE cells have not yet been successful,[42] but to date only a few diseased cell lines have been established.

One of the most striking features of the retinal dystrophies is the migration of pigment into the retina secondary to photoreceptor degeneration (**Fig. 4-8**). This is seen as free melanin granules, melanin granules within the cytoplasm of Müller cells, melanin granules within macrophages, and melanin granules within displaced RPE cells. These cells are most commonly found in large clumps or masses around the retinal vessels and the basement membrane complexes of atrophic vessels, but in some patients they become oriented beneath the inner limiting membrane.[69,117] Fluorescence microscopy gives a strong indication that the pigmented

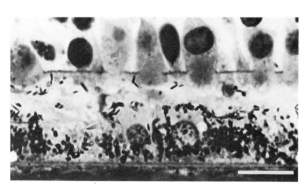

A

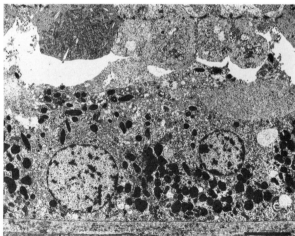

B

FIG. 4-23. *(A)* Light and *(B)* electron micrographs of the RPE of a 4-year-old boy with Laurence-Moon-Bardet-Biedl syndrome. Note the massive accumulation of lipofuscin granules, very atypical for an individual of this age, and the loss of melanin granules. (The bar markers are *[A]* 10 μm and *[B]* 5 μm.)

cells responsible for bone-spicule formation in the neural retina emanate solely from the peripheral epithelium which is relatively devoid of lipofuscin and is hence nonfluorescent as opposed to the fluorescent lipofuscin-rich epithelium near the fovea.[106] However, electron microscopy reveals that the melanin granules within these cells are predominantly spheroidal, like choroidal melanin, and not fusiform like those of normal RPE.[108]

In some cases columns or clusters of RPE cells can be seen extending from the RPE layer through the glial scar, that has replaced degenerate retina, and on to either retinal vascular element or to the outer aspect of the inner limiting membrane.[111] The RPE cells seem happy to colonize the outer aspect of the basement membrane of retinal vascular elements or inner limiting membrane, since in these locations they repolarize with a basal convoluted border adjacent to the vessel or the vitreous, and a distal surface develops with microvilli.[111]

Further, these translocated cells develop desmosomal and gap junctions along their lateral borders. These findings are not surprising because in tissue culture experiments human RPE cells have been shown to grow on artificial membranes with or without pretreatment with collagen, and even on suitably prepared substrates of Descemet's membrane.[42,45]

CHORIOCAPILLARIS

Reports on the histopathology of the choriocapillaris and choroidal vasculature in RP vary, and to some extent this apparent conflict between the presence[111,128] and absence[130] of changes must reflect variation in time course and the type of RP examined. In a study of 14 eyes from 7 patients, Gartner and Henkind concluded that since the choriocapillaris was intact in most locations even opposite degenerate retina and that since it was only lost where both RPE and photoreceptor cells were absent, then changes in this layer were secondary to disease and not causal. By contrast, Rayborn and colleagues[111] have shown in an atypical form of RP that while central choriocapillaris may be normal, that of the bone spicule zone may be reduced or absent, and where present may be abnormal in not having fenestrated endothelium. It is also interesting to note that fundus photographs of their patients clinically showed areas resembling choroidal sclerosis, and thus their cases may not be representative of typical autosomal dominant RP.

Clinically, in RP patients, the appearance of choroidal sclerosis is often seen as the pigment epithelium disappears and exposes the underlying choroid to view; however, choroidal arteriolar sclerosis is a common finding in the elderly.

THE INNER RETINA

Degenerative changes in the neural retina are highly variable, with retention of relatively unchanged ganglion cell and nerve fiber layers in some eyes long after the eye has become blind (**Fig. 4-9**), while in others it is frequently impossible to recognize any retinal architecture (**Fig. 4-8**). In all cases, the retinal vessels show atrophy with loss of endothelium and invasion of basement membrane tubes by both macrophages and glial elements.

With the increasing loss of neurons, secondary changes take place in the retinal glia. In areas of photoreceptor loss, the Müller fibers increase in size and lie in contact with the RPE. At such regions the complex villi of the Müller cells interdigitate with those of the apical surface of the epithelial cells, a phenomenon that has been reported in a variety of conditions where photoreceptor degeneration has been induced.[80] The outer limiting membrane of the retina is preserved long after photoreceptor cells are lost but becomes less clear in areas where Bruch's membrane is covered by nonpigmented epithelial cells or cells that look like macrophages. There is often a migration of nuclei of Müller cells into regions between the inner nuclear layer and RPE.

In those eyes in which the inner retinal layers appear to have a relatively normal morphology, there may be some selective loss of specific neurons. Recent metabolic studies using radioactive tracers on incubated samples of retina from different retinal locations from a donor with a dominantly inherited chorioretinal degeneration showed a loss of specific subtypes of cellular activity.[134] In this study a marked reduction was seen in both GABAergic and dopaminergic activity which indicated that few of the cells responsible remained.

REFERENCES

1. Experimental Eye Research Symposium: The pigment epithelium: Its relationship to the retina in health and disease. I. Exp Eye Res 22:395–568, 1976
2. Young RW: Visual cells. Sci Am 223:80–91, 1970
3. Young RW: The renewal of rod and cone outer segments in the rhesus monkey. J Cell Biol 49:303–312, 1971
4. Young RW: Visual cells and the concept of renewal. Invest Ophthalmol 15:700–725, 1976
5. Peymann GA, Spitznas M, Straatsma BR: Perioxidase diffusion in the normal and photocoagulated retina. Invest Ophthalmol 10:181–189, 1971
6. Bok D, Heller J: Transport of retinol from the blood to the retina: An autoradiographic study of the pigment epithelial cell surface receptor for plasma retinol binding protein. Exp Eye Res 22:395–402, 1976
7. Lake N, Marshall J, Voaden MJ: The entry of taurine into the neural retina and pigment epithelium of the frog. Brain Res 128:497–503, 1977
8. Heller J, Bok D. Transport of retinol from the blood to the retina: The involvement of high molecular weight lipoproteins as intracellular carriers. Exp Eye Res 22:403–410, 1976
9. Saari JC, Futterman S. An intracellular retinol binding protein isolated from bovine retina: Isolation and partial characterization. Exp Eye Res 22:425–433, 1976
10. Wiggert BD, Bergsma R, Chader GJ: Studies on the intracellular binding of retinol in the retina and pigment epithelium. Exp Eye Res 22:411–418, 1976
11. Ocumpaugh DE, Young RW: Distribution and synthesis of sulfated mucopolysaccharides in the retina of the rat. Invest Ophthalmol 5:196–203, 1966
12. Rohlich P: The interphotoreceptor matrix: Electron microscopic and histochemical observations on the vertebrate retina. Exp Eye Res 10:80–96, 1970
13. Young RW: Visual cell renewal systems and the problem of retinitis pigmentosa: Retinitis pigmentosa clinical implications of current research. Adv Med Biol 77:93–223, 1977
14. Young RW: Passage of newly formed protein through the connecting cilium of retinal rods in the frog. J Ultrastruct Res 23:462–473, 1968
15. Young RW: Shedding of discs from rod outer segments in the rhesus monkey. J Ultrastruct Res 34:190–203, 1971
16. Marshall J: The retinal receptors and the pigment epithelium. In Perkins ES, Hills DW (eds): Scientific Foundations of Ophthalmology, pp 8–17. London, William Heinemann, 1977
17. Bassinger S, Hoffman R, Matthes M: Photoreceptor shedding is initiated by light in the frog retina. Science 194:1074–1076, 1976
18. Lavail MM: Rod outer segment disk shedding in rat retina. Relationship to cyclic lighting. Science 194:1071–1074, 1976
19. O'Day WT, Young RW: Rhythmic daily shedding of outer segment membranes by visual cells in the gold fish. J Cell Biol 76:593–604, 1978
20. Spitznas M, Hogan MJ: Outer segments of photoreceptors and the pigment epithelium; interrelationship in the human eye. Arch Ophthalmol 84:810–819, 1970
21. Custer NV, Bok D: Pigment epithelium photoreceptor interactions in normal and dystrophic rats. Exp Eye Res 21:15–166, 1975
22. Hollyfield JG: Phagocytic capabilities of the pigment epithelium. Exp Eye Res 22:457–469, 1976
23. Hollyfield JG, Ward A: Phagocytic activity in the retinal pigment epithelium of the frog *Rana pipiens*. I. Uptake of polystyrene spheres. J Ultrastruct Res 46:327–338, 1974
24. Reich-d'Almeida FB, Hockley DJ: In situ reactivitiy of the retinal pigment epithelium: II. Phagocytosis in the dystrophic rat. Exp Eye Res 21:347–357, 1975
25. Cohen AI: Further studies on the question of the patency of saccules in outer segments of vertebrate photoreceptors. Vision Res 10:445–453, 1970
26. Steinberg RH, Wood I, Hogan MJ: Pigment epithelial ensheathment and phagocytosis of extrafoveal cones in human retina. Proc R Soc Lond (Biol) 277:459–471, 1977
27. Franceschetti A: Über tapeto-retinale Degeneration in Kindersalter. In Entwicklung und Fortschritt in der Augenheilkunde. Stuttgart, Enke Verlag, 1963
28. Marshall J: Ageing changes in human cones. In Shimizu K (ed): Proceedings of the 23rd International Congress of Ophthalmology, Kyoto, 1978, pp 375–378. Amsterdam, Excerpta Medica, 1979
29. Ishikawa T, Yamada E: The degradation of the photoreceptor outer segments within the pigment epithelial cell of rat retina. J Electron Microsc 19:85–91, 1970
30. Marshall J: Acid phosphatase activity in the retinal pigment epithelium. Vision Res 10:821–824, 1970
31. Marshall J, Ansell PL: Membranous inclusions in the retinal pigment epithelium: Phagosomes and myeloid bodies. J Anat 110:91–104, 1971
32. Feeney L: The phagolysosomal system of the pigment epithelium. A key to retinal disease. Invest Ophthalmol Vis Sci 23:635–638, 1973
33. Feeney-Burns L, Hilderbrand ES, Eldridge S: Ageing human RPE: Morphometric analysis of macular, equatorial and peripheral cells. Invest Ophthalmol Vis Sci 25:195–200, 1984
34. Feeney L: Lipofuscin and melanin of human retinal pigment epithelium: Fluorescence, enzyme cytochemical and ultrastructural studies. Invest Ophthalmol Vis Sci 17:583–600, 1978
35. Streeten BW: The sudanophilic granules of the human retinal pigment epithelium. Arch Ophthalmol 66:125–132, 1961
36. Wing GL, Blanchard GC, Weiter JJ: The topography and age relationship of lipofuscin concentration in the retinal pigment epithelium. Invest Ophthalmol Vis Sci 17:601–607, 1978
37. Hogan MJ: Role of the retinal pigment epithelium in macular disease. Trans Am Acad Ophthalmol Otolaryngol 76:64–80, 1972
38. Ghadially FN: Ultrastructural Pathology of the Cell. A Text and Atlas of Physiological and Pathological Alterations in Cell Fine Structure, pp 306–308. London, Butterworths, 1975
39. Travis DF, Travis A: Ultrastructural changes in the left ventricular rat myocardial cells with age. J Ultrastruct Res 39:124–148, 1972
40. Leuenberger PM, Novikoff AB: Studies on microperoxisomes. VII. Pigment epithelial cells and other cell types in the retina of rodents. J Cell Biol 65:324–335, 1975
41. Marsden CD: Brain melanin. In Wolman M (ed): Pigments in Pathology, pp 396–420. New York, Academic Press, 1969
42. Boulton ME, Marshall J, Mellerio J: Human retinal pigment epithelial cells in tissue culture: a means of studying inherited retinal diseases. In Cotlier E, Maumanee IH, Berman ER (eds): Genetic eye disease: Retinitis pig-

mentosa and other inherited eye disorders, vol 18, pp 101–118. New York, Alan R Liss

43. Flood MT, Gouras P, Kjeldbye H: Growth characteristics and ultrastructure of human retinal pigment epithelium in vitro. Invest Ophthalmol Vis Sci 19:1309–1320, 1980

44. Flood MT, Haley JE, Gouras P: Cellular ageing of human retinal epithelium in vivo and in vitro. Dev Biol 17:80–93, 1984

45. Boulton ME, Marshall J: The effects of increasing numbers of phagocytic inclusions on human retinal pigment epithelial cells in culture: A model for ageing. Exp Eye Res (in press)

46. Berson EL, Hayes KC, Rabin AR et al: Retinal degeneration in rats fed casein. II. Supplementation with methionine, cysteine or taurine. Invest Ophthalmol Vis Sci 15:52–58, 1975

47. Hayes KC, Carey RE, Schmidt SY: Retinal degeneration associated with taurine deficiency in the cat. Science 188:949–951, 1975

48. Schmidt SY, Berson EL, Hayes KD: Retinal degeneration in cats fed casein. I. Taurine deficiency. Invest Ophthalmol Vis Sci 15:47–52, 1975

49. Hecht S, Mandelbaum J: The relation between vitamin A and dark adaptation. JAMA 112:1910–1916, 1939

50. Hume EM, Krebs HA: Vitamin A requirements of human adults. Spec Rep Ser Med Res Coun Lond 264, 1949

51. Walt RP, Kemp CM, Lyness L et al: Vitamin A treatment for night blindness in primary biliary cirrhosis. Br Med J 288:1030–1031, 1984

52. Dowling JE, Gibbons IR: The effect of vitamin A deficiency on the fine structure of the retina. In Smelser G (ed): The Structure of the Eye, pp 85-89. New York, Academic Press, 1961

53. Hayes KC: Retinal degeneration in monkeys induced by deficiencies of vitamin E or A. Invest Ophthalmol Vis Sci 13:499–510, 1974

54. Campbell DA, Tonks EL: Biochemical findings in human retinitis pigmentosa with particular relation to vitamin A deficiency. Br J Ophthalmol 46:151–164, 1962

55. Krachmer JH, Smith JL, Tocci PM: Laboratory studies in retinitis pigmentosa. Arch Ophthalmol 75:661–673, 1966

56. Bergsma DR, Wolf ML: A therapeutic trial of vitamin A in patients with pigmentary retinal degenerations: A negative study. Adv Exp Med Biol 77:197–209, 1977

57. Chatzinoff A, Nelson E, Stahl N et al: Eleven-*cis* vitamin A in the treatment of retinitis pigmentosa. A negative study. Arch Ophthalmol 80:417–419, 1968

58. Muller-Limmroth W, Kuper J: Über den Einfluss des Adaptinols auf das elektroretinogramm bei tapetoretinalen Degenerationem. Klin Monatsbl Augenheilkd 138:37–41, 1961

59. Rahi AHS: Retinol-binding protein (RBP) and pigmentary dystsrophy of the retina. Br J Ophthalmol 56:647–651, 1972

60. Maraini G, Fadda G, Gozzoli F: Serum levels of retinol-binding protein in different genetic types of retinitis pigmentosa. Invest Ophthalmol Vis Sci 14:236–237, 1975

61. Ripps H, Brin KP, Weale RA: Rhodopsin and visual threshold in retinitis pigmentosa. Invest Ophthalmol Vis Sci 17:735–745, 1978

62. Kemp CM, Faulkner DJ, Jacobson SG: Visual pigment levels in retinitis pigmentosa. Trans Ophthalmol Soc UK 103:453–457, 1984

63. Gouras P, Carr RE, Gunkel RD: Retinitis pigmentosa in abetalipoproteinemia—effects of vitamin A. Invest Ophthalmol Vis Sci 10:784–793, 1971

64. Foulds WS: The retinal pigment epithelial interface. Br J Ophthalmol 63:71–84, 1979

65. Baum JL, Tannenbaum J, Kolodny EH: Refsum's syndrome with corneal involvement. Am J Ophthalmol 60:699–708, 1965

66. Anderson RE, Benolken RM, Dudley PA et al: Polyunsaturated fatty acids of photoreceptor membranes. Exp Eye Res 18:205–213, 1974

67. Anderson RE: Essential fatty acid deficiency and photoreceptor membrane renewal—a reappraisal. Invest Ophthalmol Vis Sci 17:1102–1104, 1978

68. Cummings JN: Inborn errors of metabolism in neurology (Wilson's disease, Refsum's disease and lipidoses). Trans R Soc Med 64:313–322, 1971

69. Wolter JR: Retinitis pigmentosa. Arch Ophthalmol 57:539–553, 1957

70. Lolly RN, Farber DB, Rayborn ME et al: Cyclic GMP accumulation causes degeneration of photoreceptor cells: Simulation of an inherited disease. Science 196:664–666, 1977

71. Farber DB, Lolley RN: Enzymatic basis for cyclic GMP accumulation in degenerative photoreceptor cells of mouse retina. J Cyclic Nucleotide Res 2:139–148, 1976

72. Aguirre G, Farber DB, Lolley RN et al: Rod cone dysplasia in Irish setters: A defect in cyclic GMP metabolism in visual cells. Science 201:1133–1134, 1978

73. Bitensky MW, Miki N, Keirns JJ et al: Activation of photoreceptor disc membrane phosphodiesterase by light and ATP. Adv Cyclic Nucleotide Res 5:213–240, 1975

74. Fletcher RT, Chader GJ: Cyclic GMP: Control of concentration by light in vertebrate photoreceptors. Biochem Biophys Res Commun 70:1297–1302, 1976

75. Lolley RN, Farber DB: A proposed link between debris accumulation, guanosine 3′, 5′ cyclic monophosphate changes and photoreceptor cell degeneration in retina of RCS rats. Exp Eye Res 22:477–487, 1976

76. Noell LWK, Walker VS, Kang BS et al: Retinal damage by light in rats. Invest Ophthalmol Vis Sci 5:450–473, 1966

77. Noell WK, Albrecht R: Irreversible effects of visible light on the retina: Role of vitamin A. Science 172:76–80, 1971

78. Noell WK, Delmelle MC, Albrecht R: Vitamin A deficiency effect on the retina: Dependence on light. Science 172:72–76, 1971

79. Grignolo A, Orzalesi N, Castellazzo R et al: Retinal damage by visible light in albino rats. An electromicroscope study. Ophthalmologica 157:43–59, 1969

80. Kuwabara T, Gorn RA: Retinal damage by visible light: An electron microscopic study. Arch Ophthalmol 79:69–78, 1968

81. Lawwill T: Effects of prolonged exposure of rabbit retina to low-intensity light. Invest Ophthalmol Vis Sci 12:45–51, 1973

82. Marshall J, Mellerio J, Palmer DA: Damage to pigeon retinae by moderate illumination from fluorescent lamps. Exp Eye Res 14:164–169, 1972

83. O'Steen WK, Shear CR, Anderson KV: Retinal damage after prolonged exposure to visible light. A light and electron microscopic study. Am J Anat 134:5–22, 1972

84. Tso MOM: Photic maculopathy in the rhesus monkey; a light and electron microscopic study. Invest Ophthalmol Vis Sci 12:17–34, 1973

85. Dowling JE, Sidman RL: Inherited retinal dystrophy in the rat. J Cell Biol 14:73–109, 1962

86. Herron WL Jr, Riegel BW: Production rate and removal of rod outer segment material in vitamin A deficiency. Invest Ophthalmol Vis Sci 13:46–53, 1974

87. Herron WL Jr, Riegel BW: Vitamin A deficiency-induced "rod thinning" to permanently decrease the production of rod outer segment material. Invest Ophthalmol Vis Sci 13:54–59, 1974

88. Berson EL: Light deprivation for early retinitis pigmentosa: An hypothesis. Arch Ophthalmol 85:521–529, 1971

89. Harwerth RS, Sperling HG: Prolonged color blindness induced by intense spectral lights in rhesus monkeys. Science 174:520–523, 1971

90. Sperling HG, Johnson C: Histological findings in the receptor layer of primate retina associated with light-induced dichromacy. Mod Probl Ophthalmol 13:291–298, 1974

91. Tso MOM, Wallow IHL, Powell JO. Differential susceptibility of rod and cone cells to argon laser. Arch Ophthalmol 89:228–234, 1973

92. Marshall J: Retinal injury from chronic exposure to light and the delayed effects from retinal exposure to intense light sources. In Tengroth B (ed): Current Concepts in Ergophthalmology. Stockholm, Societes Ergophthalmologica Internationalis, 1974

93. Kuwabara T: Photic damage to the retina. In Shimizu K, Oosterhuis JA (eds): Proceedings of the 23rd International Congress of Ophthalmology, Kyoto, 1978, pp 369–374. Amsterdam, Excerpta Medica, 1979

94. Marshall J: Light damage and the practice of ophthalmology. In Rosen ES, Haining WM, Arnott EJ (eds): Intraocular Lens Implantation, pp 182–207. St Louis, CV Mosby, 1984

95. Tso MOM, Fine BS, Zimmerman LE: Photic maculopathy produced by the indirect ophthalmoscope. Am J Ophthalmol 73:686–699, 1972

96. Marshall J: Radiation in the ageing eye. J Physiol Ophthalm Optics 5:241–263, 1985

97. Bok D, Hall MO: The role of the pigment epithelium in the etiology of inherited retinal dystrophy in the rat. J Cell Biol 49:664–682, 1971

98. LaVail MM, Sidman RL, O'Neil D: Photoreceptor pigment epithelial cell relationships in rats with inherited retinal degeneration. J Cell Biol 53:185–209, 1972

99. Herron WL Jr, Riegel BW, Myers OE et al: Retinal dystrophy in the rat–a pigment epithelial disease. Invest Ophthalmol 8:595–604, 1969

100. Custer NV, Bok D: Pigment epithelium photoreceptor interactions in normal and dystrophic rats. Exp Eye Res 21:153–166, 1975

101. Ansell PL, Marshall J: Laser induced phagocytosis in the pigment epithelium of the Hunter dystrophic rat. Br J Ophthalmol 60:819–828, 1976

102. Mullen RJ, LaVail MM: Inherited retinal dystrophy: Primary defect in pigment epithelium determined with experimental rat chimeras. Science 192:799–801, 1976

103. LaVail MM, Mullen RJ: Experimental chimeras: A new approach to the study of inherited retinal degeneration in laboratory animals. Adv Exp Med Biol 77:153–173, 1977

104. Chaitin MH, Hall MO: Defective ingestion of rod outer segments by cultured dystrophic rat pigment epithelial cells. Invest Ophthalmol Vis Sci 24:812–820, 1983

105. Eagle RC, Lucier AC, Bernardino VB et al: Retinal pigment epithelial abnormalities in fundus flavimaculatus. Ophthalmology 87:1189–1200, 1980

106. Kolb H, Gouras P: Electron microscopic observations of human retinitis pigmentosa, dominantly inherited. Invest Ophthalmol 13:489–498, 1974

107. Lahav M, Albert DM, Buyukmihci N et al: Ocular changes in Laurence Moon Bardet Biedl syndrome: A clinical and histopathologic study of a case. Adv Exp Biol 77:51–84, 1977

108. Szamier RB, Berson EL: Retinal ultrastructure in advanced retinitis pigmentosa. Invest Ophthalmol Vis Sci 16:947–962, 1977

109. Sarks SH: Ageing and degeneration in the macular region: A clinicopathological study. Br J Ophthalmol 60:324–341, 1976

110. Szamier RB, Berson EL, Klein R et al: Sex-linked retinitis pigmentosa: Ultrastructure of photoreceptors and pigment epithelium. Invest Ophthalmol Vis Sci 18:145–160, 1979

111. Rayborn ME, Moorhead LC, Hollyfield JG: A dominantly inherited chorioretinal degeneration resembling retinitis pigmentosa. Ophthalmology 89:1441–1453, 1982

112. Runge P, Calver D, Marshall J et al: The histopathology of two distinct pigmentary retinopathies: One associated with the Kearns-Sayre syndrome the other with Laurence-Moon-Biedl syndrome. Br J Ophthalmol 70:782–796, 1986

113. Bunt-Milam AH, Kalina RE, Pagon RA: Clinical-ultrastructural study of a retinal dystrophy. Invest Ophthalmol Vis Sci 24:458–469, 1983

114. Cogan DG: Symposium: Primary chorioretinal aberrrations with night blindness. Pathology Trans Am Acad Ophthalmol Otolaryngol 54:629–661, 1950

115. Deutschmann R: Einseitige typische Retinitis Pigmentosa mit pathologisch anatomischem Befund. Beitr Augenheilkd 1:69–80, 1891

116. Eicholtz W: Histologie der Retinopathia pigmentosa cum et sine Pigmento. Klin Monatsbl Augenheilkd 164:467–475, 1974

117. Gonin J: Examen anatomique d'un oeil atteint de retinite pigmentaire avec scotome zonulaire. Ann Ocul 129:24–48, 1903

118. Kolb H, Gouras P: Electron microscopic observations of human retinitis pigmentosa, dominantly inherited. Invest Ophthalmol Vis Sci 13:489–498, 1974

119. Lucas DR: Retinitis pigmentosa: Pathological findings in two cases. Br J Ophthalmol 40:14–23, 1956

120. Mizuno K, Nashida S: Electron microscopic studies of human retinitis pigmentosa. Am J Ophthalmol 63:791–803, 1967

121. Muller H: Anatomische Betrage zur Ophthalmologie Albrecht von Graefes Arch Ophthalmol 4:1j–54, 1858

122. Verhoeff FH: Microscopic observations in a case of retinitis pigmentosa. Arch Ophthalmol 5:392–407, 1931

123. Wolter JR: Retinitis pigmentosa. Arch Ophthalmol 57:539–553, 1957

124. Taylor D, Lake BD, Marshall J et al: Retinal abnormalities in ophthalmoplegic lipidosis. Br J Ophthalmol 65:484–488, 1981

125. Szamier RB: Ultrastructure of the preretinal membrane in retinitis pigmentosa. Invest Ophthalmol Vis Sci 21:227–236, 1981

126. Meyer KT, Heckenlively JR, Spitznas M et al: Dominant retinitis pigmentosa: A clinicopathologic correlation. Ophthalmol 89:1414–1424, 1982

127. Reme CE: Autophagy in visual cells and pigment epithelium. Invest Ophthalmol Vis Sci 16:807–815, 1977

128. Kroll AJ, Machemer R: Experimental retinal detachment in the owl monkey. III. Electron microscopy of retina and pigment epithelium. Am J Ophthalmol 66:410–427, 1968

129. Duvall J, McKechnie NM, Lee WR et al: Extensive subretinal pigment epithelial deposit in two brothers suffering from dominant retinitis pigmentosa: A histopathological study. Graefes Arch Ophthalmol (in press)

130. Gartner S, Henkind P: Pathology of retinitis pigmentosa. Ophthalmology 89:1425–1432, 1982

131. Bird AC, Marshall J: Retinal receptor disorders without known metabolic abnormalities. In Garner A, Klintworth GK (eds): Pathobiology of Ocular Disease: A Dynamic

Approach, pp 1167–1220. Marcel Dekker, New York, 1982

132. O'Malley P, Allen RA, Straatsma BR et al: Pavingstone degeneration of the retina. Arch Ophthalmol 73:169–182, 1965

133. Ashton N, Sorsby A: Fundus dystrophy with unusual features, a histological study. Br J Ophthalmol 35:751–764, 1951

134. Hollyfield JG, Frederick JM, Tabor GA et al: Metabolic studies on retinal tissue from a donor with a dominantly inherited chorioretinal degeneration resembling sectoral retinitis pigmentosa. Ophthalmology 91:191–196, 1986

135. Rodrigues MM, Wiggert B, Hackett J et al: Dominantly inherited retinitis pigmentosa; ultrastructure and biochemical analysis. Ophthalmology 92:1165–1172, 1985

136. Rayborn ME, Moorhead LC, Hollyfield JG: A dominantly inherited chorioretinal degeneration resembling sectoral retinitis pigmentosa. Ophthalmology 89:1441–1454, 1982

137. Hollyfield JG, Frederick JM, Tabor GA et al: Metabolic studies on retinal tissue from a donor with a dominantly inherited chorioretinal degeneration resembling sectoral retinitis pigmentosa. Ophthalmology 91:191–196, 1984

138. Szamier RB, Berson EL: Retinal histopathology of a carrier of x-chromosome-linked retinitis pigmentosa. Ophthalmology 92:271–278, 1985

139. Rodrigues MM, Battlintine EJ, Wiggert BN et al: Choroideremia: A clinical, electron microscopic, and biochemical report. Ophthalmology 91:873–883, 1984

140. McCulloch C: Choroideremia: A clinical and pathological review. Trans Am Ophthalmol Soc 67:142, 1969

141. Krill AE. In Krill AE, Archer DB (eds): Krill's Hereditary Retinal and Choroidal Diseases, pp 1036–1037. Hagerstown, Harper & Row, 1977

142. Stanescu B, Nereantu F: Laurence-Moon-Bardet-Biedl Syndrome with Juvenile Macular Degenerescence Stargardt: Clinical and Pathological Study. Ophthalmologica 162:76–81, 1971

143. Levin PS, Green WR, Victor DI et al: Histopathology of the eye in Cockayne's syndrome. Arch Ophthalmol 101:1093–1097, 1983

144. McKechnie NM, King M, Lee WR: Retinal pathology in the Kearns-Sayre syndrome. Br J Ophthalmol 69:63–75, 1985

145. Toussaint D, Danis P: An ocular pathologic study of Refsum's syndrome. Am J Ophthalmol 72:342–347, 1971

5

Clinical Findings in Retinitis Pigmentosa

JOHN R. HECKENLIVELY

A large number of retinal diseases meet the definition of retinitis pigmentosa (RP), that is, a set of hereditary diseases in which there is a progressive degeneration of the photoreceptors and retinal pigment epithelium (RPE). One of the reasons that the majority of these patients have been lumped together under a single diagnostic name is that, as a group, they have many similar features which give a commonality and sense of identity to the group. Frequently, the dissimilarities are ignored, taken as atypical features, or considered to arise from a different stage of the disease, which in some cases is correct. There is no question that the clinical features vary considerably with duration of disease. While generalizations about a large set of different diseases have limited usefulness, there are some common findings in RP patients that can be mentioned in a general fashion. Likewise, there are differences in clinical findings that are more characteristic of some types of RP compared with others, which will be reviewed. Composite descriptions of the clinical features of the genetic types of RP will be presented in the relevant chapters.

EARLY CLINICAL FEATURES OF RP (GENERALIZED TO ALL TYPES)

The most common early feature of the rod-cone or diffuse rod involvement form of RP is early night blindness, often noticed by parents within the first year of life. While cone-rod patients are not subject to profound night blindness (unless their disorder is quite advanced), they too often report problems with adapting to dark or light conditions.

Both rod-cone and cone-rod RP degenerative types demonstrate a generalized diffuse depigmentation of the RPE, resulting in a blond or tigroid retinal appearance. Many patients show granularity and tiny focal depigmented spots of the equatorial RPE where the edge is hyperpigmented (**Fig. 5-1A&B**). Many patients have relatively normal-appearing retinal vessels in this stage, but usually the electroretinogram (ERG) is abnormal, and careful visual field testing will document field loss. *Rarely,* a screening ERG in an individual at risk who has very early RP (e.g., the offspring of an affected person with autosomal dominant RP) may be normal, al-

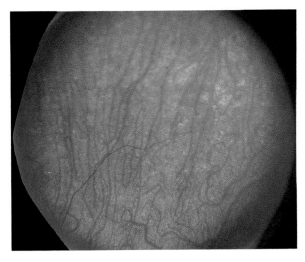

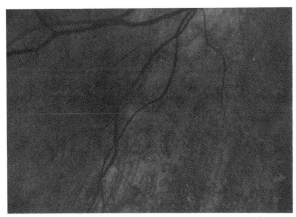

A   B

FIG. 5-1. Early fundus changes in RP: *(A)* focal depigmented spots and granularity in retinal pigment epithelium in a 17-year-old man with early dominant RP; *(B)* early equatorial pigmentation in a 29-year-old woman with multiplex rod-cone degeneration. Several tiny pigment dots are surrounded by a "halo" of depigmentation.

though more sophisticated testing will detect abnormalities.

MIDDLE STAGES

As the degeneration progresses, the most marked changes occur in the RPE. Some patients have patchy loss of the RPE, while others have a diffuse atrophy. Most patients have pigment dispersion which adheres to smaller arteriolar vessels creating a characteristic "bone spicule" pattern of retinal pigmentation. Fewer patients have subretinal clumps of pigment, and occasional patients have mixtures of pigment clumps and bone spicules.

Virtually all patients go through a stage in which there is little to no pigment deposition. This stage is more persistent in some types of RP than others, and for many years these patients would present with typical findings of RP except for no pigmentary changes; they were called "retinitis pigmentosa sine pigmento" to mark them as an atypical type. Recently, the majority of these patients have been found to have the cone-rod degeneration pattern on the ERG.[1] Most patients, however, develop pigment clumps recognizable on indirect ophthalmoscopy.

Occasionally, the retina may have a refractile

edematous appearance (Fig. 7-3*B*), but with time this is lost as the retina and RPE degenerate.

In the middle stages, the retinal vessels, particularly the arteries, show narrowing. Interestingly, some patients with RP, when compared with other types of RP in which the visual field is constricted the same amount, show patency and preservation of retinal vessels into areas of pigment deposits while most RP patients have atrophy of vessels in the areas of pigmentation. The most notable example of this is preserved para-arteriolar retinal pigment epithelium (PPRPE) RP (see Chapter 9 for details).

The optic nervehead in the early to middle stages is generally pink, although it may not look completely normal, often having a ground-glass or "creamy" hue. Disc capillaries are frequently dilated or telangiectatic; these conditions can be detected on direct ophthalmoscopy as beading or focal dilatations and are easily demonstrated on early phases of the fluorescein angiogram. Temporal optic atrophy, or disc tissue missing temporally, may be seen in all types of RP but is more common in the cone-rod varieties. Most RP patients have smaller cup-to-disc ratios and greater nerve fiber loss than normal.

Slit lamp examination invariably demonstrates pigmented flecks in the anterior vitreous space, which may be the first diagnostic clue the ophthalmologist sees on a routine examination. Some patients develop posterior subcapsular cataracts. Early syneresis of the vitreous is common.

Visual fields usually demonstrate partial or full-ring scotomata, and there may be other deficits such as baring or enlargement of the blind spot, pseudoaltitudinal defects, arcuate loss, or generalized constriction without ring scotomata (see Chapter 3).

LATER STAGES

As the retina degenerates, many patients develop large midperipheral areas of RPE mottling, which has a "reticular" or lobule structural appearance that can be mistaken for the flecks seen in fundus flavimaculatus (**Fig. 5-2**; see also Figs. 13-13, 13-23*B*). A similar RPE-choriocapillaris pattern was demonstrated by Hayreh in young monkeys examined by fluorescein angiography.[2] He found that each terminal choroidal arteriole centrally supplies an independent segment of choriocapillaris which is drained by venules lying on the periphery of this segment. The segments are polygonal and form a mosaic. This mosaic pattern is seen frequently in RP and other retinal degenerative diseases. The term *lobule pattern* is reasonable to describe this mottled

appearance because of the structural similarity to pulmonary lobules.

Retinal vessels in most forms of RP become quite constricted, often confined to the immediate posterior pole area. In advanced stages the optic nervehead develops a waxy pale appearance that is more marked on direct than indirect ophthalmoscopy. Many nerveheads have a thin white rim that may encompass the edge of the nervehead partially or 360° (**Fig. 5-3*A&B***). On careful examination, this thin white rim occurs in two situations; some patients have a subtle peripapillary withdrawal of RPE and uvea, leaving a thin scleral edge, while other patients have a definite edge of optic nervehead atrophy with 360° of glistening white granular material that shows lack of filling on early phases of fluorescein angiography. Late frames may show hyperfluorescent staining similar to that seen in retinal or choroidal scar formation and may represent areas of atrophied nerve fibers. This hypothesis has yet to be correlated on histopathology.

Some patients have such severe RPE loss that their choroidal vessels are exposed and appear yellow or white, typical of choroidal sclerosis (**Fig. 5-4**). Confirmation of this latter finding, however, can only be made on fluorescein angiography, and most of these patients will demonstrate patency of their choroidal

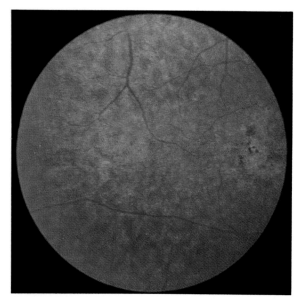

FIG. 5-2. Lobule RPE change in a 23-year-old woman with simplex rod-cone degeneration. This degenerative pattern of loss is common to many RP types and is primarily seen in the near to midequatorial regions.

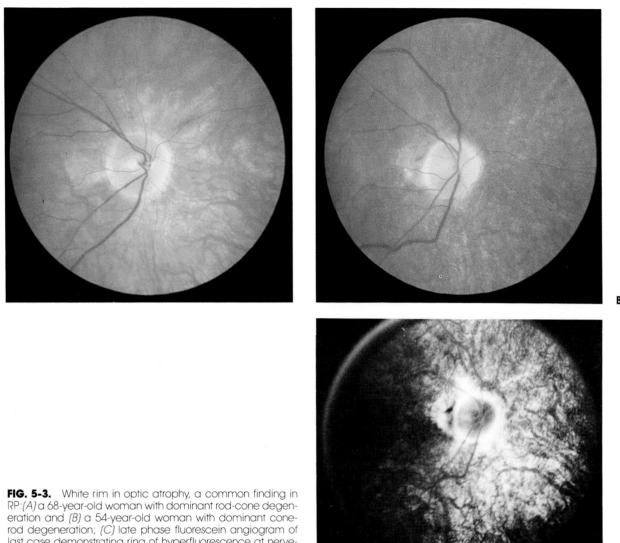

FIG. 5-3. White rim in optic atrophy, a common finding in RP:*(A)* a 68-year-old woman with dominant rod-cone degeneration and *(B)* a 54-year-old woman with dominant cone-rod degeneration; *(C)* late phase fluorescein angiogram of last case demonstrating ring of hyperfluorescence at nervehead in region of white rim.

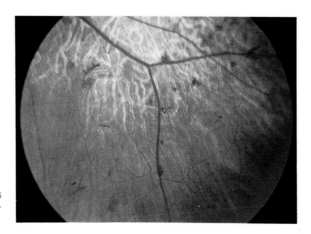

FIG. 5-4. RPE atrophy with appearance of choroidal sclerosis in a 67-year-old man with simplex RP. Fluorescein angiography demonstrated patency of vessels.

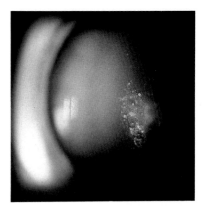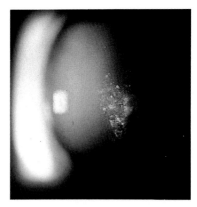

FIG. 5-5. Stereographic photograph: posterior subcapsular cataract in a 43-year-old man with simplex RP.

vessels despite their atrophic appearance. Some patients have diffuse or patchy choriocapillaris filling.

Biomicroscopy often reveals a posterior subcapsular cataract (**stereographic Fig. 5-5**) and vitreous syneresis and stranding.[3] Other types of cataracts are less frequent. This topic is covered in greater detail in the cataract section of this chapter.

Visual fields often show small central fields with temporal islands, or remnants of vision. A few patients have a rim of anterior retina which sees large targets, while in reality they have 10° or less of "useful" central vision. Catching this rim of anterior retina and missing the huge midperipheral scotomata has resulted in a number of RP patients being denied social security disability status even though they are entitled to it. Static perimetry such as the Octopus field test used in conjunction with the Goldmann visual field examination will help alleviate this problem and will demonstrate the patient's deficit more clearly to disability examiners.

MEDICAL HISTORY

The medical history is an extremely valuable tool in gaining an understanding of the functional deficits that the patient is experiencing, and frequently the derived information helps focus the patient evaluation so that appropriate testing is performed. The type of common helpful information that may be obtained includes the age at onset of symptoms, both visual field and night blindness, a family history, and

any associated medical problems such as deafness, polydactyly, kidney problems, heart block, and/or neurological problems. In listening to the speech of an RP patient, one may note a nasal intonation suggestive of congenital partial hearing loss or the diagnosis of type II Usher's syndrome.

In a preliminary analysis of reported age of onset and duration of disease in 215 RP patients at UCLA, the following information was found (Table 5-1); data are divided by whether the patient had a recordable or nonrecordable ERG, and visual acuities of each group are included.

As might be expected, the majority of patients had nonrecordable ERGs, and this group, with a few exceptions, had a longer duration of symptoms, smaller visual fields, and poorer visual acuities compared with patients with recordable ERGs.

The reliability of historical reports of symptoms in RP can be diverse, since, for a variety of reasons, the patient's account may not correlate with disease onset. Patients who are not night-blind, or even those who are night-blind but live in an urban environment may not complain of difficulty in darkened areas. Other patients have such slow onset of the disease that the visual field has to become quite limited (e.g. 12°) before they fully realize something is wrong with their vision; years prior to this time, though, relatives may note clumsy behavior and signs of visual field loss. Other patients who are night-blind from birth do not have a normal reference, learn to adapt, and may regard their vision as

TABLE 5-1

AGE AT DIAGNOSIS, DURATION OF DISEASE (BY ONSET OF SYMPTOMS), VISUAL FIELD SIZE, VISUAL ACUITY BY WHETHER ERG IS RECORDABLE OR NONRECORDABLE (215 RP PATIENTS)

DIAGNOSIS	ERG RECORDABLE	N	AGE AT DX	DURATION (YEARS)	VISUAL FIELD	VISUAL ACUITY
Dominant	Yes	11	32.4	14.4	3.4	20/30 +
rod-cone	No	20	36.5	21.8	2.5	20/40 +
Recessive	Yes	9	19.8	10.2	4.1	20/40 +
rod-cone	No	22	35.9	17.1	2.0	20/60 +
X-linked	Yes	0				
rod-cone	No	8	40.1	30.3	2.3	20/60 − 2
Choroideremia	Yes	2	32.0	17.0	3.0	20/20
	No	8	30.8	22.0	2.4	20/30 − 2
Simplex	Yes	27	30.3	14.6	2.9	20/30 − 2
rod-cone	No	37	33.1	13.9	2.2	20/40 − 2
Dominant	Yes	6	22.7	3.3	3.9	20/30 +
cone-rod	No	5	39.8	1.9	1.9	20/50 − 2
Recessive	Yes	5	37.6	5.2	3.8	20/60 + 2
cone-rod	No	1	44.0	23.0	3.0	20/25
X-linked	Yes	3	29.7	17.6	3.8	20/40
cone-rod	No	1	36.0	4.0	4.0	20/40 + 2
Usher's	Yes	7	25.3	17.4	3.4	20/40 −
	No	17	24.6	15.7	2.6	20/50 + 2
Simplex	Yes	19	38.7	9.6	3.7	20/30 −
cone-rod	No	7	45.9	16.7	2.3	20/30 − 2

ERG: yes = some aspect of the ERG was recordable
    no = the ERG was nonrecordable by single flash technique

n = sample size

Age = age at which testing was performed

Duration = number of years since patient first noted visual symptoms, whether field loss or night blindness

Visual field = reported in units representing ranges of size with IV-4 Goldmann isopter, 1 = field <5°, 2 = field 5°–15°, 3 = field 16°–30°, 4 = field 31°–50°, 5 = field >50°. Each field was measured from fixation to the edge of the field in each quadrant and averaged.

Visual acuity = best corrected Snellen score, group average

Diagnosis of cone-rod degeneration in patients with a nonrecordable ERG was made on the basis of the patient being part of an established cone-rod pedigree or having a final rod threshold <2.0 log units above normal.

normal. Determining onset can be biased in favor of early ascertainment by family examinations prompted by finding RP in another family member.

"GOOD DAYS, BAD DAYS"

A common complaint of patients with more advanced disease in all types of RP is that they note fluctuation in their vision such that they experience good and bad days. Some patients report that their vision is "crystal clear" first thing in the morning but soon becomes fuzzy. Initially, this may throw the patient into a panic that their RP is suddenly worse. Visual fields occasionally may show the same variability, a finding documented by Ross, Fishman, and colleagues.[4] They found intervisit and interexaminer variability in both normal subjects and RP patients. RP patients showed 2 to 3 times the intervisit variability compared with normal controls. The causes of these fluctuations are not clear, one association that is commonly reported to cause vision loss is stress or being under pressure.

NIGHT BLINDNESS

One of the hallmarks of RP is night blindness. It is commonly assumed that it begins at birth or early in childhood. However, when patients are closely questioned on this point, many RP patients deny that they are night-blind or that they have any particular problem in darkened areas. When this apparent discrepancy is analyzed, most of these patients are found to have cone-rod or regional degeneration of the retina. Cone-rod degeneration patients usually maintain reasonable night vision until the visual field contracts to less than 10°, at which point they begin to complain of night-blindness and symptoms referable to visual field loss.

Several retrospective studies have been done at UCLA looking at the age of onset of night blindness by RP type, and these results can be found in Table 5-2. As expected, patients with rod-cone degeneration have an earlier onset of night blindness, while patients with cone-rod patterns have a later onset.

The effect of visual field size on night blindness in cone-rod degenerations was analyzed several ways. In a study of 76 cone-rod degeneration patients of all inheritance types, symptomatic night blindness was checked against visual field size, and was correlated with the patients' best final rod threshold. As would be expected, those patients with smaller visual fields were more night-blind (Table 5-3, **Fig. 5-6**), but most patients had final rod thresholds 2.0 log units of elevation or better.[4a]

REFRACTION IN RP

A refraction, basic to ophthalmologic examination, is often overlooked in RP patients because clinicians believe that "nothing can be done" for RP. However, most RP patients are myopic and, with age, also develop presbyopic problems. Some patients develop cataracts, and their vision may be improved with refraction.

TABLE 5-2

AVERAGE AGE REPORTED FOR ONSET OF SYMPTOMS (USUALLY NYCTALOPIA)

TYPE OF RP	AGE OF ONSET (NO. OF PATIENTS)
Dominant RC	15.9 (31)
Recessive RC	16.1 (31)
X-linked RC	8.7 (9)
Simplex RC	17.7 (64)
Choroideremia	10.0 (10)
Dominant CR	20.0 (11)
Recessive CR	30.5 (6)
X-linked CR	22.3 (3)
Simplex CR	29.1 (26)

TABLE 5-3

VISUAL FIELD SIZE AND NIGHT BLINDNESS

	VISUAL FIELD (IV-4 TARGET)
Symptomatic	28.2°*
Asymptomatic	43.5°*

* p <.003 analysis of covariance controlling for age

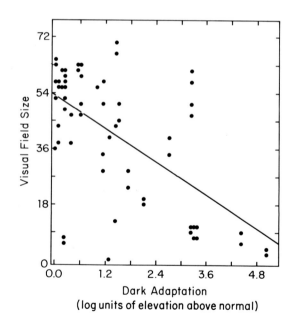

FIG. 5-6. Graph correlating visual field size to final rod threshold in 76 patients with cone-rod degeneration of the RP type. Final rod thresholds were measured across the horizontal meridian, and the best value was chosen within the area of visual field, which was measured in degrees by quadrant and the values averaged. While there is scatter, patients with smaller fields tend to be more night-blind.

TABLE 5-4

REFRACTIONS IN RP

DIAGNOSIS	NO. OF PATIENTS EVALUATED	SPHERE	CYLINDER	AXIS	SPH EQUIV
Dominant rod-cone	20	−1.29	+1.02	×102	−0.78
Recessive rod-cone	18	−1.82	+1.17	×93	−1.23
X-linked rod-cone	14	−2.91	+1.12	×101	−2.35
Choroideremia	15	−3.53	+0.76	×89	−3.30**
Simplex rod-cone	35	−2.71	+1.14	×96	−2.14
Dominant cone-rod	8	−4.13*	+1.20	×79	−3.52*
Recessive cone-rod	4	−3.25	+1.56	×92	−2.47
X-linked cone-rod	4	−4.59	+1.91	×93	−3.64
Simplex cone-rod	8	−4.09	+1.52	×97	−3.34
All cone-rod	24	−4.05**	+1.48	×89	−3.30**
Usher's syndrome	27	−1.09*	+1.12	×97	−0.53*
Bardet-Biedl	9	−2.99	+2.07*	×96	−1.95
Leber's amaurosis	7	+4.50	+1.88***	×90	+5.44***
PPRPE RP	5	+3.30***	+0.92	×101	+3.76***

Axis = right eye; left axis recalculated to right axis
Analysis of variance for all groups: * = $p < .05$, ** = $p < .01$, *** = $p < .001$

Interestingly, certain refractive errors appear to be characteristic of certain RP types: the most striking examples are PPRPE and forms of congenital RP, including typical Leber is congenital amaurosis, in which patients are quite hypermetropic, and Bardet-Biedl syndrome in which patients have increased astigmatism (Table 5-4).

The difference between right and left eyes and the patient's age and sex were found not to be statistically significant with refraction.

Cone-rod degeneration patients appear to be significantly more myopic than rod-cone degeneration patients. Table 5-4 suggests that patients with X-linked recessive disease (rod-cone, cone-rod, choroideremia) may be slightly more myopic than other patients in general. The only type of RP with a significantly different power in cylinder were the Bardet-Biedl and Leber's patients. Refractive errors in RP patients were studied by Sieving and Fishman[5]; in 134 patients they found mean refractive error of −1.86 diopters for the group which was more myopic by −2.93 diopters than the normal population ($p < 0.001$). They also found that the X-linked RP group was more myopic than non–X-linked RP, and there was a bimodal distribution to the X-linked spherical errors.

BIOMICROSCOPY IN RP

The two main findings on biomicroscopy in RP are posterior subcapsular cataracts, and pigmented flecks and syneresis of the anterior vitreous. A few patients will have white amorphous vitreal condensates, and rarely midvitreal round white cyst-like objects which may be better visualized with indirect ophthalmoscopy (see Figs. 13-3 and 13-6A).

The frequency and severity of posterior subcapsular cataracts (**Fig. 5-5**) were analyzed in 291 patients from the UCLA RP Registry (Table 5-5).[6] The overall frequency was 41%, and was less common in cone-rod degeneration and choroideremia.

Of affected patients, 73% (237 of 582 eyes) were

TABLE 5-5

POSTERIOR SUBCAPSULAR CATARACTS IN RP (291 patients)

DIAGNOSIS	PERCENTAGE OF PATIENTS WITH POSTERIOR SUBCAPSULAR CATARACTS
Dominant rod-cone	47%
Recessive rod-cone	49%
X-linked rod-cone	31%*
Simplex rod-cone	39%
Usher's syndrome	42%
All cone-rod	33%†

* The lower frequency in the X-linked recessive rod-cone group may reflect the lower mean age of those patients examined.

† A division into genetic types was not performed in this earlier study.

minimally affected, that is, had trace to 1-mm cataracts compared with 27% of patients who had posterior subcapsular cataracts 2 mm or larger or who were aphakic[6]; the latter group constituted 6% (34 eyes). The data suggest that there is an influence of age on posterior subcapsular cataract presence, since groups showed a tendency to have more severe cataracts with increasing age. However, there were older individuals in all types of RP who had clear lenses, so not every patient with RP will develop a cataract.

While other types of cataracts were not studied in a comprehensive fashion, incidental findings were noted; simplex RP patients were the only group noted to have anterior subcapsular cataracts, and in this category the frequency of nuclear sclerotic cataracts was much higher. Simplex RP was the only group in which gender was significant; females were significantly affected more often ($p<.002$). These results are similar to those reported by Pruett: in 384 eyes with RP, 178 (46.4%) had cataracts, and of these, 93% were posterior subcapsular cataracts.[7]

The etiology and pathophysiologic mechanisms of posterior subcapsular cataract formation in the progressive hereditary pigmentary degenerations are unknown. One histologic study showed distorted lens fibers, aberrantly migrated epithelial cells, and duplicated lens capsule posteriorly.[8] Fagerholm and Philipson analyzed seven RP cataracts and found lenses with extensive extracellular vacuolization, focal degeneration of epithelial cells, epithelial cell mitochondrial swelling, and hydrated posterior lens fibers.[9] It is this author's experience that anterior capsules at the time of extracapsular cataract extraction are often more elastic or tougher than those of many non-RP patients. In addition, these patients more frequently develop postoperative wrinkling of the posterior capsule requiring YAG capsulotomy.

CATARACT SURGERY IN RP

Two retrospective studies at UCLA have look at the efficacy of cataract surgery in RP patients. In 30 patients (54 eyes) who had undergone intracapsular and extracapsular surgery, 83% demonstrated improvement in visual acuity of at least two lines on the Snellen chart, and 52% achieved a visual acuity of 20/50 or better. Most patients felt that they saw better after surgery. The preoperative and postoperative visual fields were unchanged, suggesting that the surgery did not exacerbate the disease process.

Criteria for surgery include establishing:

1. History of glare phenomena or

2. Decreased vision from an axial cataract; direct ophthalmoscopy along the visual axis greatly aids in estimating the level of deficit attributable to cataract.

3. Fundus evaluation to ensure that macular RPE/function is present; visual acuity interferometry may assist in this evaluation. Occasionally, fluorescein angiography may be useful in evaluating the macular RPE status.

4. Adequate central visual field

The second retrospective study at UCLA evaluated the efficacy of intraocular lenses (IOLs) in RP cataract surgery. Seventeen RP patients of all types (23 eyes) had 19 posterior chamber and 4 anterior chamber IOLs implanted following cataract extraction. Patients were evaluated preoperatively and postoperatively for effects of surgery on visual acuity, intraocular pressure, visual fields, posterior capsules, and macular status. Sixteen of 17 patients reported definite visual improvement, and 21 of 23 eyes had better visual acuity. Patients with tiny visual fields (<5° using large isopters) tended to derive less benefit from the operation. YAG capsulotomies were performed in nine patients necessitated by capsular wrinkling and opacities. In general, RP patients with significant cataractous opacities on the visual axis and retained macular health are good candidates for extracapsular surgery with posterior chamber intraocular lenses. Increased wrinkling of the posterior capsule in these cases is consistent with experience in performing intracapsular extractions in RP patients in which zonules were not found to be tightly adherent to the lens capsule.10 (A further discussion on the management of RP cataracts is found in Chapter 6).

VITREAL CHANGES IN RP

The results of biomicroscopic study of the vitreous gel in 58 RP patients were reported by Pruett.[3] Vitreous degeneration was seen at all ages, and the severity of vitreal changes parallelled the amount of retinal destruction as determined by visual field testing. The vitreous degeneration was categorized into four stages: (1) tiny, dust-like reflective particles uniformly distributed throughout the gel; (2) particles plus complete posterior separation of the vitreous from the retina; (3) the above changes plus formation of a posterior matrix of dense white opacities and interconnecting fibers; and (4) particles, posterior separation, and coarse posterior matrix collapse and reduced volume of the residual gel.

Takahashi investigated the vitreous status in 21 RP patients of all types; 14% (6 eyes) had no vitreous detachment, 12% (5 eyes) had a partial vitreous detachment, and 74% (31 eyes) had complete vitreous detachment. "Cottonball-like" or spindle-shaped opacities were present in 91% of eyes, while interwoven filaments were present in 71%.[11]

RETINAL DETACHMENT IN RP

It might be supposed that because of retinal scarring, RP patients would not be subject to retinal detachment. However, in the UCLA RP Registry five cases have been seen, and Pruett[7] reported six patients with various types of RP who have experienced retinal detachment. Most cases appeared to arise from atrophic retinal breaks and were not highly myopic (**Fig. 5-7A-C**).

VISUAL ACUITY IN RP

One of the most interesting aspects of the natural history of RP is the relative preservation of central vision in most patients for prolonged periods, even though there is progressive peripheral visual field loss. Histologic studies by Zamier and Berson in a patient with X-linked RP, as well as cone spatial density studies by various authors,[12,13] strongly suggest that there is such a high concentration of cones in the fovea that even with a loss of 50% of foveal cones, patients may still have near-normal vision. Furthermore, many of the cones still present are shortened or disoriented, yet patients have functional vision. Sandberg found that cone increment thresholds in RP patients with visual acuity 20/25 or better were elevated two times above normal in the foveola and ten times above normal in the parafovea, suggesting that cone spatial density was reduced 50% below normal in the foveola and 90% below normal in the parafovea.

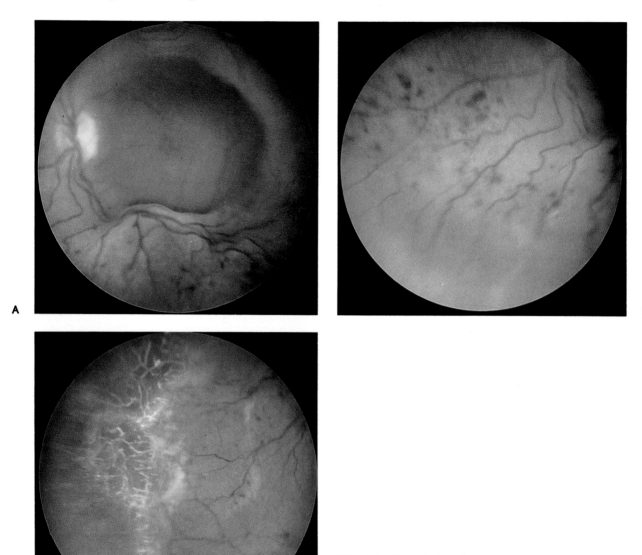

FIG. 5-7. Retinal detachment, left eye, in a 33-year-old woman with dominant rod-cone degeneration: *(A)* posterior pole surrounded by bullous retinal detachment, *(B)* superior nasal to disc showing pigment deposits, and *(C)* lattice-like degeneration with atrophic holes. (Photographs courtesy of Professor A. C. Bird)

Greenstein and colleagues suggest that early foveal sensitivity loss may be due to a decreased responsiveness of retinal elements and not to a decrease in quantum catching ability of functioning photoreceptors.[15]

Pearlman analyzed visual acuity in 250 RP patients for the relationship of visual acuity to duration of night vision loss in the three mendelian types of RP. He found no significant difference among the slopes of the regression curves by RP type.[16]

We looked at visual acuity in autosomal recessive and dominant RP in the Navaho Indian (**Fig. 5-8**); both RP types are likely to represent distinct genetic forms. There was a significant difference between

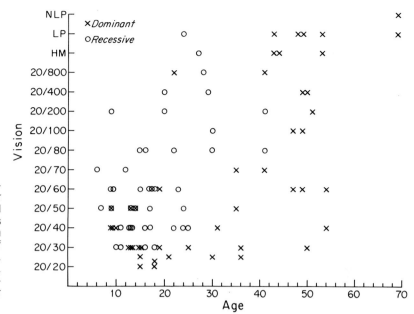

FIG. 5-8. Scattergram of visual acuities plotted against age of patient for Navaho autosomal recessive and dominant RP groups. Each eye was plotted separately. Analysis of data confirmed a significant difference of visual acuity between the two groups, but once age was taken into account, the rate of deterioration was not significantly different. (Metab Pediatr Syst Ophthalmol 5:205,1981)

the two groups; while the regression slopes were not statistically different, the age of onset differed, with the recessive patients showing earlier visual loss.[16]

Fishman evaluated central visual loss in 174 RP patients; the degree of loss was mildest in autosomal dominant RP and most severe in X-linked recessive inheritance.[17] His study found that one-third of 347 eyes had central acuity of 20/200 or less, while 55% had 20/60 or better, and only one-third had vision 20/30 or better.

Visual acuity data from the UCLA RP Registry are presented in Table 5-1. Patients with nonrecordable ERGs had visual acuities and visual fields worse than those patients of the same RP type who had recordable ERGs; the severity was related to duration of the disease.

Marmor presented data on 91 patients of all types of RP, many of whom had multiple examinations.[18] Autosomal recessive patients clearly had less preserved visual acuity with increased age, compared with autosomal dominant patients. His data suggests that once the best corrected visual acuity is 20/40 or poorer from macular changes, the visual acuity is

unstable and tends to regress to 20/200 or worse within 6 years. The issue of fluctuating vision is discussed above in the section entitled "Good days, bad days."

Concurrently, many of these patients have visual fields that are constricted to 10° or less, and the question of disability eventually arises; the visual acuity loss (often macular degeneration) with a small field is the critical factor that suddenly motivates the patient to apply for disability compensation.

MACULAR CHANGES IN RP

Even though the central vision tends to be preserved in RP, the appearance of the macula in RP patients is frequently abnormal. Pruett carefully evaluated the macular status in 383 RP eyes and concluded that only 25.8% maculae were normal[7]; his data are presented in Table 5-6. Note that frequently many of the findings coexisted, and only the main finding was recorded.

Surface wrinkling was described as a cellophane-like, irregular light reflex which was associated with fine corrugations of the inner sensory retina that

TABLE 5-6

MACULAR MORPHOLOGY

MACULAR APPEARANCE	SIMPLEX (230)	A-R (92)	A-D (50)	X-L (11)
Normal	28.7%	21.7%	20%	25.8%
Surface wrinkling	19.1%	23.9%	20%	20.4%
Cystic	13.9%	14.1%	22%	15.1%
Bull's-eye	37%	31.5%	40%	35.8%
Atrophic	12.5	29.3	16%	18.2%

AR = autosomal recessive, AD = autosomal dominant, X-L = X-linked recessive
Numbers of patients studied are in parentheses.
(Pruett: Trans. Am Ophthalmol Soc 81:720, 1983)

assumed parallel radial or whorl-like configurations (see Figs. 5-9, 7-3A, 8-14, and 10-6). Pruett found no vitreous adhesions to these areas on examination. Bull's-eye lesions were described as a halo of pallor at the level of the RPE, resulting in a circular window defect on fluorescein angiography (e.g., Fig. 8-8A–C). A single or cluster of macular cyst-like formations were recorded in the single category of "cystic"; of 37 eyes with cysts, only 29 (78%) had fluorescein angiographic evidence of macular leak-

TABLE 5-7

FLUORESCEIN ANGIOGRAPHIC FINDINGS IN RP: AVERAGE PERCENTAGE OF PARAMETER BY DIAGNOSIS

DIAGNOSIS (NUMBER OF EYES)	MACULAR HYPOFLOURESENCE	MACULAR WINDOW DEFECT	PARAMACULAR WINDOW DEFECT	CYSTOID MACULAR EDEMA
Dominant rod-cone degeneration (28)	83%	7%	11%	27%
Autosomal recessive rod-cone degeneration (9)	60%	20%	0%	0%
X-linked recessive rod-cone degeneration (8)	63%	13%	0%	13%
Choroideremia (25)	61%	21%	0%	0%
Dominant cone-rod degeneration (9)	80%	20%	0%	10%
Autosomal recessive cone-rod degeneration (8)	63%	50%	0%	0%
X-linked recessive cone-rod degeneration (4)	50%	0%	0%	0%
Usher's (23)	58%	29%	14%	8%
Simplex rod-cone degeneration (97)	61%	24%	1%	16%
Simplex cone-rod degeneration (26)	69%	15%	0%	15%
All types (237) (Mean value)	64%	21%	3.7%	12.9%

(Thomas L. Hauch is gratefully acknowledged for help in compiling these data.)

age. This is documentation of the phenomenon, also observed at UCLA, that some patients with macular cysts are really demonstrating a breakdown, or possibly a schisis-like condition, of the macular region (see Figs. 13-5*A&B* and 13-8*A&B*). Fluorescein angiography does not demonstrate cystoid edema in these cases.

Fishman, Maggiano, and Fishman in a study of 110 RP patients found that patients without fluorescein dye accumulation in a cyst lacked an inner limiting membrane and that the fluorescein was diffusing into the vitreous.[19] However, their finding and hypothesis neither supports nor refutes the possibility that some patients have a degeneration of macular structure with schisis-like changes in the macula. These changes tend to occur in more advanced stages of the RP process. Fishman found that patients with partial-thickness macular holes or cysts showed preretinal membranes or cellophane surface wrinkling.[18]

Fishman also evaluated visual loss and foveal lesions in Usher's syndrome in 48 patients; he found that 21 (44%) had either atrophic or cystic-appearing bilateral macular lesions.[18]

Merin emphasized the importance of considering the possibility of panretinal degeneration in patients presenting with macular cysts or holes.[21] Electrophysiologic testing, and often a careful examination of the peripheral retina, will establish the correct diagnosis. More data on macular changes in RP can be found in the section on Fluorescein Angiography below.

FLUORESCEIN ANGIOGRAPHY IN RP

Fluorescein angiography commonly is used to investigate the integrity of the RPE, the choroid, and the retinal vessels, as well as to study the circulatory dynamics of the retina. This test is particularly help-

VASCULAR ARCADE EDEMA	PARAPAPILLARY EDEMA	OPTIC NERVE TELANGIECTASIA	TEMPORAL ATROPHY
17%	18%	64%	50%
20%	30%	70%	50%
0%	25%	75%	75%
15%	8%	50%	29%
10%	10%	90%	75%
0%	38%	88%	75%
0%	0%	90%	50%
33%	42%	29%	21%
30%	27%	50%	50%
27%	15%	54%	58%
23%	23.6%	52.9%	48%

ful in looking for subretinal and other types of neovascularization and in establishing the presence of retinal edema.

With a few exceptions such as checking for choroideremia, cystoid macular edema, and RPE competence, fluorescein angiography is not commonly performed to evaluate RP, but the technique has been useful in clinical investigations. Preliminary evidence suggests that there are some differences on the fluorescein angiogram among various RP types (Table 5-7).

Early reports on fluorescein angiography in RP noted that the retinal blood flow was reduced such that the retinal capillaries could not be visualized. Changes in the RPE and choriocapillaris could be more easily visualized.[22] Krill, Archer, and Newell investigated the fluorescein angiogram in 23 patients with various types of RP, noting that the test was valuable in establishing the absence or presence of disease in the macula and other areas of the retina and might be helpful in differentiating RP from other diseases with similar ophthalmoscopic appearances.[23] An additional finding by fundus examination in some RP patients with severe choroidal sclerosis

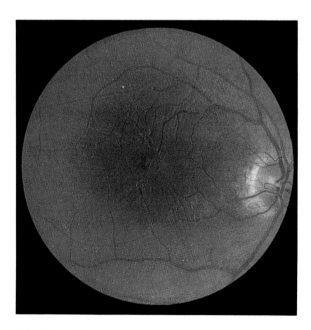

FIG. 5-9. Surface wrinkling retinopathy; 24-year-old man with simplex RP. Retinal striae of posterior pole and macular disturbance are apparent.

(Fig. 5-4) was increased fluorescein angiographic visualization of these vessels in some cases, which may help to distinguish RP patients from patients with generalized choroidal sclerosis. A unique feature of Navaho Indians with autosomal recessive RP is that while they have a diffuse atrophy of the RPE, their fluorescein angiograms demonstrate a patent choriocapillaris.[16]

Notting and Deutman demonstrated that the fluorescein angiogram was useful in establishing the amount and extent of RPE disturbance and choriocapillaris atrophy, as well as in documenting the source and types of retinal edema in hereditary retinal degeneration patients.[24]

One of the more important uses of the fluorescein angiogram is in the diagnosis of early choroideremia, or cases of choroideremia which present with minimal fundus findings of RPE loss (see Choroideremia Fundus Type III, Chapter 10). Young patients from X-linked recessive pedigrees may present initially where the type of retinal degeneration is not known to the family, and the patient has mottling and fine pigment deposits in the midperipheral retina (see Fig. 10-2A&B). A fluorescein angiogram will show whether the scalloped loss of RPE and choriocapillaris of choroideremia is present (see Figs. 10-21D, 10-23B, 10-24B & D, and 10-25D & E) or whether there is more diffuse atrophy without confluent choriocapillaris involvement.

Fish and associates noted the important angiographic finding that some retinal dystrophies exhibit an absence of normal background fluorescence or the "dark choroid" effect.[25] One cause of this phenomenon was shown by Eagle when he and his associates demonstrated intracellular lipofuscin staining deposits in the RPE of a young patient with fundus flavimaculatus.[26] It is reasonable to assume that other retinal dystrophies exhibiting the "dark choroid" effect also have a buildup of RPE intracellular materials blocking choroidal fluorescence.

The fluorescein angiograms of 125 UCLA RP patients of all types (239 eyes) were studied to establish characteristic findings (Table 5-7). Various fluorescein angiographic parameters were rated on a scale of 0 to 2 in which *0* was not present and *2* was markedly present. Fluorescein findings evaluated included presence of macular hypofluorescence, mac-

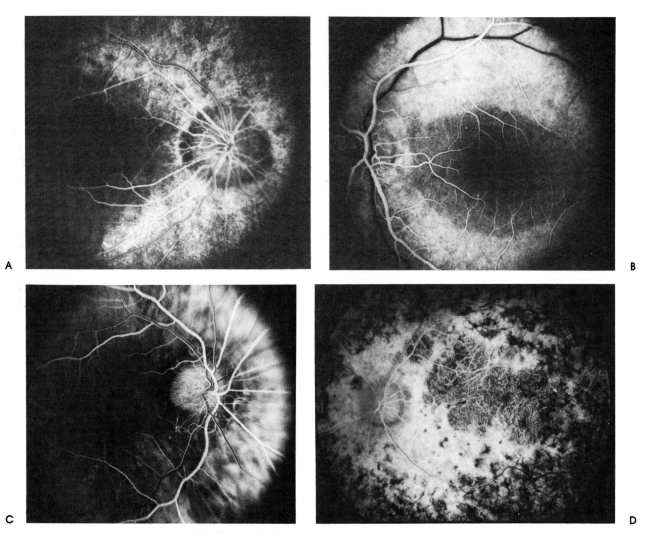

FIG. 5-10. Fluorescein angiograms: *(A)* macular hypofluorescence, disc telangiectasia, and diffuse retinal atrophy in simplex RP; *(B)* macular hypofluorescence, diffuse staining of RPE outside macula in a 12-year-old girl with dominant cone-rod degeneration; *(C)* disc telangiectasia in simplex cone-rod degeneration; *(D)* RPE staining and macular atrophy in a 14-year-old girl with Leber's congenital amaurosis; *(continued)*

ular and paramacular window defects; macular, disc, peripapillary, and vascular arcade edema; disc telangiectasia, or dilation of previously existing small vessels of the optic nervehead; and temporal optic atrophy which was distinguished by hypofluorescent areas on the transit phases of the fluorescein angiogram (Fig. 5-10*A–H*). Some cases involved the whole temporal aspect of the disc or, occasionally, the maculopapillary bundle.

The fluorescein angiographic findings in the various RP subtypes are presented in Table 5-7. One of the interesting findings in the study is that a majority of RP patients have macular hypofluorescence (see Fig. 3-6*D&E* and **5-10***A&B*), suggesting that abnormal material may be accumulating in macular RPE and blocking choroidal fluorescence, although in some cases the macula appears hypofluorescent because surrounding retina demonstrates fluorescein staining. Macular window defects were seen about 20% of the time, with autosomal recessive cone-rod degeneration patients demonstrating the highest occurrence (50%).

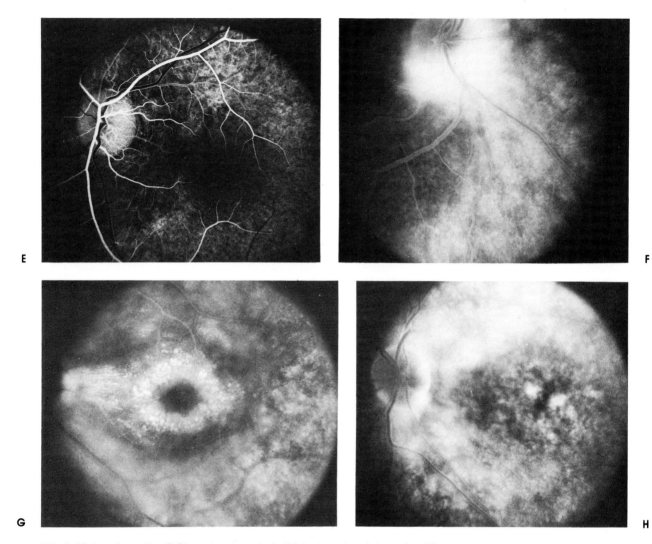

FIG. 5-10 *(continued)*. *(E)* Disc telangiectasia in X-linked cone-rod dystrophy; *(F)* peripapillary edema and diffuse retinal atrophy in a patient with atypical RP and total deafness; *(G)* cystoid macular edema in a 51-year-old woman with simplex rod-cone degeneration; *(H)* vascular arcade edema and diffuse retinal edema in a 22-year-old woman with simplex early-onset RP.

Despite one report (from a fluorescein angiography service) in which cystoid macular edema was present in half the RP patients studied,[27] we found an overall frequency of macular edema in 13% of patients. A pattern of diffuse hyperfluorescence was more common, while cystoid edema was less common in the macular area. Statistical analysis revealed that autosomal dominant and simplex rod-cone degeneration had macular edema significantly more often ($p<.05$).

Treatment of RP macular edema by scatter or grid laser photocoagulation has been suggested. This idea is untested and controversial. Since macular edema often is a feature of patients having advanced RP disease, in whom the visual field is usually severely constricted, lasering the remaining seeing retina in order to minimally improve visual acuity may not be a reasonable tradeoff. Clearly, this problem needs careful study before laser is generally offered to RP patients.

Telangiectasia of the disc was present in the majority of patients, which may help to explain why patients often have pink but abnormal-appearing discs. Disc telangiectasia was seen most frequently in cone-rod patients, while Usher's syndrome patients had disc telangiectasia the least (29%). The reason for disc telangiectasia in RP patients is not known, but it may be a subtle response to transsynaptic degeneration and neuronal loss, or a response to the retinal degeneration. X-linked carriers of various types of RP often have mild to severe disc telangiectasia, which aids in establishing their carrier status.

Analysis of temporal atrophy among RP types reveals that choroideremia and Usher's syndrome patients have temporal atrophy less frequently ($p<.05$), while X-linked rod-cone, autosomal dominant, and recessive cone-rod patients have temporal atrophy the most frequently ($p<.05$).

A potential use of the fluorescein angiogram is to aid in recognizing subtypes of RP and to look at the effects of degeneration on the RPE. Some patients have patchy loss of RPE, while others have confluent preservation of the RPE which stains, often brilliantly, on late frames of the test. Other patients have confluent loss of the RPE. Many patients lose the RPE/choriocapillaris complex altogether, while others may lose one or the other component.

FLUORESCEIN ANGIOGRAPHY AND ANTI-RETINAL ANTIBODIES

One study at UCLA correlated fluorescein angiographic findings with the presence or absence of antiretinal antibodies in 59 RP and 29 non-RP patients who had other retinal diseases.[28] The fluorescein parameters studied included disc staining, edema of the macula, vascular arcades, and peripapillary area, and focal vascular staining on late phases of the fluorescein angiogram.

Numerous significant correlations were found for both groups, but the non-RP retinal disease patients had a larger number of significant correlations. The rod-cone degeneration patients demonstrated a near significant correlation between arcade edema and the lymphocyte stimulation test ($p<.067$). To look for a cumulative effect, antiretinal immunoglobulin G and M, as well as the lymphocyte stimulation test results, were combined and analyzed with focal vascular staining; the findings were suggestive in cone-rod patients ($p<.069$) and correlated significantly with arcade edema in rod-cone patients ($p<.011$).

The above results suggest that the immune system may be playing a role in various retinal degenerations; however, it is likely that the fluorescein angiographic correlations, in the main, represent a secondary response rather than a primary disease effect.

RETINAL VASCULATURE

Vascular attenuation is one of the characteristic findings in RP; Faber found that 87% of 300 RP patients showed narrowing,[29] and Pruett found that 96.3% of 192 patients had vascular attenuation.[7] As early as 1901 various theories had been hypothesized suggesting a vascular etiology for RP[30]; however, it is generally agreed that the vascular attenuation is a secondary rather than a causal effect. It has been assumed that as the retina degenerates and thins, it needs less oxygen. Inner segments, if present, are nearer the choroidal circulation and thus would be less dependent on the retinal circulation. Fluorescein angiographic studies in RP patients have demonstrated prolonged circulation times with decreased perfusion pressures.[31,32] Differences in the degree of vascular narrowing between types of RP have not been studied, but, clearly, patients with choroideremia have less vascular attenuation than those with other forms of RP, and, as a group, cone-rod degeneration patients appear to have less attenuation.

OPTIC NERVE ALTERATIONS IN RP

The typical description of an RP disc as demonstrating "waxy pallor" was derived from examinations with the direct ophthalmoscope, often in cases in which there were more advanced changes. With the advent of indirect ophthalmoscopy, it is possible to screen the equatorial and peripheral retina, and early cases of RP are often found in the asymptomatic state; in these cases discs are pink.

Waxy pallor inadequately describes the many changes of the optic nervehead in response to the RP degenerative process. Pruett noted "normal-colored" discs in his series,[7] and on fundus photographs of RP patients at UCLA, about 70% of patients have pink-appearing though not necessarily normal discs. Many patients have a creamy or possibly a waxy appearance to the nervehead even though it is pink.

Others have a white rim on the edge of the disc. As noted in the fluorescein section, large numbers of patients have fine telangiectasia of surface disc vessels, which probably accounts for some of the pink hue.

Temporal optic atrophy is seen frequently and in the cone-rod group is correlated with increased implicit times on the ERG.[33]

Significantly smaller cup-to-disc ratios (**Fig. 5-11, composite**) and nerve fiber changes have been found in all types of RP.[34] The presence of nerve fiber layer change inversely correlated with the size of the cup (i.e., the larger the cup, the less nerve fiber layer changes seen). The size of the cup was also age-related, with older RP patients demonstrat-

ing larger (though still smaller than normal) cup-to-disc ratios (**Fig. 5-12**). Normal patients also have enlarging cup-to-disc ratios with increasing age.

It is interesting to note that most patients who have cup-to-disc ratios larger than those found in the typical RP patient frequently have no family history of RP. This could imply a noncongenital and possibly nonhereditary etiology, but this hypothesis has not been established or proven.

OPTIC DISC DRUSEN IN RP

Globular excrescences or hyaline bodies of the optic nervehead (**Fig 5-13A–D**; also see Fig. 9-4) are occasionally seen in RP patients and have been inter-

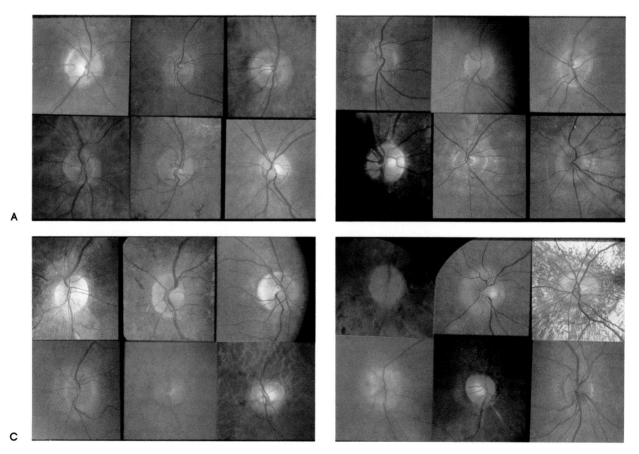

FIG. 5-11. Cup-to-disc ratio (composite) from left to right *(top row)*: simplex RC, simplex RC, dominant RC, simplex RC, dominant RC, simplex CR; *(second row from top)*: multiplex CR, autosomal recessive CR, Usher's, autosomal recessive RC, Usher's, atypical simplex RP; *(third row from top)*: simplex RC, simplex RC, multiplex CR, Usher's, simplex RC, dominant RC; *(bottom row)*: simplex RC, autosomal recessive RC, simplex RC, choroideremia, simplex RC, Usher's. (RC = rod-cone, CR = cone-rod)

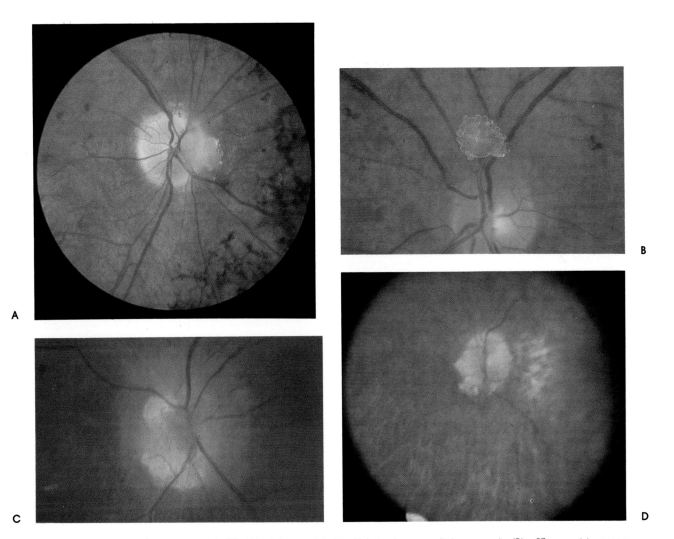

FIG. 5-12. Mean cup-to-disc ratio and percent of patients demonstrating nerve fiber layer loss graphed against all types of RP by age grouping. RP patients of all ages have significantly smaller cup-to-disc ratios compared with age-matched normal controls, even though there is an increase in cup size with age. Younger RP patients demonstrate nerve fiber layer loss more frequently, suggesting that this is an early funduscopic sign of RP.

FIG. 5-13. Optic nervehead drusen in RP: *(A)* a 14-year-old girl with Leber's congenital amaurosis; *(B)* a 37-year-old woman with simplex RP; *(C)* a 28-year-old woman with autosomal dominant RP; *(D)* a 36-year-old man with Senior-Loken syndrome.

preted as "drusen" by some authors[35,36] and as astrocytic hamartomas by others.[37,38] Spencer suggested that their pathogenesis was similar to that occurring in familial optic nervehead drusen, which he related to aberrant axoplasmic transport at the disc.[39]

Histopathologic studies have not yet settled the issue; Puck and colleagues in an autopsy report found globular bodies in the nerve fiber layer of the optic nervehead which had increased calcium and phosphorus content consistent with drusen.[40] Similar findings were reported by Novack and Foos, whose patient also had asteroide hyalosis.[41] Their study, however, does not directly address the issue of patients with vitreal epipapillary excrescences demonstrated by Robertson and others.

REFERENCES

1. Heckenlively JR, Martin DA, Rosales TR: Telangiectasia and optic atrophy in cone-rod degenerations. Arch Ophthalmol 99:1983–1991, 1981
2. Hayreh SS: The choriocapillaris. Graefes Arch Clin Exp Ophthalmol 192:165–179, 1975
3. Pruett RC: Retinitis pigmentosa: A biomicroscopical study of vitreous abnormalities. Arch Ophthalmol 93:603–608, 1975
4. Ross DF, Fishman GA, Gilbert LD et al: Variability of visual field measurements in normal subjects and patients with retinitis pigmentosa. Arch Ophthalmol 102:1004–1010, 1984
4a. Heckenlively JR: Studies in RP cone-rod degeneration. Trans Am Ophthalmol Soc (accepted)
5. Sieving PA, Fishman GA: Refractive errors in retinitis pigmentosa patients. Br J Ophthalmol 62:163–167, 1978
6. Heckenlively JR: The frequency of posterior subcapsular cataract in the hereditary retinal degenerations. Am J Ophthal 93:733–738, 1982
7. Pruett RC: Retinitis pigmentosa: Clinical and observations and correlations. Trans Am Ophthalmol Soc 76: 693–735, 1983
8. Eshaghian J, Rafferty NS, Goossens W: Ultrastructure of human cataract in retinitis pigmentosa. Arch Ophthalmol 98:2227–2230, 1980
9. Fagerholm PP, Philipson BT: Cataract in retinitis pigmentosa. An analysis of cataract surgery results and pathological lens changes. Acta Ophthalmologica 63:50–58, 1985
10. Carr RE: Discussion of retinitis pigmentosa cataracts. Ophthalmology 89:883–884, 1982
11. Takahashi M, Jalkh A, Hoskins J et al: Biomicroscopic evaluation and photography in liquefied vitreous in some vitreoretinal disorders. Arch Ophthalmol 99:1555–1559, 1981
12. Sandberg MA, Berson EL: Visual acuity and cone spatial density in retinitis pigmentosa. Invest Ophthalmol Vis Sci 24:1511–1533, 1983
13. Meel van GJ, Norren van D: Foveal densitometry in retinitis pigmentosa. Invest Ophthalmol Vis Sci 24:1123–1130, 1983
14. Greenstein VC, Hood DC, Siegel IM et al: Retinitis pigmentosa: A psychophysical test of explanations for early foveal sensitivity loss. Invest Ophthalmol Vis Sci 25:118–120, 1984
15. Pearlman JT: Mathematical models of retinitis pigmentosa: A study of the rate of progress in the different genetic forms. Trans Am Ophthalmol Soc 77:643–655, 1979
16. Heckenlively JR, Friederich F, Farson C et al: Retinitis pigmentosa in the Navajo. Metab Pediatr Syst Ophthalmol 5:201–206, 1981
17. Fishman GA, Vasquez V, Fishman M et al: Visual loss and foveal lesions in Usher's syndrome. Br J Ophthalmol 63:484–488, 1979
18. Marmor MF: Visual loss in retinitis pigmentosa. Am J Ophthalmol 89:692–698, 1980
19. Fishman GA, Maggiano JM, Fishman M: Foveal lesions seen in retinitis pigmentosa. Arch Ophthalmol 95:1993–1996, 1977
20. Fishman GA, Fishman M, Maggiano J: Macular lesions associated with retinitis pigmentosa. Arch Ophthalmol 95:798–803, 1977
21. Merin S: Macular cysts as an early sign of tapeto-retinal degeneration. J Ped Ophthalmol 7:225–228, 1970
22. Hyvarinen L, Maumenee AE, Kelley J et al: Fluorescein angiographic findings in retinitis pigmentosa. Am J Ophthalmol 71:17–26, 1971
23. Krill AE, Archer D, Newell FW: Fluorescein angiography in retinitis pigmentosa. Am J Ophthalmol 69:826–835, 1970
24. Notting JGA, Deutman AF: Leakage from retinal capillaries in hereditary dystrophies. Doc Ophthalmologica Proc Ser 9:439–447, 1976
25. Fish G, Grey R, Sehmi KS et al: The dark choroid in posterior retinal dystrophies. Br J Ophthalmol 65:359–363, 1981
26. Eagle LRC, Lucier AC, Bernardino VB et al: Retinal pigment epithelial abnormalities in fundus flavimaculatus. Ophthalmology 87:1189–1200, 1980
27. Fetkenhour CL, Choromokos E, Weinstein J et al: Cystoid macular edema in retinitis pigmentosa. Trans Am Acad Ophthalmol Otolargyngol 83:515–521, 1977
28. Heckenlively JR, Solish AM, Chant SM et al: Autoimmunity in hereditary retinal degenerations. II. Clinical studies: Antiretinal antibodies and fluoresceinangiogram findings. Br J Ophthalmol 69:758–764, 1985
29. Merin S, Auerbach E: Retinitis pigmentosa. Surv Ophthalmol 20:304, 1976
30. Gonin J: Lescotome annulaire dans la degenerescence pigmentaire de la retine. Ann Ocul 125:101–130, 1901
31. Best M, Galin MA, Blumenthal M et al: Fluorescein angiography during induced ocular hypertension in retinitis pigmentosa. Am J Ophthalmol 71:1226–1230, 1971
32. Best M, Toyofuku H, Galin MA: Ocular hemodynamics in retinitis pigmentosa. Arch Ophthalmol 88:123–130, 1972
33. Heckenlively JR: The cone-rod degenerations (accepted) Trans Am Ophthalmol Soc
34. Rajacich GM, Parelhoff ES, Heckenlively JR: The cup-disc ratio in retinitis pigmentosa subgroups. Invest Ophthalmol Vis Sci 22(suppl):55, 1982
35. Lorentzen SE: Drusen of the optic disc: A clinical and genetic study. Acta Ophthalmol 90:1–180, 1966
36. Walker CH: Diseases of the retina and optic nerve: A case

of hyaline bodies at the disc. Trans Ophthalmol Soc UK 35:366–370, 1915

37. Robertson DM: Hamartomas of the optic disk with retinitis pigmentosa. Am J Ophthalmol 74:526–531, 1972
38. Pillai S, Limaye SR, Saimovici LB: Optic disc hamartoma associated with retinitis pigmentosa. Retina 3:24–26, 1983
39. Spencer WH: Drusen of the optic disc and aberrant axoplasmic transport. Ophthalmology 85:21–38, 1978
40. Puck A, Tso MOM, Fishman GA: Drusen of the optic nerve associated with retinitis pigmentosa. Arch Ophthalmol 103:231–234, 1985
41. Novack RL, Foos RY: Drusen of the optic disk in retinitis pigmentosa. Am J Ophthalmol 103:44–47, 1987

6

Management and Treatment of Retinitis Pigmentosa

JOHN R. HECKENLIVELY
JANET SILVER

When confronted with a case of retinitis pigmentosa (RP), it is important for the ophthalmologist or other eye care professional to assume that *there is something that can be done* for the patient. Many RP patients have remediable ocular-related problems such as errors in refraction, presbyopia, reading difficulty, headaches, photophobia, and on occasion cataracts, all of which eye specialists are well trained to handle. In addition, many patients have severe anxiety over their disease and need reassurance that they will not suddenly go blind. At other times the ophthalmologist may be able to relieve the anxiety that the patient's activities or medications may make the RP worse.

Unfortunately, many RP patients do not receive the usual ophthalmic services because of a perception about RP that "nothing can be done." On occasion, a distinct disservice is performed, for example, when an ophthalmologist unfamiliar with the disease suggests that the patient "buy a white cane" or "learn braille," when in reality the disease course typically takes 30 to 40 years or more from onset. Another common misstatement is that because RP is a hereditary disease, affected persons should not have children. This statement may be ill-advised since about three-quarters of patients with RP are not at risk to have children with the disease but will either pass a normal gene or pass the gene in a carrier state mode. These questions are complicated and should be considered on an individual basis; they are best discussed with professionals who are trained in genetic counseling.

There are a number of myths about RP, concepts that are incorrect for most patients (Table 6-1), which can be dispelled by the ophthalmologist. Invariably, patients hear about various RP syndromes. These syndromes tend to be rare, and often the systemic disease precedes any ocular symptoms. Deafness is one of the more common concerns of RP patients, but since Usher's syndrome is congenital, this type of RP can usually be recognized on the initial visit. Some older RP patients develop mild deafness which is seldom severe. However, RP patients who are not born deaf will not normally go deaf.

Most patients have a deep fear that they will suddenly go blind; the ophthalmologist can do a great service, particularly in early to intermediate cases of

TABLE 6-1
MYTHS ABOUT RP (THAT ARE USUALLY INCORRECT FOR MOST PATIENTS)

Nothing can be done about RP.

Most RP patients go deaf.

RP patients will suddenly go blind.

All RP patients are night-blind from an early age (see discussions on cone-rod degeneration).

All RP is inherited from the mother.

The cause of RP is that pigment gets in the way of the light.

RP, by emphasizing the chronicity of the disease. It is always a mistake for the doctor to give a patient a time when the patient "will go blind" because he will undoubtedly be wrong. Even estimates are taken literally and should be avoided. Educating the patient about the disease and relating the steps by which he can help himself is the key to good patient care in RP.

In general, RP patients should receive routine ophthalmic care including visual field tests, refrac-tion, biomicroscopy, intraocular pressures, and brief retinal examination. Many patients are reassured when field size does not change dramatically over the years. If there are severe problems, many pa-tients and relatives want a realistic idea of what is happening. A few patients and relatives prefer not to be told about their disease, and clinical judgment will help guide the practitioner. Since most RP pa-tients are myopic, loss of vision may be due to re-fractive changes; patients who may assume that their disease is worse are pleased when a lens change corrects the problem. A retinal examination may dis-close new problems such as macular cystoid edema or early macular degeneration, or, rarely, a Coats' reaction which may call for special attention.

ROUTINE WORKUP OF A PATIENT WITH PIGMENTARY RETINOPATHY

When a patient presents with a partially diagnosed or undiagnosed pigmentary retinopathy, a basic eval-uation (Table 6-2) is recommended. These sugges-tions have been found by the first author to be useful. Other clinicians may believe other tests or approaches to be helpful for a particular patient.

TABLE 6-2
DIAGNOSTIC WORKUP OF A NEW RP PATIENT

1. Careful ocular and medical history, date of onset of symptoms.
2. Family history with pedigree (Fig. 2-6).
3. Best corrected visual acuity (refraction for distant and near vision).
4. Baseline visual field (Goldmann or tangent fields are superior, automatic screening fields less helpful)
5. Biomicroscopy, applanation tonometry, indirect ophthalmoscopy.
6. ERG, full-field Ganzfeld stimulus.
7. Final rod threshold in several fields.
8. Fundus photographs, in selected cases fluorescein angiogram.
9. Audiogram in patients with nasal or slurred speech, or with partial deafness (see Chapter 13, Usher's syndrome).
10. FTA-ABS blood test to rule out luetic chorioretinitis, and history recheck of possible past uveitis or retinitis in cases of simplex RP or cases with marked asymmetry of retinal involvement.
11. Unilateral cases should be checked for signs of blunt trauma (e.g., examining for angle recession between eyes) vascular occlusion, retained metallic foreign body, and parasites.
12. Medical, pediatric, otolaryngologic, neurologic or medical genetics consultation if nonocular problems are present and need evaluation.

Marmor and colleagues have published articles on the management and evaluation of RP which may be of additional interest.[1,2]

The main purpose behind these recommendations is to aid the ophthalmologist in diagnosing as accurately as possible the *type of RP*. While treatments for ocular-only forms of RP are currently unavailable, future management may benefit from a differentiation of the type in the earliest stages of the disease.

Although clinicians are thoroughly familiar with history taking, they need to recognize that RP patients have a few unique problems. Despite common belief, not all RP patients are night-blind in the early stages of the disease; those with cone-rod degeneration have late-onset night-blindness but may present with symptoms referable to visual field loss or problems of their cones dark-adapting in lighted areas (e.g., in the city) at night. Many RP patients complain of light flashes not unlike patients with ongoing retinal detachment, but indirect ophthalmoscopy will rule out the possibility of the latter. Retinal detachment in an RP patient should not be discounted initially although it rarely occurs. Once a baseline retinal status is established, then the photopsia may be less alarming since many RP patients experience flashes or rolling waves of light on a chronic basis.

A number of RP patients with moderate to advanced disease complain of having "bad days" during which they note that everything is fuzzy or less clear, and other days when they wake up and see everything crystal clear. The cause of this variation is unknown, but short-term multiple visual field testing in RP patients does demonstrate a great deal of variability from test to test.[3]

Patients who are legally blind on presentation (U.S.A. standards: visual field <20° with 3-mm target and visual acuity 20/200 or worse in both eyes), can be gently informed of their status; it is important to emphasize that the term refers to establishing that they have a disability, not that they are blind! The U.S. government, as well as many American state governments, provides an extra exemption on income taxes for legal blindness, and various governmental and community services are available to visually disabled persons (see Appendix, end of this chapter). A few RP patients with advanced disease and some other medical problem may need disability parking permits.

Many RP patients are afraid that they will lose their driving licenses if they activate their legal blindness status with the government. Fortunately, this precipitous action has not been initiated by U.S. authorities. It should be noted, however, that patients who apply for social security disability may be asked to give up their driving licences. Because these regulations vary depending on location and nationality, interested readers should check on local laws and policies.

Studies by Fishman and colleagues[4] comparing RP driving performance with normal controls found that 50% of patients were not involved in any accident during their most recent 5-year driving period. They did find a higher number of RP patients who were involved in isolated road accidents, however, mainly among a subgroup of female RP patients who had a disproportionately higher number of accidents compared with controls. The investigators had no immediate explanation for this higher accident rate. They pointed out that 74% of patients reported that they voluntarily restricted their driving to daylight hours, when fewer accidents occurred. Most RP drivers compensate for their loss of peripheral vision by using mirrors and turning their heads more. In other countries different criteria may apply; for example, in the United Kingdom there is a catch-all clause that prohibits anyone from driving who has a field loss or any other disability that would present a hazard. It is generally accepted that a field less than 60% would, therefore, prohibit someone from driving in the U.K. Even more stringent conditions apply in some other European countries. Fonda has suggested vision standards for partially sighted drivers and suggests that driver's licenses with limitations may be one solution for dealing with the problem.[5]

Of particular interest to RP patients, depending on residential area, are special or lower rates on telephone service, directory assistance calls, bus passes, and in some localities lower rates on electricity. This last service is quite important to the RP patient (as well as others with macular degeneration) who frequently have every light in the house turned on at night.

The family history is extremely important in sorting out the RP type in most instances. Examination of other family members is often advisable and may help to establish the inheritance pattern. Simplex or multiplex cases should not be assumed to be autosomal recessive (see Chapter 2).

The electroretinogram (ERG) should be performed with a full field Ganzfeld stimulus and a standardized protocol. Extremely useful information is provided by an evaluation of cone function (photopic and flicker ERG) and rod function (scotopic ERG with dim blue or white light below cone threshold); on occasion, a dark-adapted bright flash ERG with a white stimulus may be recordable, although it adds little diagnostic information. A dark-adapted bright red stimulus may give information on the cone and rod systems.

It is not normally necessary to perform a time-consuming dark adaptation curve, but a final rod threshold with a 2° target from several retinal locations, such as 12°, 20°, and 30° after at least 30 minutes of dark adaptation is important in distinguishing those patients with diffuse rod disease or rod-cone degeneration from those patients with residual rod function or (usually) cone-rod degeneration.

Fundus photography is useful in establishing a baseline record of the retina. On subsequent examinations, many patients specifically ask if there are any changes from the previous visit, and retinal photographs are extremely helpful in this evaluation. Photographs may be especially helpful in following macular changes.

The indications for fluorescein angiography (FA) are more limited; the characteristic FA pattern in choroideremia is helpful in cases in which there is any question of the diagnosis. Questions of visual loss from macular edema or possibly atrophy may be aided by FA, and the diagnosis of preserved para-arteriolar retinal pigment epithelium (PPRPE) RP may be clarified by FA. Eventually, the FA may be a standard diagnostic test in all RP patients if the FA is shown to differentiate between RP types and proves useful in diagnosis; currently, it is helpful only in selected cases (see Chapter 5).

Light Toxicity

Some concern has been expressed about photographing patients with RP or other types of retinal degeneration for fear that the camera flash will cause retinal damage. There is currently no information to verify this possibility in any substantial way. There is some historical evidence from the occasional patient who complains that his vision is affected after having ERG and fundus photographs. The latter complaint has been in cases of advanced RP, but fortunately the occurrence has been rare, and all patients have recovered preexamination visual levels.

There has been concern also that chronic exposure to sunlight may exacerbate the RP process. This was tested by Berson[4] but was not found to make any difference in the progression. A similar study, performed by Jerome Pearlman, M.D., using red contact lens occlusion in RP patients (unpublished data), also failed to support this theory.

Despite these studies, which were difficult to control, there is historical as well as some scientific evidence to support the notion that high-energy sunlight (ultraviolet to blue spectrum) may exacerbate the disease. In large autosomal dominant RP families in which all members have the same gene defect, variable expressivity is found, and in several pedigrees, members working outdoors have had a more severe disease course than those working indoors. This is difficult to document scientifically. That the ultraviolet spectrum of light can cause retinal damage is well established; the question that arises is whether RP patients have as good a reparative mechanism to light damage as non-RP patients, and whether high energy light can make their disease worse. Of particular concern recently is the destructive role of radical oxygen which may be created when ultraviolet (UV) light hits the tissue.

Whether UV-screening lenses prolong eyesight in RP has not been proven, yet many patients report quite positively that they tolerate sunlight better in UV screening and/or tinted lenses. Interestingly, even though cautioned about potential harmful effects, a few patients throw UV-screening lenses away and appear to want extra energy from the blue end of the spectrum.

Because of their potential benefits, UV-screening lenses are often recommended to RP patients. UV screens may be added to prescription lenses or may be purchased as nonprescription sunglasses. Some UV-screening lenses are reported to lose effectiveness after a year or two, and wearers should ascertain the normal life span of their purchase. For the above reasons, vitamin E, a known radical oxygen "quencher" also may be recommended. If vitamin E is prescribed, 400 IU b.i.d. is a reasonable dose.

CATARACT SURGERY IN RP PATIENTS

In the first author's experience, 41% of RP patients can be expected to present with posterior subcapsular cataracts,[7] but in most patients the cataract is small and seldom causes significant visual loss. Because these patients have a concurrent retinal degeneration, it cannot be assumed that the cataract is causing the visual loss, and careful evaluation must be done to avoid needlessly taking out insignificant cataracts (Table 6-3). In a few patients, however, the centrally located opacity causes a light scatter-glare with visual loss, and the patient will benefit from cataract extraction.

A combination of methods has to be employed to establish the efficacy of cataract extraction, and in general the same criteria used for non-RP cataracts applies; a determination of best corrected undilated and dilated visual acuity will frequently give an idea whether removing posterior opacity will improve vision, and dilation can be used as a clinical trial. Some RP patients are content to use daily mydriatics for visual improvement, and phenylephrine 10% in patients without cardiovascular problems once or twice a day may improve vision; plus additions may be needed for near vision.

In looking at a series of RP patient cataract extractions, we found no evidence that any patient was made worse or that the disease was exacerbated by the surgery. Careful selection of patients for surgery must be employed. The criteria noted above should be closely followed, since RP patients with advanced disease are easily given false hope that cataract extraction will restore vision.

In comparing RP patients who underwent intracapsular cataract extraction with those who had extracapsular cataract surgery with posterior chamber intraocular insertion, it is the primary author's impression that the latter procedure gave better results from the patient's point of view. YAG posterior capsulotomies are more common due to capsular wrinkling. Because of the potential for postoperative intraocular inflammation which could exacerbate the RP process, insertion of anterior chamber lenses should be avoided in this patient group.

When results of surgery were analyzed in the RP cataract group, it became apparent that patients with significant cataracts in whom the central visual field was less than 4° had a less favorable outcome than those with significant cataracts with larger fields.

TABLE 6-3

GUIDELINES FOR RP PATIENT CATARACT EXTRACTION—CRITERIA AND EXAMINATION PROCEDURE

1. History of glare phenomena, visual loss unexplained by retinal appearance.
2. Best corrected distant and near visual acuity, undilated and dilated.
3. Examination of macula by direct ophthalmoscopy for effect of cataract on visualization, for health of macular RPE, and signs of macular atrophy.
4. Examination of macula by indirect ophthalmoscopy.
5. Evaluation of visual field size. Patients with less than 4° of central field should be cautioned that although they may have some improvement, the visual result may not be as great as for other patients.
6. In cases in which macular RPE is disrupted, the visual potential can be assessed by testing visual acuity with laser interferometry.
7. Rarely, fluorescein angiography may assist in evaluating macular health.
8. Possible clinical trial of dilating drops.

Even still, several of these latter patients were pleased with the results of their operation, stating that objects looked clearer and brighter to them.

COUNSELING THE PATIENT AND FAMILY

Because there is no known effective therapy for RP (except for vitamin A deficiencies), counseling the patient plays a major role in delivery of care, which markedly contrasts with much of ophthalmic care in which patient interaction may be less extensive. In order that the patient and his family may deal adequately with the disease, it is important that they have a basic understanding of what is occurring. Many patients will wish to seek additional opinions, since in this age of modern medicine it is hard to accept the lack of treatment for any disease. The primary ophthalmologist can greatly aid the referral process by sending their patients to retinal specialists knowledgeable about and sympathetic to patients with retinal dystrophies.

BE POSITIVE

It is important to discuss the prognosis from a positive point of view. Emphasis that the disease course extends over many years, that there are normally no sudden changes in vision, and that the patient often develops compensatory strategies, such as scanning, for dealing with the disability are important points for reassuring the patient. While some patients will eventually experience severe disability from the disease, even those patients who become severely disabled usually retain some degree of sight.

If the ophthalmologist is not comfortable counseling the patient, there are a number of options. If genetic counseling is sought, a referral to a genetic counselor should be arranged. In such cases it is absolutely essential that the correct retinal diagnosis has been made, since the genetic counselor has no way to validate the diagnosis.

Many patients find it useful to communicate with other RP patients through support groups. These are frequently sponsored by local RP societies or, occasionally, low vision centers. The National RP Foundation in Baltimore, Maryland, RP International in Woodland Hills, California, the Texas Association for Retinitis Pigmentosa in Corpus Christi, and the British Retinitis Pigmentosa Society all maintain newsletters for members, as well as other services. Addresses for these organizations can be found in the Appendix at the end of this chapter.

Psychological Consultation

The two most psychologically stressful periods for RP patients are usually upon initially learning the diagnosis and when the disease has advanced to the stage where the patient is forced to be formally described as legally blind or disabled, often accompanied by such significant events as giving up driving. While most RP patients do not have the grieving reaction of a patient who suddenly loses his vision, often severe depression occurs. Other patients have anxiety or anger toward relatives, their physician, or even God for having allowed the disease to happen. These issues are discussed in an excellent chapter on "Reaction to the Loss of Sight" by Paul Schultz in *Psychiatric Problems in Ophthalmology*.[8] Unfortunately, psychiatric training seldom deals with patient problems caused by blindness, and psychiatric assistance to the ophthalmologist in this area appears to be limited; for these reasons, an ophthalmologist who has patience and skill in counseling can be of great help to his patient.

Most patients with advanced RP fear the loss of independence, and one of the major patient care goals should be to ensure that the patient is introduced to low vision skills such as mobility training, utilizing residual vision with low vision aids, and learning skills for the nonsighted for dealing with household chores. Many of these skills and aids are discussed in more detail below. Patients with enough vision to read are not motivated to learn braille, and suggesting this possibility inappropriately or too early can be very destructive psychologically to the patient. It should also be remembered that many RP patients will have useful vision throughout their normal life.

Parents frequently ask how to handle children with the disease. Special schooling is seldom needed except in cases of Type I Usher disease, and even individuals with visual acuity as low as 20/200 may do well in a regular school using low vision aids as necessary. Parents are well advised to treat an RP child like their other children, and to avoid being overprotective. On the other hand, there may be a tendency to blame the child's shortcomings on the eye problem; in particular, children of poor academic ability have this excuse made for them, even in the presence of relatively good acuity. Children with visual difficulties are amazingly adaptive. School authorities need to be aware of the visual disorder so that gym activities can be suited to the child's abilities and vocational direction can be assisted.

Another difficult area in the psychology of the disease is the extreme guilt that many parents feel on learning that RP is a genetic disease. Even though these parents rationally understand that there is no way that they could have known ahead of time that they were giving the disease to their child, and that the occurrence was random, many parents, particularly mothers (if the disease is X-linked), feel extreme guilt about the situation. Genetic counselors are well acquainted with this phenomenon and can assist the ophthalmologist with the problem. On occasion a patient may exhibit anger toward the parent(s), but often other psychological dynamics appear to be active, and in extreme cases psychological counseling can be recommended.

Many parents are told incorrectly that RP is X-linked which creates unnecessary guilt in the mother, when in fact X-linked RP is among the rarer types.

LOW VISION AIDS (PRACTICAL HELP FOR THE PATIENT WITH RP)

Often the different types of disability associated with RP are classified together despite the different impairments they cause. It is convenient to consider the impairments under five headings, although they tend to occur severally rather than separately.

1. *Classic tunnel vision:* Central vision is preserved at perhaps 20/30 level with a field that may be less than 7° in diameter.
2. *Central scotoma type:* A relatively good visual field of perhaps 30° to 40° or more is preserved, but with a central loss and visual acuity of 20/200 or poorer.
3. *Cataract:* Posterior subcapsular opacities cause a

degradation of the retinal image. The cataract is often seen as a positive scotoma, due to the position of the opacity very close to the nodal point.

4. *Light adaptation problems:* There are two main types; the most common difficulty is the lack of rod function in rod-cone patients or cone-rod patients with advanced disease. These patients are profoundly night-blind in dim to dark environments. The second problem that many patients have is abnormal cone adaptation; this may manifest itself in a "white out" effect on going outdoors on a bright day, in problems of adjustment to dimly lighted areas at night in urban areas, or in difficulty walking into a dimly lighted restaurant (also reflecting rod disease).

5. *Other disabilities:* The most common disability is deafness, which is covered in the discussion of Usher syndrome. Most RP patients have no other disability other than visual loss. There are rare secondary RPs with associated mental retardation and neurologic deficits.

GROUP 1. TUNNEL VISION

This group can read and perform competently in a familiar environment. They are at some risk outdoors from their lack of peripheral visual field; obstructions such as overhanging branches, low-lying objects, traffic, and steps may be difficult to manage. People with tunnel vision become very orderly in order to stabilize their environment.

Several devices have been suggested to improve RP visual fields, which are described in the hardware section below. Although sound theoretically, in practice these aids are rarely used. Their appearance and weight act as a disincentive, and since the onset of the impairment is insidious, the patient usually acquires techniques of scanning as the impairment develops. The minification effect of the devices is often found to be disorienting, and the aids are less effective to the degree that cataracts or macular atrophy exacerbate the loss associated with tunnel vision.

GROUP 2. MACULAR ATROPHY

The central scotoma precipitates a demand for help with reading. The second most frequent complaint is, "I can't recognise my friends in the street." Rarely remarked but probably more significant is that visual clues are lost in normal conversation, which can lead to at best confused communication and at worst severe alienation and feelings of isolation.

The visual problems are more easily solved. Young patients need a good working distance in order to encourage the widest range of activities; therefore, the appliance of choice tends to be telescopic lenses for distance and near, although such generalizations must always be placed second to the patient's choice.

An Amsler's chart is frequently used to discover where the most useful areas of vision are. The patient should be encouraged to direct his gaze so that the visual axis arrives at this point (i.e., eccentric gazing).

GROUP 3. CATARACTS

While cataract surgery can be recommended to RP patients who meet standard criteria (Table 6-3), some patients with cataracts may present who do not wish surgery or who may not benefit from it.

Patients with cataract present special problems. Retinoscopy is frequently difficult, and while some guidance may be obtained from a previous prescription, it frequently gives only historical information. It is unwise to dilate the pupils as part of low vision assessment because this presents an abnormal situation. If there is central lens sclerosis, refractive myopia may be present. This information may be readily elicited simply by putting −2.00 over the old distance correction working on a chart at 10 feet. If this fails to produce any useful acuity, the examiner can work on correcting near vision.

The near point (i.e., the point at which print is clearest) should be checked with the patient's present glasses, stressing that the vision will not be adequate for reading and starting on perhaps 36-point print. It is likely that the patient has been wearing no more than a +3.00 addition. If the clear point is at 12 cm, it is therefore reasonable to assume that the extra 5.00 diopters needed to focus to that point is caused by refractive myopia, and a distance subjective refraction can commence from that position. It must be remembered that the pupil tends to constrict for near and that lens sclerosing will increase myopia more in the central area; therefore, an ab-

solute correlation between near and distance correction may be unlikely. If the patient presents without any glasses, a +10.00 in a trial frame can be used as a basis for the same calculation. For example, if with a +10.00 the clear point is at 5 cm, there may be 10.00 diopters of myopia. This number is, of course, an average sphere and can be refined with a high-powered crossed-cylinder lens.

Hand lenses, often with built-in illumination, tend to be the appliance of choice in patients with senile cataract. The situation is dynamic, and long-term solutions are rarely indicated. The primary need in this group is often for good contrast levels, and unexpectedly good results can be obtained with a dome type magnifier (Visolet loupe).

Several useful general references to low vision optics include Mehr and Fried,[9] Faye,[10] Jose,[11] and Silver.[12]

For people with posterior subcapsular cataract, it is sometimes an advantage to dilate the pupil chronically, although this exacerbates the light problem and any accommodation that is present is lost.

With any opacity of the media, there is considerable inconvenience in bright light, especially if the light source is in the field of vision (e.g., the setting sun). The situation is analogous to the view through a dirty windshield, a description readily recognized by the patient.

GROUP 4. LIGHT ADAPTATION

Apart from tinted lenses to aid adaptation when light levels can be expected to change (e.g., going outdoors on a bright day,) the important priority is to protect the eye from strong oblique light. Particular problems are recorded for patients walking toward the setting sun or in the early morning, and seeing car lights straight on. Some patients report that riding higher, such as in a pickup truck, helps alleviate this problem. Tinted lenses have little effect, but some sort of solid visor or a hat with a shady brim can make a huge difference to comfort. The patient rapidly learns to angle his head to cut off the strong beam.

A number of RP patients find that problems of light adaptation are helped by tinted UV-screening lenses which are purchased according to the patient's needs and are widely available commercially;

some are photochromatic, while others may be plano with tint or clear with UV screen.

It is only in this century that visually handicapped people have been encouraged to use residual vision and to employ optical and other appliances to maximize it. Many imaginative devices are available to help.[13,14] Although most of the principles have been well understood for centuries, within the last 25 years, aids have become significantly less expensive in real terms and far more acceptable in weight and performance. These developments have coincided with changes in attitude both from patients and clinicians.

The function of the clinician can no longer be considered simply as supplying every medical and surgical technique for the preservation of sight, but must also encompass the supply of services that will allow the visually handicapped person to function to the limit of his capability. The intelligent prescribing of low vision aids will enable many employed people with an acquired visual disability to use previous experience skills and training, and allow many visually handicapped children to remain in open education.

Much benefit can be derived from simple strategies, such as the creative use of contrast. Steak will be difficult to see on a brown plate, cooked fish disappears on a white plate; reverse them and add a green vegetable, and a common task is made easier. Apart from the purely practical application of these ideas themselves, their main function is to encourage the patient to think creatively about his everyday life. It should be stressed that major changes are not necessary, that simple adjustments improving contrast aid vision (e.g., that red or green striped toothpaste is easier than white to see on the toothbrush and not significantly more expensive). Since RP patients frequently have partial color deficits, using strong contrasts in colors can be very beneficial to their daily living.

The simple strategy of enlargement is often neglected. Nearly all libraries hold a reasonable selection of books in large print; telephones with large numerals are available, as are typewriters with enlarged typeface.

The simplest way of gaining magnification is simply to move closer to the object. Holding a book closer or sitting closer to the television is an effective method for improving vision. But when this is not possible, optical and other appliances, while never able to replace normal vision, may enable a visually handicapped person to continue to use what vision remains.

APPLIANCES

Effective prescribing for the low-vision patient depends on the skill of the prescriber and the availability of a comprehensive range of aids. Several manufacturers, notably, Designs for Vision, using methods and instruments devised by William Feinbloom,[15] or the intelligent and flexible system devised by Charles Keeler[16] and marketed under his name, have produced "fitting sets" that cover many functions. Every type of aid has different characteristics, and ultimately the function of the practitioner is to prescribe for the individual patient the aid that confers the greatest advantage combined with the minimum disadvantages.

Near Vision

There are many alternatives for helping near vision; the simple magnifier is probably the most widely used and best accepted aid (**Fig. 6-1**). Hand and stand magnifiers are available in an enormous variety of power, quality, and material.[17] Hand lenses are usually held well within their focal length, and the resultant magnification may in practice be considerably less than the stated power would suggest.

Hand and stand magnifiers meet different needs. For both types, built-in illumination may be an advantage; both have a relatively small field unless the patient can be persuaded to use the appliance close to the eye. Stand magnifiers (**Fig. 6-2**) are often bulky but they have applications in industry if low power is adequate, and may allow a task requiring both hands. Stand magnifiers have particular advantages when there are additional handicaps or a need for extra light (**Fig. 6-3**), or when a large field is essential and low power acceptable. Even if other aids are used, a hand lens is a great advantage in pocket or handbag.

High-powered convex lenses, sometimes called hyperoculars or microscopes, may be mounted in

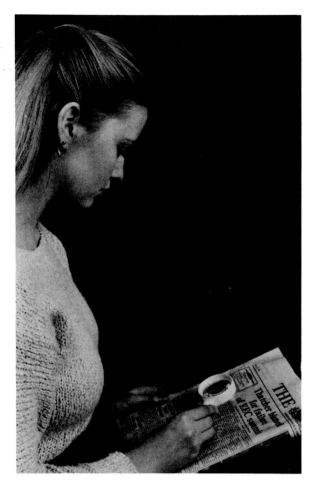

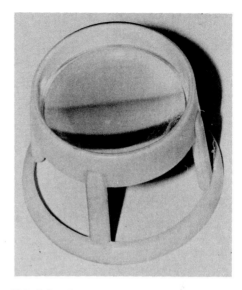

FIG. 6-2.. Simple stand magnifier. Similar to a simple hand magnifier but it is very easily managed if there is an extra disability or the patient is a small child.

FIG. 6-1. Simple hand magnifier (5×) (+20.00D). This device is useful as an extra reading aid to look up a telephone number and read other fine print.

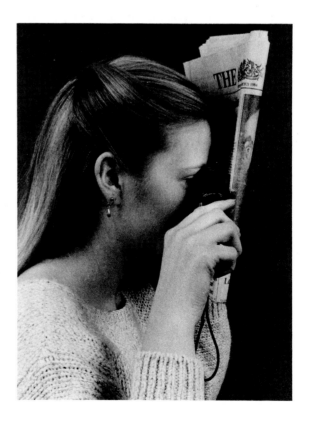

FIG. 6-3. Illuminated magnifier (15×). The field is much better if used very close to the eye. Generally, this device is used to acquire information rather than for reading for pleasure, but it can make a big difference between independence or dependence for the patient.

spectacle frames, attached to them with clips, or simply used as watchmaker's loupes.[18] Such lenses, which may be spherical or aspheric, are normally described by magnification powers. A 4× spectacle magnifier will have the power of 16 diopters, a 9× of 36 diopters, and so on. However, it is generally accepted that the main function of the lens is to focus the image at the retina, most of the magnification is due to proximity of the object.

It must be remembered that both magnification and working distance will be modified by the patient's own refractive error. If a 5× spectacle magnifier is used by an aphakic patient where 12 diopters is used to correct the surgical hypermetropia, only 8 diopters will remain for the near vision correction. This will give 2× magnification and a working distance of 12 cm. Conversely, if a similar lens is put before a 12 diopter myopic eye the total positive power would be 32 diopters, the working distance 3 cm, and the actual magnification 8×.

Spectacle magnifiers are excellent cosmetically and have a relatively good field. They are also produced in bifocal form, which is often an advantage. Disadvantages are the short working distance in higher powers and the inevitable decision to abandon binocular vision where more than about 2× magnification is indicated. Spectacle magnifiers are usually single lenses (**Fig. 6-4A**), although sometimes two or more lenses are used in combination (**Fig. 6-4B&C**). Powers available at the time of writing are up to about 20×, and built-in illumination is available for some high-powered aids.

If high reading additions are to be given binocularly, problems will arise with convergence. In practice, patients rarely cope with more than 10 or 12 diopters addition, and then base-in prism is needed to relieve the convergence. Fonda suggests that it is appropriate to incorporate one prism diopter in each eye for each diopter of addition and it must be borne in mind that normal convergence will reduce

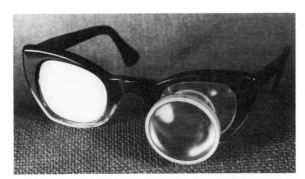

A

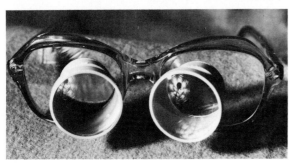

B

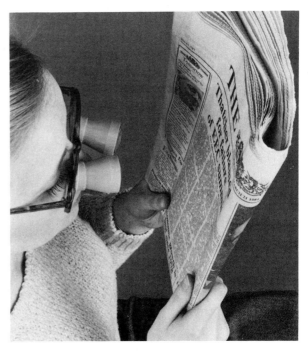

C

FIG. 6-4. Monocular 3× telescopic spectacle *(top left)* for near vision; the device shown has a good working distance, allowing 30–35 cm with a field of close to 15°. It is useful for tasks that require some manipulative skills (e.g., for sewing or handicrafts). Distances are difficult to judge and it requires practice. *(B,C)* Binocular 5× telescopic spectacle for near vision *(bottom left and right).* This type of aid is expensive, can incorporate an aphakic correction or a deep minus lens. The working distance is about 15 cm, but the appliance must be fitted by a skilled low vision specialist.

the interpupillary distance[19]; therefore, spectacles with small eye sizes are essential. Inevitably, chromatic aberrations are increased and a heavy, thick lens is created.

Telescopes

For a larger working distance, that is from 25 cm to infinity, only telescopic systems are in normal use. The major disadvantages of telescopes are that they reduce field, are heavy, have a bizarre appearance, disrupt normal spatial relationships, and are relatively expensive.[20]

Simple binocular sports spectacles are mass-produced with adjustable interpupillary distances and are often focusable. One of the elements is movable to allow for the correction of spherical refractive errors up to perhaps plus or minus 6 diopters and magnification of up to 3×.

Several manufacturers (Designs for Vision, Hamblin, Keeler, Stigmat, Zeiss, etc.) produce monocular or binocular telescopes that can incorporate a correction for ametropia (**Fig. 6-5**). They can sometimes be mounted high on a carrier spectacle lens to allow normal vision below; the head is dropped slightly to allow vision along the tubes (**Fig. 6-6**). These devices are called bioptic telescopes, and their magnification is also no more than 3×. They have obvious applications in the classroom.

For practical purposes, few face-mounted aids are made at more than 3× magnification for distance use, although up to about 12× monocularly and 8× binocularly are available for near use. Contact lens telescopes, consisting of a contact lens eyepiece which is a high minus contact lens and a high plus objective lens carried in a spectacle frame, are available; the back vertex distance forms the space between the elements. However, its magnification is

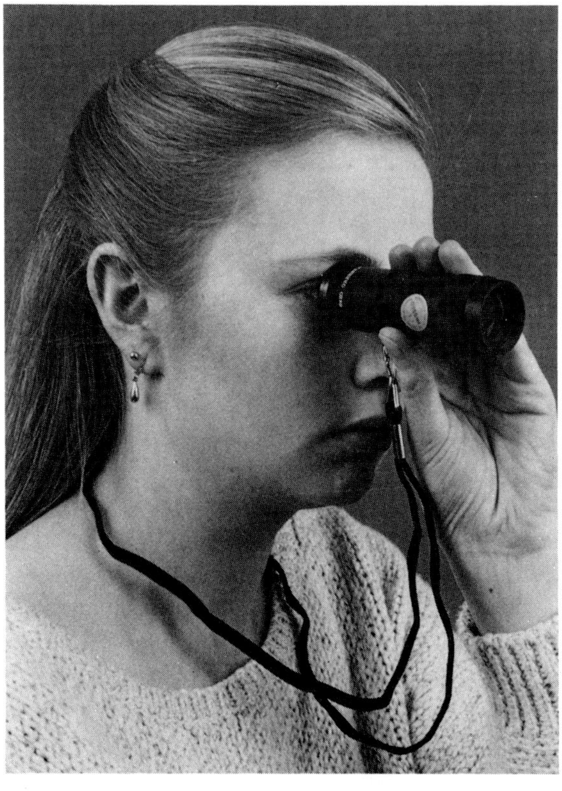

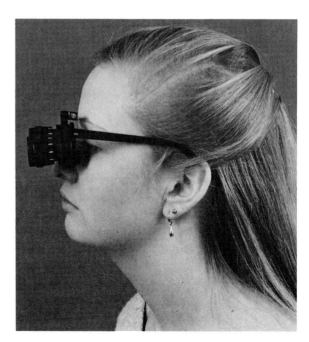

FIG. 6-5. 8× roof prism telescope (for distance). This device is no substitute for a guide dog or a white cane, but this type of aid will allow the discrimination of the number on a bus, the prices in a shop window, and the platform at which a train is located. It takes practice to use, but after a time focusing becomes second nature.

FIG. 6-6. Nonprescription 3× telescopic spectacle for distance. This device is relatively inexpensive and available off the shelf. This device could be used commonly for watching television if the user does not sit close to the set, and it is good for watching sports and theater. It is difficult to use for walking.

never more than 2×, and although perfectly sound theoretically, these aids are very rarely practical, and few cases are on record of prolonged use.

Various devices have been suggested for improving the field of vision; these are either variants on a reversed Galilean telescope (with the disadvantages of such systems) or use prisms or mirrors that allow a lateral view. Although these instruments are effective in the laboratory, in normal use patients prefer to scan. Various devices have also been designed specifically for RP patients, with very limited success.

Electronic Aids

Aids utilizing closed-circuit television techniques (CCTV) have become widely used as low vision aids (**Fig. 6-7**). They produce far higher levels of magnification (up to 50×) than can be obtained optically, and they allow image reversal (i.e., white print on black background) and have a normal reading position with the distance from the screen selected by the subject. Pictures from two cameras can be combined onto a split screen to permit copying. CCTV aids are enormously flexible, particuarly when a

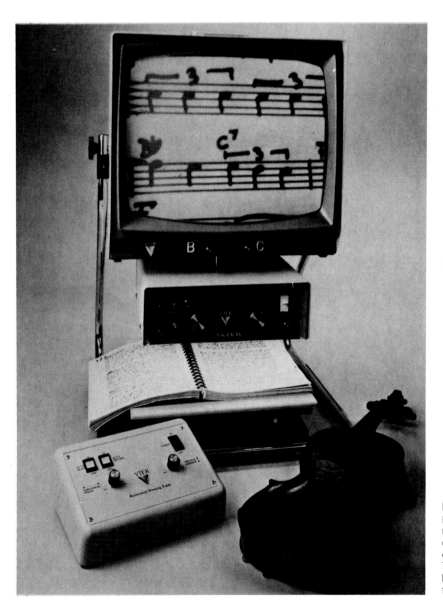

FIG. 6-7. Close circuit television (CCTV). Very high levels of magnification are available with white on black imaging which may be easier for some patients to see. The model demonstrated here has an automated viewing table for scanning material.

zoom lens is incorporated, providing a wide range of magnification by a simple adjustment. Disadvantages are the cost, currently at least $1000, and the bulk, which limits the portability.

Many patients with RP are able to read using CCTV long after they have been forced to abandon reading with optical aids, possibly because of the high contrast and their ability to build up information by multiple scanning.

Recently, a new device has been introduced, a hand-held multiple photoreceptor that is moved across the line of print. The image is orange on very dark red, and the fidelity of the image is limited by the number of receptors. The machine is about briefcase size and allows magnification up to 64×. Several electronic reading machines are now compatible with computer systems.

In the U.S.A., some patients' insurance policies will cover optical aids, and in some American states, departments of rehabilitation will help patients with the cost. In the U.K. and some other countries, low vision aids are supplied on loan and are updated, replaced, or recycled. Often employers are willing to purchase equipment if its effectiveness can be demonstrated. Philanthropic organizations often will help patients purchase these devices, and in some localities the state makes a contribution.

Image Intensifiers

In the early 1970s there was great excitement in the field of RP because of the development of night vision aids using image intensifiers (**Fig. 6-8A&B**).[21] These civilian-adapted versions of military scopes are designed for monocular use, and testing demonstrated that they provided sufficient light amplification to allow cone function under dark conditions. Berson tested 14 patients with RP and 2 patients with stationary night blindness and found that they had visual acuities under scotopic conditions that were comparable to vision under photopic conditions.[20] In practical terms, however, the device is expensive (>$2000), and as with any low vision aid a patient has to have a particular task in mind to provide motivation for using the device, which is initially cumbersome. Studies by the Stanford group comparing the night vision aid to a wide-angle powerful flashlight suggested that this latter, less expensive device is more widely accepted and just as effective.[22]

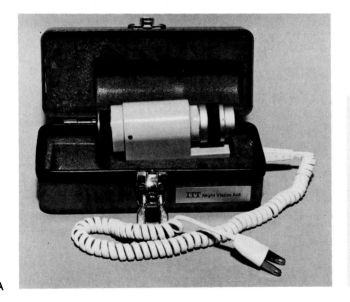

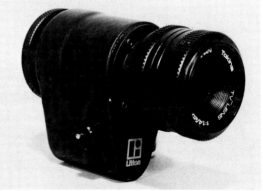

A   B

FIG. 6-8. Night vision aids by ITT *(A)* and Litton *(B)*; both are used monocularly, allowing motivated RP patients to be mobile in darkened conditions. Like any vision aid, it is necessary to develop skill in using the device and to identify specific tasks or circumstances where the aid will be helpful.

Halogen flashlights with focusable beams are now becoming available and are likely to be a valuable night aid for RP patients.

Illumination

The subject of hardware cannot be left without mention of illumination. Every practitioner needs to be familiar with the principles of lighting and to be equipped with flexible lighting in order to demonstrate ideal conditions for the patient.

A normal tungsten bulb produces an unacceptable level of heat at high wattage, but this can be reduced significantly by using a focused luminaire which at 60 watts will give 3000 lux at 30 cm compared with 500 lux for a standard tungsten bulb. The luminaire needs to be sited carefully to avoid glare.

THE LOW VISION ASSESSMENT

The patient should be seen in the low vision clinic when he wishes to perform tasks that he cannot manage with a normal spectacle correction. A complete ophthalmological report, including visual fields, greatly assists the low vision practitioner.

The patient is encouraged to describe his problem tasks as specifically as possible and to put them in order of priority. This process may be more complicated than expected since the patient may present in a complex psychological state, having been told that he is "blind," or likely to become so in the foreseeable future. Some patients react by abandoning all ambition to acquire information visually or to attempt new techniques. Such patients will state modest aims, such as "to read my bank statement and letters." Other patients present diffuse problems, stating that they want a device to "do my job and lead a normal life," a plea for a cure rather than a means to cope with their disability. In both situations the true problem must be confronted and the function of the low vision clinic explained and understood.

The importance of follow-up cannot be overestimated. Even the most experienced practitioner may not be able to prescribe the ideal appliance at the first visit. Indeed, many patients reject the "ideal" appliance, particularly if it is conspicuous or necessitates major behavior modifications. Changes in attitudes and skills may take place by the first follow-up visit, commonly at 3 months, and alternative devices may become acceptable to the patient.

A distinction must be made between disability occurring in the adult and a congenital problem. Adults, more particularly elderly adults, will need to sustain previously learned skills and habits; the congenitally disabled frequently adopt alternative strategies and activities. They listen to the news on the radio rather than read a newspaper, swim rather than play ball. Children may opt out of activities for fear of danger or failure. In the clinic the child may express himself as uninterested in "normal" activities, thereby shielding himself from rejection by the peer group.

MOBILITY TRAINING

Patients with severely constricted visual fields can derive much benefit from mobility training. Taking up a cane represents a big psychological hurdle, and the ophthalmologist can be greatly supportive in this decision. Learning to avoid obstacles, protect his own safety, and let others know that he is visually disabled are major factors in encouraging the patient to learn and use this skill. Most states give right of way to persons carrying white canes, and motorists need the visual clue in order to exercise caution. Some RP patients, even with tiny fields and reasonable acuity, may use a guide dog for increasing their mobility.

MEDICAL THERAPIES FOR RP

Various medical therapies have been advocated for "curing" or treating RP, including ribonucleic acid injections, immunologic intervention, and bee sting therapy; new ideas are constantly being tested or tried, sometimes in very unscientific ways and often to the detriment of the patient's pocketbook. There also appears to be little recognition by some practitioners giving these treatments that there are at least 14 different types of primary RP and countless secondary types; the same treatment is expected to help all of them! On the positive side, many patients receive psychological benefit from having "done something." Unfortunately, there currently is no known effective treatment for curing primary or secondary RP except for vitamin A deficiency related retinopathy. As our knowledge of RP pathogenic mechanisms improves, rational therapies undoubtedly will be developed.

APPENDIX

Agencies that offer services or information to the visually handicapped or deaf-blind are listed below; this listing is included as a public service and is not necessarily a recommendation of any specific program. Many of these organizations would appreciate self-addressed postage-paid envelopes, since they have limited budgets.

American Association for the Deaf–Blind (Membership organization)
814 Thayer Avenue
Silver Spring, MD 20910

American Council of the Blind, Inc.(Membership organization)
1010 Vermont Avenue NW
Suite 1100
Washington, DC 20005

American Foundation for the Blind (Information)
15 West 16th Street
New York, NY 10011

Australian RP Association (Information)
43 Sexton Road
Inglewood
Western Australia 5052

British Retinitis Pigmentosa Society (Overseas newsletter, information; please include return postage)
Greens Norton Court
Greens Norton, Towcester, Northants.
England, U.K.

Canada, National RP Foundation (Information)
1 Spadina Crescent
Suite 115
Toronto, Ontario
Canada

Center for Services for Deaf–Blind Children (Information and services)
Bureau of Education of Handicapped
Department of Education
400 Maryland Ave. SW
Washington, DC 20202

German RP Society (Information)
An den Muhlen 21
4400 Munster
West Germany

Helen Keller National Center for Deaf–Blind Youths and Adults (Services)
111 Middle Neck Road
Sands Point, NY 11050
(516) 944-8900 (TTY and voice)

Library of Congress (Information and services)
Division for the Blind and Physically Handicapped
1291 Taylor Street NW
Washington, DC 20542

The Lighthouse (Low vision aids and information)
New York Association for the Blind
111 East 59th St.
New York, NY 10022

National Association for Visually Handicapped (Information)
305 East 24th St.
New York, NY 10010

National RP Foundation (Information, services, fund raising for research; other International Society addresses available)
1401 Mount Royal Avenue
Baltimore, MD 21217
(301) 225-9400

National Society to Prevent Blindness (Information)
16 East 40th Street
New York, NY 10016

Public Services Program (Deaf-blind)
Gallaudet College
Washington, DC 20002

RP International (Information, services, fund raising)
PO Box 900
Woodland Hills, CA 91365
(818) 992-0500

Royal National Institute for the Blind (Services and Aids for the blind)
Great Portland St.
London, W1
England, U.K.

Texas RP Society (TARP, Inc) (Information, library services)
PO Box 8388
Corpus Christi, TX 78412-0388

State Commissions for the Blind and Visually Handicapped and Vocational Rehabilitation—consult your local telephone directory

REFERENCES

1. Marmor MF: The management of retinitis pigmentosa and allied diseases. Ophthalmol Digest 41:13–29, 1979
2. Marmor MF et al: Retinitis pigmentosa: A symposium on terminology and methods of examination. Ophthalmology 90:126–131, 1983
3. Ross D, Fishman G, Gilbert L et al: Variability of visual field measurements in normal subjects and patients with retinitis pigmentosa. Arch Ophthalmol 102:1004–1010, 1984
4. Fishman FA, Anderson RJ, Stinson L et al: Driving performance of retinitis pigmentosa patients. Br J Ophthalmol 65:122–126, 1981
5. Fonda G: Suggested vision standards for drivers in the United States with vision ranging from 20/175 (6/52) to 20/50 (6/15). Ann Ophthalmol 18:76–79, 1986
6. Berson EL: Light deprivation for early retinitis pigmentosa. Arch Ophthalmol 85:521–529, 1971
7. Heckenlively JR: The frequency of posterior subcapsular cataract in the hereditary retinal degenerations. Am J Ophthalmol 93:733–738, 1982
8. Pearlman JT, Adams GL, Sloan SH: Psychiatric Problems in Ophthalmology. Springfield, IL, Charles C Thomas, 1977
9. Mehr EB, Fried AN: Low Vision Care. Chicago, The Professional Press, 1975
10. Faye E: Clinical Low Vision. Boston, Little, Brown & Co, 1984
11. Jose RT: Understanding Low Vision. New York, American Foundation for the Blind, 1983
12. Silver J, Jackson J: Visual disability, Parts 8 & 9: Setting up the clinic and the work-up. Ophthalmic Optician 23:699–706, 804–813, 1983
13. International guide to aids and appliances. New York, The American Foundation for the Blind (Similar guides are published by the Royal National Institute for the Blind, London)
14. Silver J, Gould E, Thomsitt J. The provision of low vision aids to the visually handicapped. Trans Ophthalmol Soc UK 94:310, 1974
15. Optical Aids for the Partially Sighted. Designs for Vision, Inc., 120 East 23rd St, New York, NY 10010
16. Helping the partially sighted. Published by Keeler, Ltd, Clewer Hill Road, Windsor, Berk., England, 1979
17. Silver J, Jackson J: Visual disability, Part 2: Hand magnifiers and Part 3: Stand magnifiers. Ophthalmic Optician 23:29–35, 85–95, 1983
18. Silver J, Jackson J: Visual disability, Part 4: Spectacle and headborne magnifiers. Ophthalmic Optician 23:214–223, 1983
19. Fonda G: Management of Low vision. New York, Thieme-Stratton, 1981
20. Silver J, Jackson J: Visual disability, Part 7: Telescopic systems for near vision. Ophthalmic Optician 23:489–498, 597–610, 1983
21. Berson EL, Mehaffey L, Rabin AR: A night vision device as an aid for patients with retinitis pigmentosa. Arch Ophthalmol 90:112–116, 1973
22. Morrissette DL, Marmor MF, Goodrich GL: An evaluation of night vision mobility aids. Ophthalmology 90:1226–1230, 1983

7

Congenital and Early-Onset Forms of Retinitis Pigmentosa

JOHN R. HECKENLIVELY
SCOTT G. FOXMAN

The congenital and childhood forms of pigmentary retinal dystrophy are relatively rare, but most of these diseases can be readily distinguished by their clinical characteristics (particularly age of onset), inheritance pattern, the status of the electroretinogram (ERG) final rod threshold, visual field, and presence or absence of systemic manifestations. Entities which will be covered in this chapter include juvenile and early-onset retinitis pigmentosa (RP) and Leber's congenital amaurosis, both uncomplicated types and types with associated systemic findings; those discussed are Zellweger syndrome, Senior-Loken syndrome, and Saldino-Mainzer syndrome. A schematic approach for differentiating the various congenital and early-onset RP types is presented.

LEBER'S CONGENITAL AMAUROSIS

Leber's congenital amaurosis (LCA) is a congenital retinal dystrophy characterized by profound visual impairment at birth, coarse nystagmus, an extinguished ERG, and the eventual appearance of pigmentary and degenerative changes in the fundus. It is difficult to ascertain the incidence of LCA since many studies found in the older literature did not use comparative criteria for defining LCA and did not differentiate between LCA and other forms of early-onset RP.[1,2] The largest of these studies, by Alstrom and Olson, estimated that LCA patients constituted as many as 10% of all congenitally blind children and occurred at an incidence of 3 in 100,000 of the general population in Sweden.[1]

HISTORICAL REVIEW

In 1869, Theodore Leber described a disease which he called a "pigmentary retinopathy with congenital amaurosis".[3] In 1871, Leber emphasized the familial nature of the disease and the frequency of parental consanguinity.[4] In 1916, Leber differentiated between a "congenital" form with blindness in the first year of life and a "juvenile" form with onset between the first year and puberty. Commonly, patients with the juvenile form did not exhibit total blindness. For many years, the juvenile form did not receive attention, since it usually was classified as an early form of RP.

With the advent of the ERG in the 1950s, interest in LCA was revitalized. Franceschetti and Dieterle showed that in the absence of fundus abnormalities only the ERG could establish the diagnosis of LCA and would rule out a neurological cause of congenital blindness.[5] In 1957, Alstrom and Olson published a monograph describing 105 families containing 175 cases of LCA. Although this study did not use strict criteria for defining LCA and examined less than 50% of those cases cited, the authors established the autosomal recessive character of this condition.

CLASSIFICATION SCHEME

Many of the older studies evaluating LCA failed to differentiate between congenital retinal dystrophy and early-onset forms of classical RP. This led Krill and other authors to conclude that LCA is a syndrome in which different nosologic entities are grouped together.[6-8] In early investigations studying the clinical heterogeneity of LCA, Foxman and colleagues found a group of 11 children with LCA uniquely characterized by high hyperopia (greater than 5 diopters) and the absence of systemic abnormalities.[9,10] This finding prompted the development of a new classification system.[11]

Patients with congenital and early-onset retinal degeneration were divided into four groups based on the age of onset of visual loss, the severity of loss of visual acuity and visual field, and the presence or absence of nonocular abnormalities (Tables 7-1 and 7-2). Each group may contain several different (genetic) diseases, but the groups are meant to be an organizational scheme for rationally separating the various types of congenital and early-onset panretinal degenerations (**Fig. 7-1**).

Group 1: Uncomplicated LCA

Uncomplicated LCA patients are characterized by congenital blindness, an extinguished ERG, sluggish pupillary responses to light, and searching nystagmus. The distinguishing features of this group are the lack of systemic abnormalities and the presence of high hyperopia of greater than 5 diopters.

Most patients were noted to have visual difficulties

TABLE 7-1

CLINICAL CHARACTERISTICS OF PATIENTS WITH CONGENITAL AND EARLY-ONSET RETINITIS PIGMENTOSA

				VISUAL ACUITY	
GROUP	ONSET OF SYMPTOMS*	FIRST VISIT*	REFRACTIVE ERROR†	First visit	Most recent visit
1(n = 14)	0.1–1.0 (0.3)	0.3–1.0 (0.5)	+4.00 to +10.50 (+6.54)	No F	No F–20/400 (No F)
2(n = 5)	0.1–1.0 (0.4)	0.3–6.0 (2.3)	−3.75 to +5.50 (+0.94)	No F–20/200 (No F)	
3(n = 5)	0.1–0.9 (0.5)	1.3–7.0 (3.2)	−3.75 to +4.00 (+1.26)	20/80–CF (20/80)	20/50–CF (20/80)
4(n = 10)	2.0–8.0 (5.0)	4.0–9.0 (6.2)	−1.00 to +5.25 (+2.33)	20/20–20/80 (20/50)	20/20–20/80 (20/50)

Values are given in ranges, and mean value in parentheses.

*Age in months   † Refractive error in diopters   No F = no fixation to bright light

CF = count fingers

(Foxman: Arch Ophthalmol 103:1503, 1985)

TABLE 7-2

DIFFERENTIAL DIAGNOSIS OF CONGENITAL AND EARLY-ONSET RETINITIS PIGMENTOSA

FINDINGS ON INITIAL EXAMINATION	UNCOMPLICATED LCA (GROUP 1)	COMPLICATED LCA (GROUP 2)	JUVENILE RP (GROUP 3)	EARLY ONSET RP (GROUP 4)
Onset of symptoms	<6 mo	Difficult to determine	<2 yr	≥4 yr
Visual acuity	Poorer than 20/400	Poorer than 20/400	Better than 20/100	Better than 20/60
Refractive error	>4 diopters hyperopic	Variable	Slightly hyperopic	Slightly hyperopic
Nystagmus	Searching	Searching	Occasionally latent	Absent
Pupillary reaction	Sluggish	Sluggish	Normal	Normal
Systemic abnormalities	None	Neurologic, renal, skeletal	None	None
Electroretinographic responses	Extinguished	Extinguished or minimally recordable	Extinguished	Extinguished or minimally recordable
Fundus appearance	Normal or mild pigmentary changes	Normal or mild pigmentary changes	Variable	Typical peripheral pigmentary abnormalities
Family history	Autosomal recessive	Dependent on syndrome	Unknown	X-linked recessive; autosomal recessive; autosomal dominant
Visual fields	Unable to determine	Unable to determine	Constricted and tubular	Mild to moderate constriction

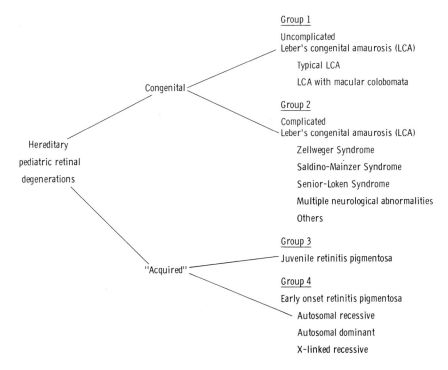

FIG. 7-1. Classification of congenital and early-onset RP. (LCA indicates Leber's congenital amaurosis.)

by seven months and were examined before 1 year of age. Parents most commonly noted visual impairment between 3 and 5 months of age. None of the children exhibit the ability to fixate to bright light on initial examination and usually do not achieve a visual acuity better than counting fingers.

Fundus examination in the earlier years is usually normal, with peripheral pigmentary stippling to occasional bone spicules and even macular pigmentary abnormalities in older individuals. An interesting subgroup which genetically is also autosomal recessive but is quite distinct are those patients who have LCA with macular colobomas. Both these types of LCA will be discussed further after the classification section.

Group 2: Complicated LCA

Complicated LCA represents several well-defined single gene defects and some less well-defined diseases in which congenital retinal dysfunction is one aspect of a generalized process that usually involves another organ system.

This group of children are often noted to have poor vision by 1 year of age. However, they may not be examined by an ophthalmologist until several years of age, since their blindness is often attributed to associated neurological abnormalities. The child usually is not able to fixate to a bright light on the initial examination and rarely achieves a visual acuity better than 20/400. No particular refractive error is associated with any of the syndromes in this group. With the exception of refractive error, the ocular findings are similar to those of group 1.

Specific syndromes which meet the criteria for group 2 patients include cerebrohepatorenal syndrome of Zellweger, Moore-Taylor syndrome, Senior-Loken syndrome, and Saldino-Mainzer syndrome. Sporadic cases of children with congenital blindness and other systemic abnormalities will be mentioned.

Group 3: Juvenile RP

Juvenile Leber's patients are children who show signs of visual impairment within the first several years of life and develop severe visual field loss and retinal degeneration by age 6 years. This entity also was described by Leber in a later article.[12] These children are frequently examined by age 3 years, although visual abnormalities may be noted by the parent as early as 6 months of age. Visual acuity on initial examination is usually better than 20/100 but progressively deteriorates, usually leading to blindness by the third or fourth decade. Many patients have tiny central fields and 20/200 level of vision through their twenties. The fundus examination reveals mild to moderate pigmentary changes, and the ERG is extinguished.

These children are differentiated from group 1 by the absence of searching nystagmus and the relatively good central visual acuity, and, while they are usually farsighted, the refraction is seldom more than a couple of diopters positive. They are differentiated from group 4 by the severity of visual loss and age of onset of symptoms (Table 7-2). No child in group 4 had the severe tubular visual field abnormalites found by age 6 in the children in group 3 (see also Autosomal Dominant Leber's Amaurosis, p. 146)

Group 4: Early-onset RP

Children categorized as having early-onset adult RP characteristically have nyctalopia by age 6 years. These children initially have good central vision and only minor visual field abnormalities. The disease course is similiar to classical adult RP, but the onset is at a younger age.

The initial visual acuity is usually better than 20/50 and rarely less than 20/80. These children have mild to moderate visual field constriction. The ERG is quite variable, with some patients demonstrating extinguished ERGs while other patients may have partially recordable ERGs. An example of early-onset adult RP is illustrated by cases VIII-7 and VIII-11 in Chapter 8.

The early-onset group encompasses a large variety of RP types; one of the intentions of including this category is to schematically account for the occasional atypical earlier-onset cases of RP from established pedigrees. It also will accommodate other less well-defined cases in which the children have early night blindness, mild visual acuity, and field defects.

If the above classification scheme is employed, the various congenital retinal blinding dystrophies which have been called LCA begin to make more sense, as they are divided into more identifiable groups. An occasional patient does not fit, however, which may be useful in further modifying and understanding the classification of these early-onset retinal dystrophies.

Uncomplicated LCA is identified early by parents as the infants develop nystagmus or roving eye movements during the first year of life. Visual acuity is usually 20/200 or worse. Examination during infancy usually reveals a normal, though frequently blond retina; hypoplastic (**Fig. 7-2A**) or slightly swollen discs[13] (**Fig. 7-2B**) and wrinkling of the inner limiting membrane may be seen (**Fig. 7-3A&B**). Nerve fiber layer dropout is an additional subtle feature (**Fig. 7-4**).

Pigmentary stippling or deposits develop later in childhood (**Fig. 7-3C**), and by the teenage years may show severe pigmentary changes (**Fig. 7-5A&B**). Yellowish to white flecks may be seen at the level of the RPE in the midperipheral retina (**Fig. 7-6**).[14]

However, children with juvenile nephronophthisis and LCA have been noted to have depigmented atrophic spots in peripheral retina,[15] which are quite different from findings of the Chew report in which the lesions were confluent and deep in the retina.[14] As the children grow older, they may develop strabismus and usually have a roving nystagmus of a sightless person. Young LCA children may induce a sensation of "phosphenes" by pushing or even hitting their eyes, a phenomenon which has been termed the "oculodigital sign of Franceschetti."[16] Many LCA patients have eyes that lie deep in their sockets, and the presence of keratoconus has been noted[7,17–19]; it has been postulated that both the enophthalmos and keratoconus may be the result of the prolonged oculodigital habit of the child. Waardenburg found keratoconus in 15% of his LCA patients, while Karel followed 40 patients with LCA and found that 16 patients (38.6%) developed keratoconus. The keratoconus is usually bilateral, and no patient developed keratoconus before the age of 7 years. The etiology of the keratoconus is unknown.

(Text continues on p. 114.)

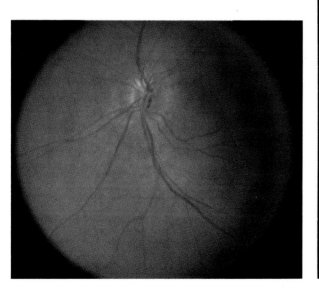

A

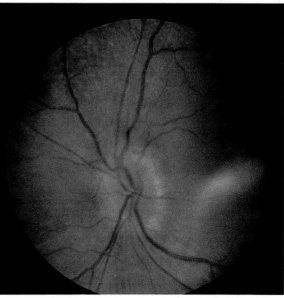

B

FIG. 7-2. Typical LCA with *(A)* slightly hypoplastic disc and mild vessel attenuation with otherwise normal fundus; *(B)* disc swelling in a 2-year-old girl. (White spot temporally is artifect.)

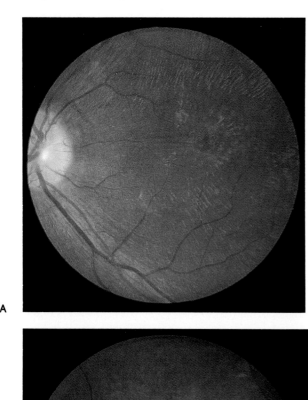

A

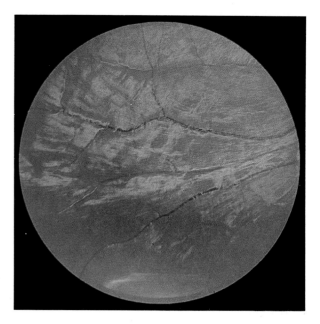

B

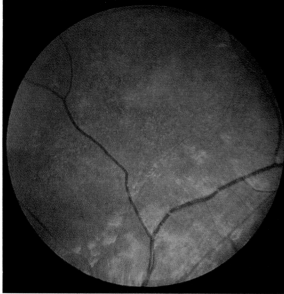

C

FIG. 7-3. LCA in a 6-year-old boy with 6°–7° central fields with the IV-4 isopter and vision of OD 1/160, OS 4/160 whose parents were first cousins, demonstrating *(A)* early macular degeneration, vessel attenuation, and *(A&B)* severe wrinkling of the inner limiting membrane with a "wet cellophane" appearance; *(C)* early granularity and fine pigment deposition in the superior equator region.

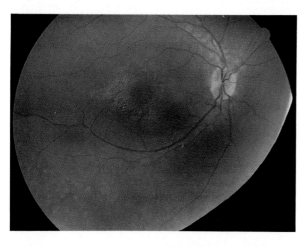

FIG. 7-4. Typical LCA in a 3-year-old girl, right eye; there are minimal fundus findings of mild attenuation of retinal vessels, wrinkling of inner limiting membrane, nerve fiber layer dropout superior to disc, and focal depigmented lesions in the RPE in the inferior equatorial region. (Photograph courtesy of Richard Weleber, M.D.)

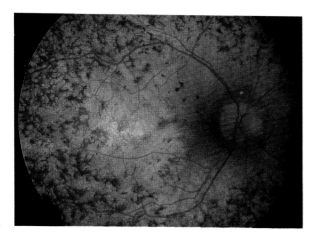

A

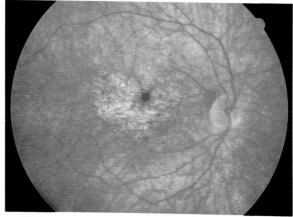

B

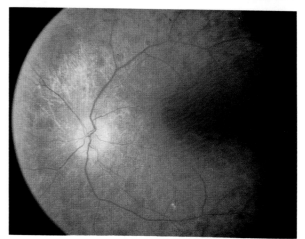

C

FIG. 7-5. Severe pigmentary alterations in adolescent children with juvenile LCA: *(A)* a 14-year-old girl with 3° visual fields and a visual acuity of OD 20/40, OS 20/70 with + 3.25 refraction showing heavy bone spicule-like pigmentary deposits and disc drusen; *(B)* a 12-year-old boy who had nystagmus and poor vision as an infant, 2° visual fields and 20/60 visual acuity O.U., demonstrating severe depigmentation and diffuse atrophy, foveal hyperpigmentation and thickening, and optic atrophy; (C) 50-year-old man with juvenile LCA with diffuse atrophy and interesting round subretinal pigmentary lesions. Vision was light perception OU.

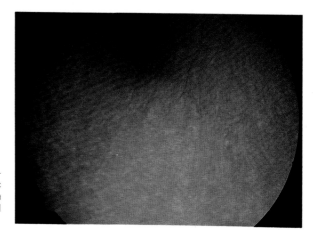

FIG. 7-6. Juvenile LCA in a 10-year-old girl with mild hyperopia and a visual acuity of OD 20/70, OS 20/50 and eccentric Goldmann visual fields with large targets of about 30° in each eye; equatorial retina shows diffuse atrophy with multiple focal depigmented lesions in the RPE.

COMPOSITE PICTURE

UNCOMPLICATED LEBER'S CONGENITAL AMAUROSIS

A 10-month-old infant was seen on referral with a history of poor vision and nystagmus first noted at the age of 10 weeks. The parents were second cousins, but there was no family history of any eye or neurological disease. On examination, the eyes appeared deep-set, and the child reacted only to a bright light stimulus and, in fact, appeared to have photophobia. Pupillary reaction was sluggish, and a random large-amplitude low-frequency nystagmus was present. There was no evidence of cataract or keratoconus. Indirect ophthalmoscopy revealed a blond fundus, and the discs were small but appeared mildly swollen. The RPE was granular, appearing with some fine "salt-and-pepper" pigment deposition throughout the fundus. Retinoscopy showed a hypermetropic error of +7.00 diopters in each eye. The electroretinogram was nonrecordable in both eyes. A neurological examination and computerized axial tomography were normal. During the examination, the child was observed to be striking his right eye with his palm.

The patient was followed for a number of years, maintaining light perception vision. The parents were able to alter the eye striking behavior by age 2 1/2. The child was enrolled in a school for the visually handicapped and did well. He presented at age 14 complaining of some discomfort in his right eye, and on examination, keratoconus with small rupture of Descemet's membrane, corneal edema, and trace posterior subcapsular cataract was seen.

Another case example of typical LCA is presented in this chapter (Baby A) emphasizing management of the blind child as well as the emotional needs of parents and siblings.

CATARACTS

Karel reported that cataracts were present in 52% of his patients with LCA.[20] He found that cataract formation usually started between the first and tenth year of life, and its frequency increased with age. In patients with cataracts, cortical cataracts were found in 68% and a posterior subcapsular cataract in 18%.

PATHOLOGY

There are few reports of histological examinations in congenital RP, and most were performed in older patients. Babel found changes of only the neuroepithelium in two cases.[21] He found the absence of a layer of cones and rods in one case and an unrecognizable mass at the level of the photoreceptors in the other. Sorsby reported on a 20-year-old patient who was blind from birth.[22] This patient exhibited advanced pigmentary retinopathy with disorganization of the retinal structure at all layers. Gillespie's cases demonstrated disappearance of photoreceptors and their replacement by a single layer of cuboidal cells.[23]

The only pathological report from an infant was reported by Mizuno and colleagues.[24] This female patient was born blind and had an extinguished ERG performed at 9 months of age. The patient also had multiple neurological abnormalities and died at 18 months of age from cardiac arrest and frequent dyspneic episodes.

Light microscopy revealed subretinal deposits corresponding to white spots and lines in the fundus. The inner layers were spared, while there were changes in the outer retinal layers and choroid. On electron microscopy (EM), the white subretinal deposits were noted to consist of loose outer segments, apical processes of RPE, and macrophages. Other EM findings included undifferentiated photoreceptor nuclei, inner segments of RPE cells, and choriocapillaris. Based on these findings, Mizuno speculated that LCA was characterized by primary dystrophic and secondary degenerative changes of the neurosensory retina, RPE, and choroid.

LEBER'S AMAUROSIS WITH MACULAR COLOBOMA

A specific form of congenital RP or LCA is associated with atrophic macular staphylomata. The disease is inhertied in an autosomal recessive pattern. The term "coloboma" has been used because of the sim-

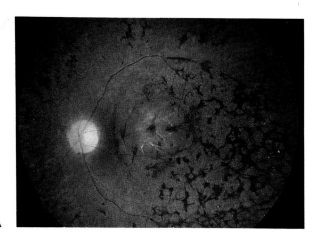
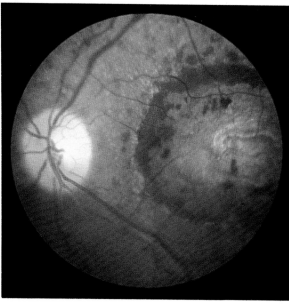

FIG. 7-7. Congenital RP with macular colobomata (staphylomata) in *(A)* a 27-year-old woman from a consanguineous marriage and *(B)* a 14-year-old male with multiplex inheritance who subsequently has developed bilateral keratoconus.

ilarity in appearance to retinal colobomata, although the usage is perhaps an unfortunate one since the defect is not due to failure of embryonic fissure closure. The macular lesions (**Fig.** 7-7*A&B*) could be confused with those seen in congenital infections with *Toxoplasma gondii* or cytomegalovirus, but the panretinal pigmentary degeneration, lack of vision from childhood, and hereditary nature of the disease establish the diagnosis. The ERG is extingished by one year of age. Keratoconus and minor skeletal abnormalities have been reported in this entity.[25–27]

COMPLICATED LEBER'S AMAUROSIS

CASE STUDY

A 7-month-old male infant was first seen with nystagmus and sluggish pupillary reactions. The parents were first cousins, but there was no family history of eye problems. The pregnancy and birth were normal, but with time, the child missed developmental milestones, clearly showing psychomotor retardation. By the age of 9 months, his pupils were dilated and nonresponsive to light, and on testing, the ERG was nonrecordable.

Retinal examination revealed thickening and graying of parafoveal retina, a hypoplastic disc, and multiple round white spots at the level of the RPE, extending from the arcades to the anterior retina. (Multiple white dots are a variable feature in complicated LCA.) The inner limiting membrane was wrinkled.

Neurological examination showed positive Babinski reflex, hyperreactive reflexes, and hearing loss. The medical workup included blood count and differential, urinalysis, serum protein, glucose, lipid profile, metabolic screen, and x-rays, the results of all of which were normal. EEG showed changes consistent with diffuse organic brain disease. By 13 months, the child was having frequent dyspneic episodes and died of cardiac arrest.

While there are a number of reports in the ophthalmic literature of infants with structural neurological and renal abnormalities, examined either post mortem, by CT scan, or by peumoencephalography, associated with complicated LCA, findings are nonspecific and do not fit established diagnostic categories.[28-31]

There have been many reports of patients with LCA having associated neurological abnormalities, including mental and motor retardation, epilepsy, microcephaly, hydrocephalus, hypertonia, hypotonia, and deaf-mutism.[32-35] In many of these cases, the neurological abnormalities were acquired, not congenital, and the exact age of onset of retinal dysfunction was not accurately documented. It has been speculated that some of these children may have had storage diseases such as ceroid lipofuscinosis. Indeed, Pinckers believes this to have been the case in many of the children that Leber classified as having juvenile RP.[36]

Several well-recognized syndromes should be mentioned. These include the Senior-Loken and Saldino-Mainzer syndromes and the cerebrohepatorenal syndrome of Zellweger.

Senior-Loken Syndrome

This autosomal recessive syndrome is manifested by a childhood onset of nephronophthisis associated with congenital-onset retinal degeneration. Both Senior and Loken with associates described an association of tapetoretinal degeneration with renal dysplasia.[37,38] In the absence of renal dialysis, the disease is fatal in the second to third decade. The patients are usually blind from birth or early childhood. They develop a pigmentary retinopathy and extinguished ERG response. Abnormal ERG and EOG responses may be of value in detecting asymptomatic carriers.[39]

Saldino-Mainzer Syndrome

The Saldino-Mainzer syndrome consists of skeletal dysplasia associated with congenital-onset retinal degeneration, familial juvenile nephronophthisis, cerebellar ataxia, and cone-shaped epiphyses of the hands with short stature.[40] Poor vision, nystagmus, and an extinguished ERG are typically present from an early age. Ophthalmoscopy shows panretinal atrophy, optic nervehead pallor, and retinal vessel attenuation (**Fig. 7-8A&B**). Midperipheral multiple focal depigmented atrophic spots in the RPE may be seen in equator regions.[41] Opinion varies as to whether Saldino-Mainzer and Senior-Loken syndromes may be one and the same disease process.

Moore-Taylor Syndrome

Moore and Taylor reported three male infants, two of whom were siblings, who presented with a syn-

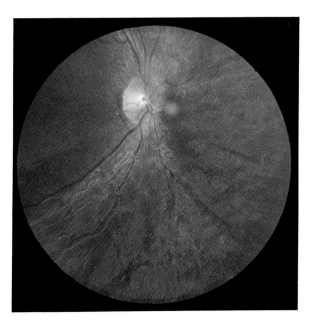
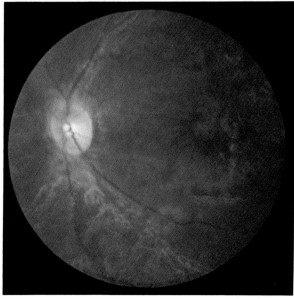

A   B

FIG. 7-8. Saldino-Mainzer (Senior-Loken) syndrome; a 13-year-old girl with LCA, familial juvenile nephronophthisis, cone-shaped epiphyses, and skeletal dysplasia, demonstrating diffuse retinal atrophy *(A)* right eye and *(B)* left eye.

drome of pendular nystagmus by 12 weeks, barely recordable to nonrecordable ERGs, low-amplitude visual evoked responses (VERs), gross defects in saccadic eye movements, and head thrusts similar to those seen in oculomotor apraxia.[42] All patients had generalized hypotonia and developmental delay, and one child was severely mentally retarded. The two patients who could be tested retained good visual fields and visual acuities ranging from 6/18 to 6/36. These two latter findings are not found in typical Leber's congenital amaurosis.

Zellweger Syndrome

This autosomal recessive, fatal syndrome consists of multiple congenital defects associated with characteristic facies, hypotonia, abnormalities of the central nervous system and liver, renal cortical cysts, and stippled irregular calcifications of the patellae and greater trochanters. Ocular abnormalities include congenital retinal degeneration manifested by RPE changes and an extinguished ERG, and corneal clouding, cataract, glaucoma, and optic atrophy.[43,44] Ultrastructural examination of the retina of an infant who died showed bileaflet inclusions identical to those seen in neonatal adrenoleukodystrophy.[45] Moser and colleagues identified increased very-long-chain fatty acid levels, particulary hexacosanoic acid and hexacosenoic acid in plasma and skin fibroblasts of 20 patients. They were able to use this finding for prenatal diagnosis.[46]

Ek reported a patient with psychomotor retardation and Leber's amaurosis congenita with an accumulation of bile acid precursors and very long chain fatty acids with impaired biosynthesis of plasmalogens and defective oxidation of phytanic acid in cultured fibroflasts. There was a virtual lack of peroxisomes in a liver biopsy specimen.[46a] Goldfischer found abnormal peroxisomal enzymatic activity in a patient clinically similar to Zellweger syndrome.[46b]

DIFFERENTIAL DIAGNOSIS

Congenital blindness may occur secondary to many different causes; the most commonly confused ones include cortical blindness, optic atrophy or hypoplasia, inflammatory retinal diseases, and neuronal storage diseases such as Haltia-Santavuori (early in-

fancy), Jansky-Bielschowsky (late infancy), and Spielmeyer-Vogt (early childhood) types of Batten disease.[47] Nystagmus is commonly seen in a number of these conditions. A further discussion of Batten disease can be found in Chapter 12.

In cortical blindness, the fundus and ERG are normal, while the cortical VER is absent or diminished. Neurological abnormalities such as hydrocephaly or microcephaly are usually present. In LCA the ERG is always extinguished.

Optic atrophy can be the potential cause of either unilateral or bilateral visual impairment in infants and children, particularly those with cerebral palsy due to perinatal anoxia, birth injury, or hydrocephalus. In optic atrophy the ERG may be subnormal, normal, or even occasionally supranormal,[48] while the VER is minimal or absent. Hereditary optic atrophy usually does not lead to complete blindness and can be differentiated on the basis of the ERG and VER response.

Optic nerve hypoplasia may occur alone or in association with midline or other cerebral structural abnormalities including porencephaly[49] and De Morsier syndrome.[50] Any infant with optic hypoplasia should be evaluated for pituitary deficiency, since an endocrine crisis may be life-threatening. A frequent finding on fundus examination is the "double ring" sign. On the basis of fundus examination alone, these patients may be difficult to differentiate from those with LCA, since both may have a normal-appearing fundus and patients with LCA have been reported to have a pigmented ring around the optic nerve.[9] However, the ERG response clearly differentiates the two entities.

Inflammatory retinal disease (e.g., congenital rubella retinopathy) is usually characterized by patchy, discrete black salt-and-pepper pigmentation, which may be variable in size and location (**Fig. 11-6A–D**). The ERG is usually normal to slightly subnormal. Other findings include cataract, glaucoma, microophthalmia, deafness, and cardiac malformations. Visual fields usually remain stable over time. Congenital syphilis can lead to diffuse pigmentary retinopathy (**Fig. 11-4**), but the retinal changes usually are late manifestations of the disease and occur after the age of 5 or 6 years (see Chapter 11, Simplex RP). The pigmentary changes seen in congenital toxoplasmosis are confined to the macular region, and the diffuse RPE seen in LCA with macular colobomas are not present.

Finally, there are two reports of a very rare autosomal dominant form of LCA which have features similar to the juvenile type (group 3) reported in this chapter.[51,52]

It is our opinion that every child who presents with congenital blindness with or without a normal fundus examination should have an ERG performed to rule out the possibility of LCA. This particularly applies to those children with neurological diseases or nystagmus.

REHABILITATION

One of the principal reasons for differentiating between group 1 and group 2 (uncomplicated and complicated LCA) is to determine which child will benefit from rehabilitation and special education programs. We found that group 1 children were of normal intelligence and responded well to special education programs. Nickel and Hoyt have also drawn attention to the educational and psychological importance of offering a good prognosis for the neurological development of group 1 LCA children.[53]

Management of Blind Infants and Their Families

TONI G. MARCY

While a lack of stimulation can have tragic consequences for any infant, the outcome is even more devastating and often irreversible for blind babies. In order to forestall deviant behavior and delay in mental development, a program has been developed at the Los Angeles Blind Children's Center to promote growth in various developmental areas during the critical first 2 years of the blind infant's life. A correspondence course is available for families who have no other resources.

Each family is seen on a monthly basis or more often if necessary. A thorough medical history is taken, which includes the family's emotional structure, giving useful information about the child's physical condition and the parents' ability to cope with the handicap. Parents are given opportunities in group meetings to ask questions and to air their anxieties, with the help of a team consisting of a social worker, a child development specialist, and a psychiatrist. Because siblings of blind children often show emotional disturbances such as acting out or withdrawal because parents' time and energy are taken up with caring for the blind child, a psychiatrist is also made available to sighted siblings.

CASE STUDY

Baby A was the product of a full-term, uncomplicated pregnancy, except that she was delivered by cesarean section because of maternal medical problems. Her birth weight was 6 pounds, 1 ounce, and she had Apgar scores of 9 at 1 minute and 10 at 5 minutes. There was no consanguinity of the parents, nor any eye problems on either side of the family.

At 2 months, her mother noticed that the infant did not follow motion or light. She became alarmed about a possible visual impairment and shared her observations with her pediatrician, who referred her to a pediatric ophthalmologist. His diagnosis was ocular albinism, but the parents asked for a second opinion. The child was examined under anesthesia. While the fundi appeared to lack pigment, the ERG was nonrecordable in both eyes. A diagnosis of LCA was made. A brain scan was normal and did not show any CNS abnormalities.

In panic, the parents immediately made an appointment with a third ophthalmologist in another city, hoping to find some "cure" for their child's visual handicap. "We needed somebody to explain the technical terms given to us and to get some direction about raising a blind baby." When their hopes were unfulfilled, both parents were in such deep depression that the mother was emotionally unavailable to her older child as well as the baby. The father found himself working longer and longer hours in his business away from home. Neither could face the prospect of telling their parents, friends, and business associates of their child's blindness, hoping the friends would find out by themselves that the baby had visual problems.

The parents described their feelings when told about their child's blindness as, "the bottom has dropped out of our world." They still had not accepted the diagnosis when they were referred 2 months later to our intervention program for blind infants and their families. Individual counseling by a social worker and a psychiatrist helped the parents through stages of guilt, mourning, and searching for answers. Group meetings with other mothers experiencing similar feelings also helped the mother to overcome her feelings of helplessness and to regroup her mental energy.

The older brother, a very sensitive child, had difficulties dealing with his sister's blindness. He was annoyed that people stared at her, and was very controlled in expressing his feelings. A child psychiatrist helped alleviate his many fears, such as that of losing his eyesight because of misbehaving.

A child development specialist saw the family on a monthly basis, helping them to reach the next developmental milestones. The parents were advised about proper stimulation, and behavioral danger signals were pointed out.

The first meeting took place when the child was 5 1/2 months old. She was seen to squint when exposed to light and had horizontal nystagmus. A bald spot was noticed on her occiput, a sign the baby was mostly left in the supine position. All the toys given to the infant were ones with auditory cues, such as rattles, bells, and musical toys. The mother reported that her child cried when placed on her tummy or in the seated position. A ball placed between the infant's legs with her hands resting on it made her tolerate the seated position more readily.

In the following months, it became evident that the gross motor milestones were delayed, while fine motor and language development were satisfactory. In spite of much encouragement, the baby never went through the creeping stage, but was finally able at 14 months to pull to a stand and to cruise, holding onto furniture. The parents were reassured that blind children often are delayed in mobility and that there was no reason to be concerned about their child's devel-

opment. At 18 months, she was able to walk by herself and also was very independent in the personal–social area, such as feeding herself and drinking from a cup. Her exploratory behavior of toys and her language development were excellent. At the age of 2 1/2 years, the child advanced to the toddler group. She adapted well to being with other children, walked freely about the room, stretching out her hands to protect herself against being hurt by obstacles. She was very cautious when moving, avoided walking on the grass, and preferred solid ground. Once she became acquainted with the school, she used her light perception in combination with auditory cues to find her way to familiar places. Her only mannerisms were walking in circles when anxious or frustrated and poking her eyes with her hands. When told to put her hands down, she cooperated readily.

The child is now 5 1/2 years old. She has begun to learn prebraille and is capable of abstract thinking and problem solving. Her verbal expression is advanced. She rides a tricycle, climbs, runs, and swims. Socially she is very adept and derives pleasure from organized games. She has made many friends in her class. Plans for the future include attendance at an integrated school program with sighted children. A resource teacher will help her with Braille.

The importance of guidance at the earliest possible date cannot be stressed strongly enough in order to maximize the sensory–motor development of a congenitally blind infant and to help the family cope with the difficult task of raising a visually handicapped child.

The following represent the goals of our management–intervention program:

First: To win the confidence of the parents and to help them accept the diagnosis of blindness. The wide range of developmental milestones of blind children is pointed out to the parents, and they are also informed that progress in one area often is followed by regression in others (e.g., when the child makes progress in the motoric area, such as walking, he very often regresses in expressive language). From this approach, parents learn what to expect for their visually handicapped child without unnecessary fear of mental retardation.

Second: To promote parent–child attachment. Many authors who have worked with blind infants have stressed the importance of a mutually satisfying relationship between parent and child during the first 2 years of life.[54] Much deviant behavior in later life can be attributed to a breakdown of nurturing interaction.[55-59] In 70% of cases of congenital blindness, the diagnosis is made during the first year of life.[60] Even though it is the mother who usually notices the visual handicap of the child, she very often cannot accept the fact once the diagnosis has been made. Helplessness and guilt feelings for having borne a "defective" baby may lead to severe depression, which in turn makes her incapable of caring for the handicapped child. Most mothers need support to cope with facing and accepting blindness as a permanent handicap.

As a rule, the blind infant is passive and a "good baby" who places few demands on his mother. Whereas the sighted child's motor activity is increased at the sight of mother's approach to the crib, the blind baby will lie more still to integrate the sounds.[61] Since his visual input is missing, his main interest is focused on his own body. To get him interested in persons and objects around him, he needs more holding, cuddling, and being talked to than a sighted child who benefits from visual stimulation.[63] If the mother prefers to bottle-feed the infant, the bottle should always be given while the baby is cradled in mother's arms. This strengthens the bond to the mother as the person who attends to his immediate needs. The blind infant is very sensitive to the way he is held and differentiates kinesthetic sensations much earlier than do sighted children.

We recommend a baby-carrying sling in which the infant faces his mother; in this fashion, it is easier to control his position, stroke his head, and talk to him. He gets used to different acoustic and olfactory stimuli while his mother goes about her household duties. Extending and flexing his arms and legs, massaging them gently, and playing "this little piggy goes to market" makes him aware of his body parts.

Baby's first smile brings one of the greatest satisfactions to parents; blind infants show responsive smiling to mother's voice or touch at approximately 6 weeks, much the same time as a sighted baby. Their smiles have been described as being more fleeting and harder to evoke.[57] Great emphasis should also be placed on the father taking an active part in handling his baby, such as mutual rubbing of foreheads to elicit an immediate smiling response.

Third: To further gross motor development. While there is no difference between sighted and blind children in the development of postural accomplishments, there is a delay in all motor areas which involve mobility, and the blind child needs assistance in this area.[61]

Sitting, first supported and then unsupported, is accomplished at the same time as for sighted children, between 6 and 9 months. Creeping sometimes is delayed with a blind child. It is replaced by scooting, which gives him a more pleasurable feeling, or is not exercised at all unless an auditory cue is used as a lure to move. Learning to pull to a stand occurs at the same time as for sighted children, but blind children often need many months to learn to walk, and few blind children walk alone before 18 months of age. Parents are instructed to stay put while the child is taking steps, since this aids the child's sense of spatial relations. During the toddler stage, blind babies will often knock against an object accidentally, and then repeat it for spatial orientation; these hurts and bumps are important learning cues for the blind child. Restraining the child's mobility is devastating to development and may lead to self-stimulatory behavior such as rocking back and forth or repetitive hitting of himself.

Fourth: Handling of objects. During the first 3 months of life, the blind child usually keeps his hands close to his shoulders with little movement. While the sighted baby is fascinated with watching his hands engaged in the midline when 3 to 4 months old, the blind baby brings his hands together only accidentally and not in a purposeful way. Blind infants have to be taught to use their hands.[63] Colorful cradle gyms (if there is some residual vision) and various toys are placed in his crib within easy reach. The first fortuitous response to touch of the toy will give him incentive to repeat the act.

As soon as the child is able to sit by himself, he should be placed in a high chair with a tray where a few objects are put within easy reach so that he can explore them by banging, pulling, matching, and mouthing. The choice of toys must be made carefully, using different textures and shapes, such as wooden spoons, plastic cubes, metal cups, rough and soft materials, and toys with auditory cues. It is important not to provide only toys with auditory cues, since this leads to self-stimulatory behavior such as ringing the bell or rattle in a repetitive way, which does not draw the child outward, but lets him dwell on his sound making. Cutsworth warns of choosing too complex or too uninteresting objects which discourages manipulation and therefore interferes with the purpose of giving mental input to the child.[64] A young blind child "sees" with his hands and his mouth, and mouthing objects should not be discouraged as antisocial behavior, since the sensory information derived in this manner is important to the child.

An important milestone in fine motor development is finger-feeding, starting at about 9 months. Some mothers object to it because it is messy and therefore will spoon-feed their child. However, it is extremely critical that the blind child learns to differentiate between edible and nonedible objects and be made independent for eating.

Many blind children do not chew properly, perhaps because they lack opportunity of watching the mother chew, and take only pureed food. Letting them feel with their hands while mother chews crunchy foods often gives the blind child the incentive to copy mother.

During the second year, placing objects into and out of containers should be encouraged. The concept of object permanence is often delayed in blind children for up to 1 year. Much patience is needed to encourage a blind child to search for the lost object because vision cannot be replaced by sound as a distance sense. This is a cause of much frustration for the child.

Fifth: Developing perceptual, cognitive, and language skills. Without vision from birth the blind child has considerable difficulty in translating perceptual experiences into mental representations.[65] During the first year, the blind baby bab-

bles like a sighted baby, but in a more subdued way. It is important to keep up a dialogue with the baby by repeating his own sounds and adding some meaningful ones, such as "ma-ma" and "da-da." Since the child cannot see mother's approving face, tactile stimulation such as stroking the infant's body will encourage more babbling. Social games such as "patty-cake" and "kissing mommie" open up a warm relationship and add to the baby's development of receptive language.

During the second year, the blind child's language development is slower than that of a sighted child. Tactual and auditory cues alone make identification of items more difficult. Many blind infants between 16 and 20 months stop using words they have previously learned and do not add new ones. This happens at a time when the child becomes more mobile and the parents are more aware of their child's handicap. The mother's depression and threats of breakdown in the marriage, common in the child's second year, lead to isolation from the child. Hospitalizations for checking his eye condition may also add to the child's regression, especially in the language area. As a more relaxed relationship between the parents is established, often through parental counseling, the child's language development progresses. One word of caution should be noted: too much verbal stimulation by the mother which does not give the child time to organize his input will lead to parrotting. The same warning also is true for the indiscriminate use of television to keep the child busy. Since the picture cannot be seen, most of the words are meaningless. A favorite pastime of many blind children is to get stimulation from the repetition of commercials or jingles. The acquisition of pronouns is delayed, and some echolalia is present in all blind children between 2 and 3 years of age; their language acquisition catches up when they are 4 years old.

CASE STUDY

A mother presented complaining that her 6-month-old blind daughter, who had previously turned from her back to her stomach, was now lying on her back only, without moving. Intense questioning about the day's events revealed that the television was playing all day long. It became apparent that the child was listening and had no reason to change position since no additional input would result. As soon as the mother used the television sparingly and used her voice as an incentive, the blind child started to roll over again.

Sixth: To prevent deviant behavior. Gesell and Amatruda state that the blind child's major problem is to achieve some degree of extroversion.[66] Unless his environment gives him enough opportunity for exploration, the blind child uses self-stimulatory measures to keep himself busy. Some of these mannerisms, called "blindisms," are noticeable in most blind children. They consist of flipping of hands, especially when there is some peripheral vision, or poking their fingers into their eyes, the oculodigital sign of Franceschetti,[16] which probably generates phosphenes. Walking with the head tilted down at an angle of 30° gives the child the best spatial information from the vestibular system's semicircular canals and should not be discouraged.[67] When the child is more confident of moving about, he will abandon this mannerism and hold his head in an upright position. Occasional walking on tiptoes supplies him with additional kinesthetic input which helps him sense where his legs are in space.[67] Swaying body movements help him evaluate spatial relations and may help to release tension. Omwake and Solnit have pointed out that children with sensory defects are more likely to develop autistic-like behavior. Some blindisms are a sign that the flooding of perceptual sensations without an appropriate visual filtering system makes it difficult for the visually deprived child to organize his input. He becomes overwhelmed and overanxious. His coping mechanism is to shut off the world around him. Many blind children lie motionless on the floor for a few minutes when they are overwhelmed by perceptual sensations such as noise bombardment.[68] They should be left alone until they recuperate from this momentary emotional trauma. On the other hand, excessive amounts of this autistic-like behavior might interfere with their learning process, and they may need psychiatric intervention. In contrast to true autism, this behavior responds well to treatment when caught early.

ROLE OF THE OPHTHALMOLOGIST

The ophthalmologist has a great impact upon the family. In fathers' and mothers' meetings, it has been expressed again and again that especially after they have learned the diagnosis of blindness, their primary focus is on the ophthalmologist. Some of the families have very positive and some very ambivalent or negative feelings. Many times, parents misinterpret the ophthalmologist's recognition of his inability to change the diagnosis of blindness as hostility or insensitivity when, in fact, parents are not aware of how difficult and painful it is to share this devastating diagnosis with the family. Many anxieties could be relieved if the door is opened for the parents to share their feelings and to have a chance to ask questions before they leave the office.

However, our experience is that the shock is so great once the parents hear that their child is blind, that they cannot absorb any explanations offered by the ophthalmologist and later on remember only the cold facts and deny they were given any specific details. A second appointment should be made at a later date to give the parents a chance to ask questions that have arisen in the intervening period. Suggestions on management of RP can be found in Chapter 6.

It is our hope that the issues raised in this section will help parents and professionals who work with blind infants to recognize the importance of early intervention so that blind children will be able to live independent, useful lives.

RESOURCES

(Further listing of other RP resources are at the end of Chapter 6.)

National Association for Parents of the Visually
    Impaired, Inc.
PO Box 180806
Austin, Texas 78718
(512) 459-6651 (Chapters in some states)

Correspondence Course for Parents of Blind or
    Partially Sighted Pre-school Children

Blind Children's Center
PO Box 21959
4120 Marathon St.
Los Angeles, CA 90029-0159
(213) 664-2153

Directors of Agencies for the Blind in the British
  Isles and Overseas
Royal National Institute for the Blind

224 Great Portland Street
London, WIN 6AA, England

Director of Agencies Serving the Visually Handicapped in the U.S.
American Foundation for the Blind
111 E. 59th
New York, NY 10022

REFERENCES

1. Alström CH, Olson O: Heredo-retinopathia congenitalis monohybrida recessiva autosomalis. Hereditas 43:1–178, 1957
2. Schappert-Kimmijser J, Henkes HE, van den Bosch J: Amaurosiscongenita (Leber). Arch Ophthalmol 61:211–218, l959
3. Leber T: Ueber Retinitis pigmentosa and angeborene Amaurose. Albrecht von Graefes Arch Ophthalmol 15:1–25, l869
4. Leber T: Ueber anomale Formen der Retinitis pigmentosa. Albrecht von Graefes Arch Ophthalmol 17:314–340, 1871
5. Franceschetti A, Dieterle P, Schwartz A: Retinitepigmentaire a virus: relation entre tableau clinique etelectroretinogramme (ERG). Ophthalmologica 135:545–554, 1958
6. Deutman AF: "Rod-cone dystrophy." In Archer D (ed): Krill's Hereditary Retinal and Choroidal Diseases, vol 2, Clinical Characteristics, pp 552–576. Hagerstown, Harper & Row, 1977
7. Waardenburg PJ: Does agenesis or dysgenesis neuro-epithelialis retinae, whether or not related to keratoglobus, exist? Ophthalmologica 113:454–461, 1957
8. Franceschetti A, François J, Babel J: Autosomal chorioretinal heredodegenerations with tapetoretinal predominance. In Chorioretinal Heredodegenerations, pp 305–325. Springfield, IL, Charles C Thomas, 1974
9. Foxman SG, Wirtschater JD, Letson RD: Leber's congenital amaurosis and high hyperopia: A discrete entity. In Henkind P (ed): Acta XXIV. International Congress of Ophthalmology, pp 55–58. Philadelphia, JB Lippincott, 1983
10. Rajacich GM, Wreagh P, Solish AM et al: The usefulness of refractive error in diagnosing RP subtypes. Invest Ophthalmol 24(suppl):294, 1983
11. Foxman SG, Heckenlively JR, Bateman JB et al: A classification of congenital and early-onset retinitis pigmentosa. Arch Ophthalmol 108:1502–1506, 1985
12. Leber T: Die Amaurose durch Tapetoretinal-degeneration. In Graefe-Saemish Handbuch der gesamten Augenheilkunde. II Aufl., Bd. 7, Teil 2, Kap. l0A. Die Krankheitem der Netzhaut, pp 1025–1035. Leipzig, Engelmann, 1916
13. Flynn JT, Cullen RF: Disc oedema in congenital amaurosis of Leber. Br J Ophthalmol 59:497–502, 1975
14. Chew E, Deutman A, Pinckers A et al: Yellowish flecks in Leber's congenital amaurosis. Br J Ophthalmol 68:727–731, l984
15. Ellis DS, Heckenlively JR, Martin CL et al: Leber's congenital amaurosis associated with familial juvenile nephronophthisis and cone-shaped epiphyses of the hands (The Saldino-Mainzer syndrome). Am J Ophthalmol 97:233–239, 1984
16. Franceschetti A: Rubeola pendant la grossesse et cataracte congenitale chez l'enfant, accompagnee du phenomene digito-oculaire. Ophthalmologica 114:332–339, 1947
17. Freedman J, Gombos GM: Bilateral macular coloboma, keratoconus and retinitis pigmentosa. Ann Ophthalmol 3:664–668, 1971
18. Godel V, Blumenthal M, Iaina A: Congenital Leber amaurosis, keratoconus, and mental retardation in familial juvenile nephronophthisis. J Pediatr Ophthalmol Strabismus 15:89–91, 1978
19. Karel I: Keratoconus in congenital diffuse tapetoretinal degeneration. Ophthalmologica 155:8–15, 1968
20. Karel I: Clinical picture of congenital diffuse tapetoretinal degeneration in 42 cases. Acta Universitatis Carolinae Medica [Mongr] (Prague) 15:259–335, 1969
21. Babel J: Constatations histologiques dans l'amaurose infantile de Leber et dans diverses forms d'hemeralopie. Ophthalmologica 145:399–402, 1963
22. Sorsby A, Williams CE: Retinal aplasia as a clinical entity. Br Med J 1:293–297, 1960
23. Gillespie FD: Congenital amaurosis of Leber. Am J Ophthalmol 61:374–880, 1966
24. Mizuno K, Takei Y, Sears ML et al: Leber's congenital amaurosis. Am J Ophthalmol 83:32–42, 1977
25. Phillips GJ, Griffiths DL: Macular coloboma and skeletal abnormalities. Br J Ophthalmol 53:346–349, 1969
26. Leighton DA, Harris R: Retinal aplasia in association with macular coloboma, keratoconus and cataract. Clin Genet 4:270–274, 1973
27. Margolis S, Scher BM, Carr RE: Macular colobomas in Leber's congenital amaurosis. Am J Ophthalmol 83:27–31, 1977
28. Mizuno K, Takei Y, Peterson WS et al: Leber's congenital amaurosis. Am J Ophthalmol 83:32–42, 1977
29. Noble KG, Carr RE: Leber's congenital amaurosis. Arch Ophthalmol 96:818–821, 1978
30. Dekaban AS: Hereditary syndrome of congenital retinal blindness (Leber), polycystic kidneys and maldevelopment of the brain. Am J Ophthalmol 68:1029–1037, 1969
31. Fulton AB, Hansen RM, Harris SJ. Retinal degenerations and brain abnormalities in infants and young children. Doc Ophthalmologica (in press)
32. Vaizey MJ, Sander MD, Wybar KC et al: Neurological abnormalities in congenital amaurosis of Leber. Arch Dis Child 52:399–402, 1977
33. McKusick VA, Stauffer M, Knox DL et al: Chorioretinopathy with hereditary microencephaly. Arch Ophthalmol 75:597–601, 1965
34. Dekaban AS: Mental retardation and neurologic involvement in patient with congenital retinal blindness. Dev Med Child Neurol 14:436–444, 1972

35. Hussels IE: Leber's congenital amaurosis and mental retardation. Birth Defects 7(3):198, 1971
36. Pinckers AJL: Leber's congenital amaurosis as conceived by Leber. Ophthalmologica 179:48–51, 1979
37. Senior B, Friedmann AI, Braudo JL. Juvenile familial nephropathy with tapetoretinal degeneration. A new oculorenal dystrophy. Am J Ophthalmol 52:625–633, 1961
38. Loken A, Hanssen O, Halvorsen S et al: Hereditary renal dysplasia and blindness. Acta Paediatr Scand 50:177–184, 1961
39. Polak CB, van Lith HMF, Delleman JW et al: Carrier detection in tapetoretinal degeneration in association with medullary cystic disease. Am J Ophthalmol 95:487–494, 1983
40. Mainzer F, Saldino R, Ozonoff M et al: Familial nephropathy associated with retinitis pigmentosa, cerebellar ataxia and skeletal abnormalities. Am J Med 49:556–562, 1970
41. Ellis DS, Heckenlively JR, Martin CL et al: Leber's congenital amaurosis associated with familial juvenile nephronopthisis and cone-shaped epiphyses of the hands (the Saldino-Mainzer syndrome). Am J Ophthalmol 97:233–239, 1984
42. Moore AT, Taylor DSI: A syndrome of congenital retinal dystrophy and saccade palsy—a subset of Leber's amaurosis. Br J Ophthalmol 68:421–431, 1984
43. Stanescu B, Draloands L: Cerebro-hepato-renal (Zellweger's) syndrome: Ocular involvement. Arch Ophthalmol 87:590–592, 1972
44. Haddad R, Font FL, Friendly DS: Cerebro-hepato-renal syndrome of Zellweger. Ocular histopathologic findings. Arch Ophthalmol 94:1927–1930, 1976
45. Cohen S, Brown F, Martyn L et al: Ocular histopathologic and biochemical studies of the cerebrohepatic renal syndrome (Zellweger's syndrome) and its relationship to neonatal adrenoleukodystrophy. Am J Ophthalmol 96:488–501, 1983
46. Moser AE, Singh I, Brown FR et al: The cerebrohepatorenal (Zellweger) Syndrome. Increased levels and impaired degradation of very-long-chain fatty acids and their use in prenatal diagnosis. N Engl J Med 3l0:1141–1146, 1984
46a Ek J, Kase BF, Reith A: Peroxisomal dysfunction in a boy with neurologic syptoms and amaurosis (Leber disease): Clinical and biochemical findings similar to those observed in Zellweger syndrome. J Pediatr 108:19–24, 1986
46b Goldfischer S, Collins J, Rapin I et al. Pseudo-Zellweger syndrome: Deficiencies in several peroxisomal oxidative activities. J Pediatr 108:25–32, 1986
47. Zeman W: Batten Disease: Ocular features, differential diagnosis by enzyme analysis. In Bergsma D, Bron AJ, Cotlier E (eds): The Eye and Inborn Errors of Metabolism, pp 441–453. New York, Alan R Liss, 1976
48. Feinsod M, Rowe H, Auerbach E: Changes in the electroretinogram in patients with optic nerve lesions. Doc Ophthalmologica 29:169–200, 1971
49. Greenfield PS et al: Hypoplasia of the optic nerve in association with porencephaly. J Pediatr Ophthalmol Strab 17:75–80, 1980
50. de Morsier G: Etudes sur les dysraphies cranio-encephaliques: III. Agenesie du septum lucidum avec malformation du tractus optique: La dysplasie septooptique. Schweiz Arch Neurol Psychiatr 77:267–692, 1956
51. François J, de Rouck A: Degenerescence tapeto-rietienne congenitale de Leber. 18 Cong Ass Pediat Langue Fr. Geneva, 1961. Cited in FRanceschetti A, François J, Babel J (eds): Chorioretinol Heredodegenerations, p 316. Charles C Thomas, Springfield, IL, 1974
52. Linstone F, Heckenlively J: Autosomal dominant Leber's amaurosis congenita. Invest Ophthalmol Vis Sci 24(suppl):293, 1983
53. Nickel B, Hoyt CS: Leber's congenital amaurosis: Is mental retardation a frequent associated defect? Arch Ophthalmol 100:1089-1092, 1982
54. Wills DM: Vulnerable periods in the early development of blind children. Psychoanal Study Child 25:461–479, 1970
55. Burlingham D: Some notes on the development of the blind. Psychoanal Study Child 16:121–145, 1961
56. Fraiberg S, Freedman DA: Studies in the ego development of the congenitally blind infant. Psychoanal Study Child 19:113–169, 1966
57. Fraiberg S, Smith M, Adelson E: An educational program for blind infants. J Special Ed 3:121–139, 1969
58. Lairy GC, Harrison-Covello A: The blind child and his parents: Congenital visual defect and the repercussion of family attitudes on the early development of the child. Res Bull Am Found Blind no. 25, 1973
59 Williams CE: Psychiatric implications of severe visual defect for the child and for the parents. Clin Dev Med 32:110–118, 1969
60. Parmelee AH, Cutsforth MG, Jackson CL. Mental development of children with blindness due to retrolental fibroplasia. Am J Dis Child 96:641–654, 1958
61. Sonksen PM, Levitt S, Kitzinger M: Identification of constraints acting on motor development in young visually disabled children and principles of remediation. Child Care Health Dev 10:273–286, 1984
62. Sandler AM, Wills DM: Preliminary notes on play and mastery in the blind child. J Child Psychotherapy 3:7–19, 1965
63. Kastein S, Spaulding J, Scharf B: Raising the Young Blind Child. New York, Human Science Press, 1980
64. Cutsforth TD: The blind in school and society, a psychological study. New York, American Foundation for the Blind, 1951
65. Omwake EB, Solnit AJ: "It isn't fair, the treatment of a blind child." Psychoanal Study Child 16:352–404, 1961
66. Gesell A, Amatruda C: Developmental Diagnosis. Boston, Hoeber, 1974
67. Parmelee AH: Personal communication
68. Als H, Tronick E, Braselton TB: Affective reciprocity and the development of autonomy, the study of a blind infant. J Am Acad Child Psychiatry 19:22–40, 1980

8

Autosomal Dominant Retinitis Pigmentosa

JOHN R. HECKENLIVELY

There are at least five forms of autosomal dominant retinitis pigmentosa (ADRP); these include autosomal dominant rod-cone degeneration, cone-rod degeneration, sector RP, and two rare forms, one with a congenital onset, and retinitis punctata albescens, both of which are usually inherited in an autosomal recessive fashion. *All forms are identified by establishing a dominant inheritance pattern and noting the characteristic clinical or electrophysiologic finding which identifies the type of RP.*

Autosomal dominant inheritance is established by taking a detailed family history and carefully noting who in the pedigree is affected or not affected. An unequivocal pattern of autosomal dominant inheritance occurs when there are three generations of affected individuals in which there is male-to-male transmission of the disease and no unaffected individual had any children with the disease. Most dominant RP patients seldom present with this ideal picture, and factors such as nonpenetrance of the gene or a lack of knowledge about prior generations such that only two generations are known to have the disease must be analyzed by the clinician. In these less than certain cases, the patient and his family must be told that from the available evidence it is likely but not confirmed that they have autosomal dominant disease. Frequently, a referral to a genetic counselor can clarify these complicated issues.

The rod-cone and cone-rod electroretinographic (ERG) patterns are established by comparing the cone and rod components of the ERG or using psychophysical testing; these are discussed extensively in Chapter 2. Sector RP and retinitis punctata albescens have distinctive fundus patterns which can be seen on indirect ophthalmoscopy. Retinitis punctata albescens, usually seen as an autosomal recessive disease, is extremely rare in autosomal dominant form, with only two examples in the literature.[1,2] There is also a rare autosomal dominant form of congenital RP which is discussed at the end of this chapter.

PREVALENCE OF AUTOSOMAL DOMINANT RP

In various surveys of the genetic types of RP, the prevalence of ADRP has ranged from 9% in Switzerland to 39% in England with a 10.1% prevalence estimated for the United States[3] (see Table 2-5). No attempt was made in these genetic studies to further characterize the type of RP (within inheritance pattern), which is true of most articles until the last several years. Because most of the available literature covers ADRP as a whole (generally lumping rod-cone, cone-rod, and other dominant RP degenerations), summary data on dominant RP will be reviewed in this first section.

VISUAL ACUITY AND MACULAR STATUS

Several studies of visual acuity in RP patients have suggested that dominant patients may have a slower loss at a later age than autosomal and X-linked recessive RP patients.[4,5] Fishman's data on RP visual acuities show that the mean for his dominant group was 20/30 compared with a range of 20/70 to 20/100 for the autosomal and X-linked recessive RP patients.[6] In his thesis on RP, Pruett noted that 58% of his ADRP patients had 20/100 vision or better. Interestingly, he also evaluated the macular status, and 80% of 50 eyes had striate, cystic bull's-eye or atrophic maculopathy.[7] In Fishman's study of macular lesions in 110 RP patients of all types, 7 of 47 patients with atrophic and 2 of 22 with cystic-appearing foveal lesions had ADRP.[8]

Most studies of visual functioning in dominant RP have been performed, of necessity, in large groups of unrelated patients, such that it can *only be assumed* that they all have the same genetic defect. Visual acuity was studied in autosomal dominant and recessive RP occurring in Navajo, presumably a relatively closed gene pool. The dominant Navajo RP group had onset of visual acuity loss significantly later than the autosomal recessive group, but once visual loss started, both RP groups had the same deterioration rate.[9]

ERG STUDIES

Various authors have reported ERG findings in ADRP; Arden and associates performed extensive testing in 57 cases.[10] In 36 of the 57 cases, called group A, only cone waves were evoked (rod-cone degeneration pattern). Static scotopic perimetry demonstrated cone-mediated function in 16 of the 36, while 20 of the 36 patients had some residual rod function. In the remaining 21 patients, called group B, rod ERGs were found and rod function was confirmed with scotopic perimetry. While the mean age of patients was the same between groups A and B, the visual fields were found to be larger in group B.

Berson and colleagues evaluated the ERG over a 3-year period in 18 patients with dominant RP. In the first year, five patients showed worse ERGs, and one had a better ERG. By the third year, no patient had a better ERG, and eight patients were worse.[11]

Berson noted that patients from autosomal dominant pedigrees with incomplete penetrance demonstrate b-wave implicit times that are delayed, although other investigators have noted that increased implicit times are generally found in more advanced disease of all hereditary types.[12]

Investigations in early dominant RP have found that rod ERG responses have reduced amplitudes and delayed implicit times while the cone ERG is normal.[13] Berson and Goldstein evaluated the recovery of early receptor potential in several families with dominant RP and found that they had faster-than-normal recovery time.[14] They hypothesized that the lack of rod function in these patients may have influenced the cones to recover more quickly compared with normal.

AUTOSOMAL DOMINANT RP WITH REDUCED PENETRANCE

While the majority of dominant RP families will demonstrate the typical pattern of inheritance, with each generation being affected and affected individuals on the average having about 50% affected children, a few pedigrees clearly show individuals who should have been affected but whom the disease skipped. Such an example is drawn in Figure 2-9. The occurrence of incomplete penetrance can play havoc with genetic counseling, since it may be assumed that an individual who is without clinical findings and presents for genetic counseling (1) does not have the disease and thus will not pass it on or (2) is from an autosomal recessive pedigree and thus would have little risk of giving the disease to his children. However, the risk to offspring is almost 50% from an individual with ADRP with reduced penetrance.

Individuals demonstrating incomplete penetrance clearly carry the RP gene, but for unknown reasons they do not express the disease. We examined one individual who was 90 years old and the patriach of a large ADRP family but who was stated to be free of the disease. On indirect ophthalmoscopy he clearly had bone spicule pigmentation in the equator and anterior retina, but still had good preservation of central retina. In his case, late expression was occurring, but the natural course of the incompletely penetrant state still must be worked out. In contrast to this example, we have examined several nonpenetrant individuals at UCLA whose ages were over 50 years who had no clinical, psychophysical, or ERG evidence of RP. Clearly, there is variability, and both normal and abnormal ERGs have been reported in incompletely penetrant individuals.[15]

PSYCHOPHYSICAL STUDIES

Massof and Finkelstein performed pioneering studies of ADRP using perimetric measures of rod and cone sensitivity. They defined two types of dominant RP, type I in which patients experience an early diffuse loss of rod sensitivity with a childhood onset of night blindness, with a later loss of cone sensitivity, and type II characterized by a regionalized and combined loss of rod and cone sensitivity with adult onset of night blindness.[16] Of the 25 patients they tested, only 10 had recordable ERGs. They analyzed the relative amplitudes using a photopic (cone) to rod (scotopic) ratio. A value less than 1.0 indicated a greater photopic loss and values larger than 1.0 a greater scotopic loss. Type I patients had ratios of 2:3, while type II patients had ratios ranging from 0.8:1.7. Four of the type II patients had ratios very close to 1, suggesting equal loss of rod and cone function. While the authors did not use the ERG terminology of "rod-cone" and "cone-rod," these results are strikingly similar to studies at UCLA in which patients with the rod-cone ERG patterns are found to have elevated final rod thresholds, while RP patients with cone-rod patterns of loss typically have final rod thresholds 2.4 log units elevated or better. Since their test techniques were not the same, however, a direct correlation of material is not possible.

Massof and Finkelstein also found clinical differences; type I patients reported childhood (<9 years) onset of night blindness, while most type II patients reported adult (>18 years) onset. Type I patient visual field areas showed a sharp drop that occurred between ages 30 and 40, while type II patients appeared to have longer preservation of peripheral field. Central cone thresholds remained good for both groups.

Lyness and colleagues performed similar studies at Moorfields Eye Hospital on 104 patients with ADRP. They also found two groups of patients, which they called "D" for "diffuse" loss of rod function and "R" in which the rod loss is regional. They found regional cone loss in both groups. The scotopic ERG was absent in D patients and was recordable in most R patients.[17]

COMPOSITE PICTURE

AUTOSOMAL DOMINANT ROD-CONE DEGENERATION (ADRC)

The mean age of patients presenting at UCLA for their initial examination was 35.0 years with a mean duration of symptoms of 19.2 years. The incidence of ADRC in the UCLA RP Registry is 7.7%. Posterior subcapsular cataracts were found in 47% and marked nuclear sclerotic cataracts in 2% of ADRC patients. The cup-to-disc ratio was 0.19 and temporal optic nervehead atrophy was present in 50% of patients. The average refraction was $-1.29 + 1.02 \times 102$ with a mean visual acuity of 20/30−. Some aspect of the ERG was recordable in 11 of 31 (35%), and the final rod threshold at 40 minutes averaged 3.45 log units of elevation. The mean visual field width from fixation was 22° with the IV-4 isopter.

Macular edema (not necessarily cystoid edema) was present in 27%, macular hypofluorescence in 83%, macular window defect in 7%, paramacular window defect in 11%, parapapillary edema in 18%, vascular arcade edema in 17%, nerve fiber layer defects in 46%, and optic nervehead telangiectasia in 64%.

This composite picture, while giving an average picture of the ADRP group, does not describe the course of the disease, which is illustrated by the following case reports.

CASE REPORTS

FAMILY ADRP-1

Case 1 A 64-year-old man has been night-blind since childhood. The family pedigree **(Fig. 8-1,** individual V-1) revealed a number of affected individuals. The patient had seven children, four of which, three males and one female, are known to have RP. He first noted problems with his side vision in his twenties, and he had severe visual difficulties by age 60. On examination, his visual acuity was hand motions in each eye. He had small posterior subcapsular cataracts in each eye, which did not appear significant clinically. On indirect ophthalmoscopy, he had heavy scattered pigment deposits, optic atrophy, and areas of diffuse retinal atrophy **(Fig. 8-2A–D)**. The fluorescein angiogram demonstrated areas of retinal pigment epithelial and choriocapillaris loss **(Fig. 8-2B)**.

Case 2 The third son of case 1 **(Fig. 8-1, Vi-3)** presented at age 31 with a history of being night-blind

"all his life" and he first noted visual field loss at age 13. His visual acuity was OD 20/30+1, OS 20/50+3, and he had an exophoria of 20 prism diopters. His Goldmann visual fields were constricted to 10° to 12° with the IV-4 isopter with a temporal island at four clock hours in each eye **(Fig. 8-3)**. On biomicroscopy, he had minor posterior capsule opacities. Indirect ophthalmoscopy revealed a blond fundus with mild pigmentary deposition in the equator regions, diffuse RPE atrophy outside the posterior pole, mild optic atrophy, and retinal vessel attenuation **(Fig. 8-4A)**. The fluorescein angiogram showed diffuse RPE staining and some paramacular hyperfluorescence, but no evidence of macular edema **(Fig. 8-4B)**.

The patient returned 2 years later, and his best corrected acuity had dropped to OD 20/60-1, OS 20/70; Goldmann field was 2° with the I-4 and 8° with the IV-4 OU.

CLINICOPATHOLOGIC CORRELATION

A clinicopathologic correlation from an ADRC family **(Fig. 8-5)** is presented below in which features seen clinically in younger members of the family are contrasted with the histological changes seen in two older members of the family.[18]

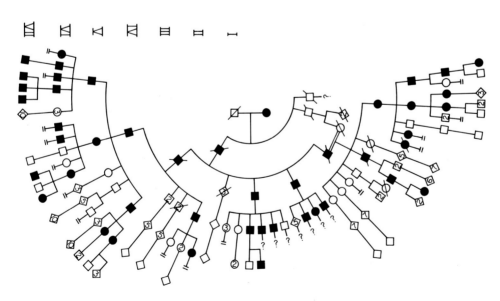

FIG. 8-1. Pedigree of ADRP-1, a large autosomal dominant family with rod–cone degeneration.

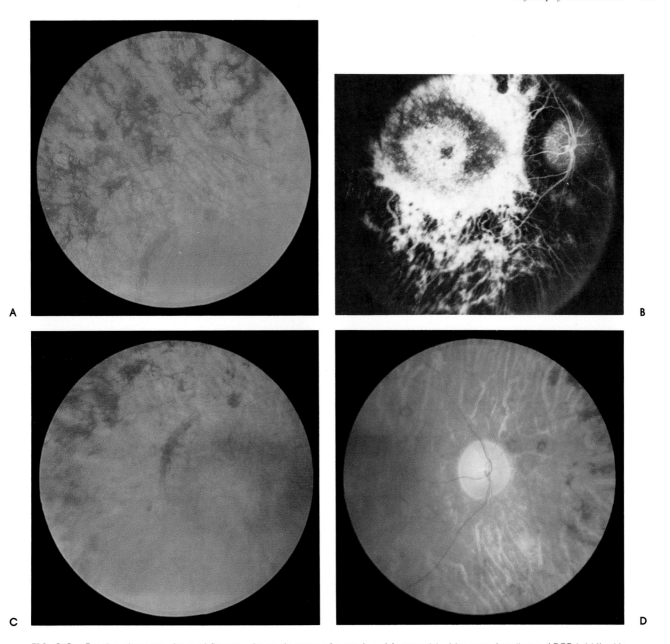

FIG. 8-2. Fundus photographs and fluorescein angiogram of case 1, a 64-year-old white man (pedigree ADRP-1, V-1) with advanced ADRP demonstrating *(A)* heavy bone spicule formation superior temporal to right macula; *(B)* fluorescein angiography demonstrates areas of loss of RPE and choriocapillaris outside of posterior pole as well as in the paramacular region, giving a partial bull's-eye appearance; RPE in macular area stains diffusely; *(C)* generalized RPE atrophy with remnant RPE in the posterior pole and macular degeneration; *(D)* optic atrophy and vessel attenuation.

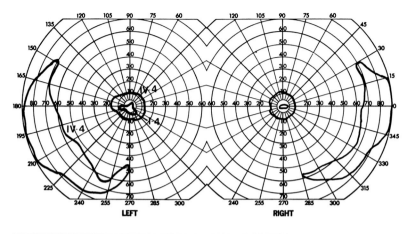

FIG. 8-3. Goldmann visual field of case 2 with moderately advanced ADRP. I-4 isopter was about 2° OD and an uneven 6° OS; IV-4 isopter demonstrates temporal islands with a 10°-to-12° field centrally.

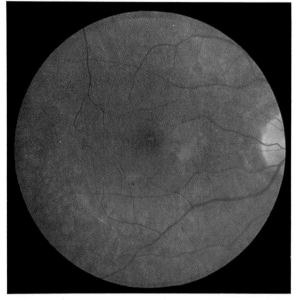

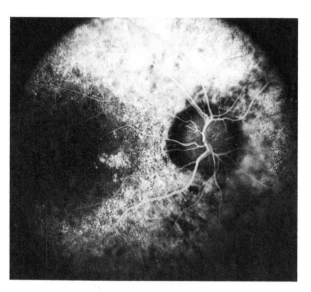

A   B

FIG. 8-4. *(A)* Fundus photograph, right eye of case 2, 31-year-old son of case 1 with moderately advanced ADRP; there is generalized RPE loss outside of the posterior pole and mild bone spicule formation in the periphery. *(B)* Fluorescein angiogram shows hypofluorescent macular RPE with diffuse staining of RPE elsewhere. Inferior to the disc are areas of missing RPE and choriocapillaris; disc telangiectasia is present.

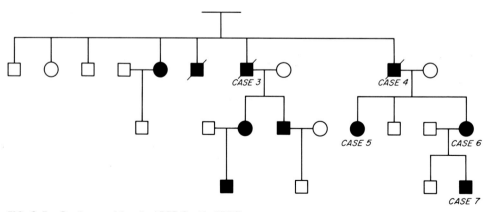

FIG. 8-5. Pedigree of family ADRP-2 with ADRC.

FAMILY ADRP-2

Case 3 A 56-year-old man **(Fig. 8-5)** developed nyctalopia and visual field loss in his midtwenties. At the time of his death in 1964 from pneumonia, he had hand motion vision. No further eye examination records were available. The eyes were obtained in the course of routine autopsy studies in March 1964.

Case 4 A 63-year-old man **(Fig. 8-5)**, brother of case 3, was first seen in 1970, 7 years prior to his death. He developed night blindness and peripheral visual field loss by age 21. Visual acuity on presentation was OD count fingers, OS 20/50. The fundi showed arteriolar attenuation and bone spicules throughout the midperiphery of each eye. The discs had waxy pallor. Visual fields were OD 2°, OS 4° with a 5-mm white target. In 1974, the visual acuity was OD count fingers, OS 20/80 with visual fields of 1° in each eye. The patient died of an acute myocardial infarction in 1977, and his eyes were donated by the family for study. The gross specimen showed areas of paving stone-like degeneration and scattered pigmented bone

spicule-like formation **(Fig. 8-6A)** while the posterior pole demonstrated atrophic macular lesions **(Fig. 8-6B&C)**.

Case 5 The 32-year-old daughter of case 4 **(Figure 8-5)** was seen in 1974 with a recent history of night blindness. Her visual acuity was OD 20/25, OS 20/20 with visual fields of OD 30°, OS 40° with I-4 isopter. Biomicroscopy was normal. The fundus showed an early pigmentary retinopathy, with tiny drusen in the posterior pole and surface wrinkling retinopathy **(Fig. 8-7A&B)**. In 1979, the visual acuity was 20/20 in each eye, and the visual fields were OD 6°, OS 10° with the I-4 isopter. The ERG demonstrated a barely recordable photopic and a nonrecordable scotopic ERG. The final rod threshold was 3.55 log units above normal.

Case 6 The 37-year-old daughter of case 4 **(Fig. 8-5)** noted night blindness in high school and visual field loss in her twenties. She was first seen in 1974, at which time her visual acuity was 20/20 in each eye. Her visual field was 9° in each eye with the I-4 isopter and 60°

FIG. 8-6. *(A)* Gross photograph, case 4, both calottes showing paving stone-like degeneration and pigmentary deposits. *(B)* Large calotte shows diffuse equator RPE atrophy and surface wrinkling of posterior pole. *(C)* Back-lighting of large calotte demonstrates macular atrophy not obvious in *B.* (Photographs courtesy of Professor Robert Foos)

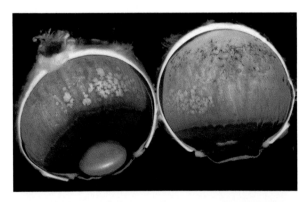

A

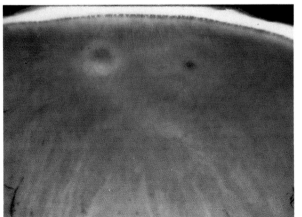

B

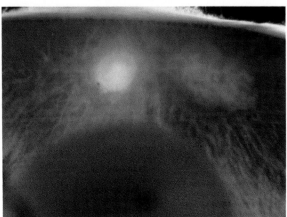

C

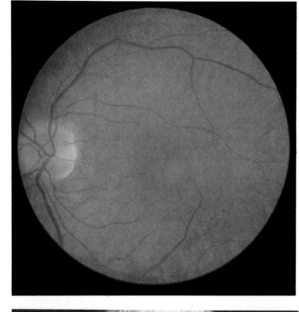

A

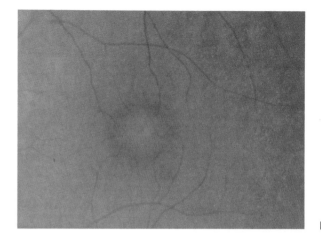

B

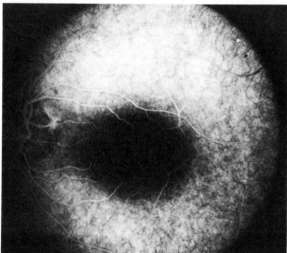

C

FIG. 8-7. *(A)* Fundus photograph, left eye, case 5, daughter of case 4, demonstrating mild vessel attenuation, a white disc rim temporally, scattered drusen, and early macular atrophy. *(B)* Magnified view of macular area shows generalized fine punctate drusen throughout posterior pole. *(C)* On fluorescein angiography, the macula is hypofluorescent with no window defects from the drusen.

with the IV-4 isopter. Funduscopy revealed a pigmentary retinopathy with bilateral bull's-eye macular lesions **(Fig. 8-8***A–C)* and tiny yellow drusen scattered throughout the posterior pole. Surface wrinkling retinopathy was also present. The ERG was nonrecordable.

In 1975, the patient attempted weight control with exogenous thyroid medication, which resulted in a precipitous loss of visual field to 3° with the I-4 isopter and 10° with the IV-4 isopter. When the exogenous thyroid medication was discontinued, the patient showed some re-expansion of field size to 20° in each eye with the IV-4 isopter. The visual acuity in 1977 was OD 20/30 and OS 20/25.

Case 7 The 15-year-old son of case 6 was noted to be clumsy and night-blind at age 11. The visual acuity was 20/25 in each eye, and the visual field was 5° in each eye with the I-4 isopter. Biomicroscopy revealed pigment flecks in the anterior vitreous space and trace posterior subcapsular cataracts. Fundus examination revealed a diffuse pigmentary retinopathy **(Fig. 8-9).**

All cases showed extensive bone-spicule formation. Case 4 had a 12-mm wide circumferential band of pigment deposition with its anterior border at the

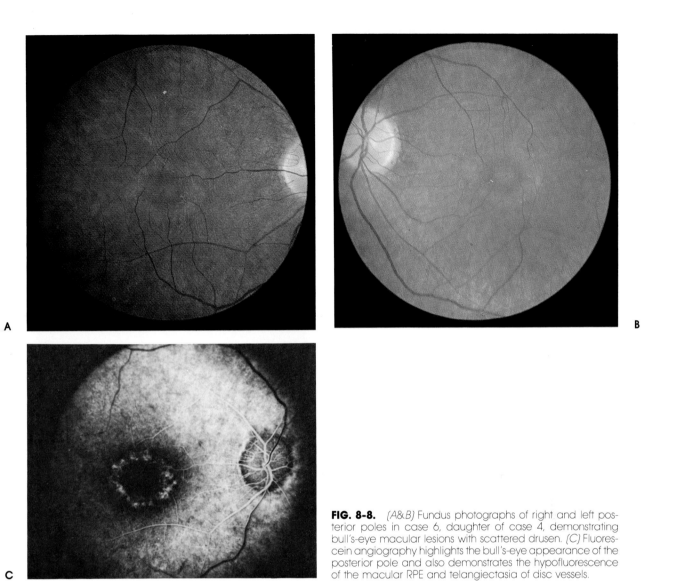

FIG. 8-8. *(A&B)* Fundus photographs of right and left posterior poles in case 6, daughter of case 4, demonstrating bull's-eye macular lesions with scattered drusen. *(C)* Fluorescein angiography highlights the bull's-eye appearance of the posterior pole and also demonstrates the hypofluorescence of the macular RPE and telangiectasia of disc vessels.

FIG. 8-9. Fundus photograph, case 7, a 15-year-old boy, showing early RPE degeneration and bone spicule formation temporal to the macular area; surface wrinkling of posterior pole inner limiting membrane is present.

TABLE 8-1

PATHOHISTOLOGIC CHANGES IN AUTOSOMAL DOMINANT RETINITIS PIGMENTOSA

STRUCTURE	BOND SPICULE AREA	INTERMEDIATE AREA	ATROPHIC AREA
Retinal vessels	Pigmented, partially sclerosed	Largely sclerosed	Sclerosed
Retinal layers	Diffusely atrophic	Diffusely atrophic	Gliotic scar
Pigment epithelium	Normal to hypopigmented	Pigmented to hyperpigmented	Absent
Pigment	RPE and vessels	In RPE cells overlying thick basal deposits	Largely absent
Basal deposits	Few	Prominent	Absent
Outer limiting membrane	Present	Present	Absent
Choriocapillaris	Intact	Intact	Attenuated

(Meyer K, Heckenlively JR, Spitznas M et al: Dominant retinitis pigmentosa: A clinicopathologic correlation. Ophthalmology 89:1418, 1982)

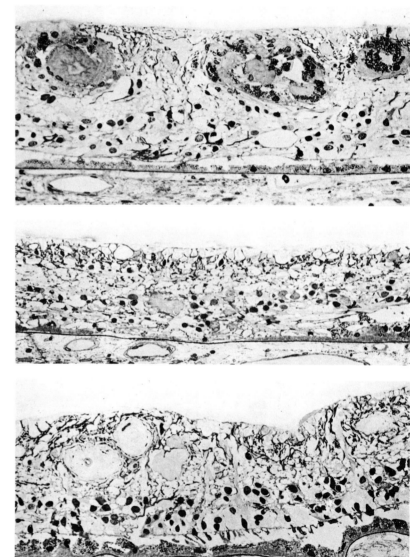

FIG. 8-10. Light micrograph, case 4: *(A)* bone spicule area, *(B)* atrophic area, *(C)* intermediate area (toluidine blue, ×450). (Meyer K, Heckenlively JR, Spitznas M et al: Dominant retinitis pigmentosa: A clinicopathologic correlation. Ophthalmology 89:1419, 1981)

equator. The pigment clumping was most dense in the superonasal quadrant of each eye, with relative sparing of the inferotemporal quadrant. Case 4 also had irregular atrophic patches resembling paving stone degeneration in the temporal preequatorial zone of each eye (**Fig. 8-6A**).

Three relatively distinct categories of histopathologic foci were identified on the basis of pigmentary, vascular and retinal changes in cases 3 and 4 (Table 8-1).

Bone spicule areas (**Figs. 8-10A** and **8-11**) were most striking for pigment accumulation in and surrounding blood vessels. Pigment was seen particularly at vascular bifurcations, and blood vessels were somewhat sclerosed. Pigment was also seen in association with the accumulations of hyalinized material that did not resemble blood vessels. The retina was diffusely atrophic with nearly total loss of the photoreceptor and nuclear layers. There was nearly normal-appearing RPE and an intact outer limiting membrane. Th RPE was moderately hypopigmented, particularly in areas subjacent to dense pigmentary accumulations. The choriocapillaris was intact.

Atrophic areas (**Fig. 8-10B**) showed full-thickness retinal scars. The choriocapillaris, RPE, outer limiting membrane, and retinal layers were involved in a gliotic scar. The retinal vessels were largely occluded and had little or no associated pigment.

Intermediate areas (**Fig. 8-10C**) showed severely hyalinized vessels with little pigmentary accumulation. These areas were similar to atrophic areas, but lacked the full-thickness gliotic scar and had more pigment in the RPE than occurred in bone spicule areas. Basal deposits, amorphous, mineralized, granular material located between the basal infoldings of the RPE cell and its basal lamina, were most prominent in the intermediate area and were found in case 2 on electron microscopy (**Fig. 8-12**).

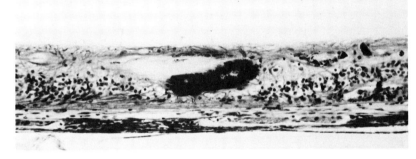

FIG. 8-11. Light micrograph, case 3. Retina at temporal equator of left eye shows heavy pigmentary deposition at a vascular bifurcation (hematoxylin-eosin, × 312). (Meyer K, Heckenlively JR, Spitznas M et al: Dominant retinitis pigmentosa: A clinicopathologic correlation. Ophthalmology 89:1420, 1981)

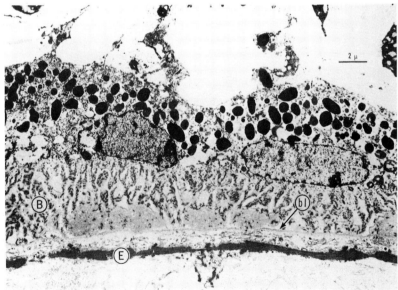

FIG. 8-12. Electron micrograph, case 4. Chorioretinal juncture, 3 mm behind the temporal ora serrata. Membranes of the RPE are poorly preserved (formalin fixation). Basal deposits *(B)* between the basal infoldings of the RPE and above its basal lamina *(arrow)*. Inner collagenous layer of Bruch's membrane, above the elastic layer *(E)* is slightly thickened (× 6000). (Meyer K, Heckenlively JR, Spitznas M et al: Dominant retinitis pigmentosa: A clinicopathologic correlation. Ophthalmology 89:1421, 1981)

All patients examined in this family demonstrated degenerative deposits beneath the retina. The cases examined clinically (5–7) showed small, yellowish subretinal dots resembling tiny drusen (**Fig. 8-7***B*). Histologically, the presence of confluent and placoid drusen was confirmed in cases 3 and 4 (**Fig. 8-13**).

Surface wrinkling was found both clinically and histologically (**Fig. 8-14**) and is a common feature in RP patients in general. Hansen and colleagues found preretinal membranes in all 10 RP sets of eyes which they examined.[19] This contrasts with a 6.4% normal incidence of surface wrinkling in an autopsy population.[20]

Pallor of the disc was noted in case 2 clinically, and both cases 1 and 2 showed optic atrophy histologically. Perhaps more striking was the extensive gliosis of the optic nervehead (**Fig 8-15**). This gliosis, which is commonly found in RP patients, may help explain why they have smaller cup-to-disc ratios than normal.

Three of the five cases (3, 4, and 6) demonstrated circumscribed atrophic lesions centered at the fovea. Clinically, a narrow ring of RPE atrophy was seen surrounding the fovea in case 6 (**Fig. 8-8***A&B*). Fluorescein angiography showed a window defect corresponding to the area of atrophy (**Fig. 8-8***C*). Histologically, the atrophic lesion consisted of an abrupt loss of the RPE, with attenuation of the choriocapillaris (**Fig. 8-16**); there was an island of central sparing within the foveal lesion in case 4 similar to that seen in case 6 clinically.

AUTOSOMAL DOMINANT CONE-ROD DEGENERATION

Cone-rod dysfunction is an electroretinographic term that has been useful in describing a degenerative pattern occurring in subgroups of RP patients who generally have late-onset night blindness, less pigment deposition, better preserved visual fields, and more recordable ERGs than rod-cone degeneration patients.[21]

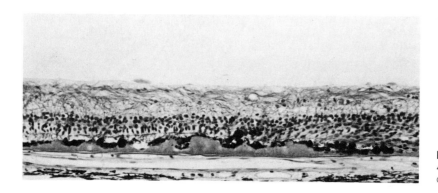

FIG. 8-13. Light micrograph, case 4. Temporal retina showing confluent drusen (hematoxylin-eosin, × 312).

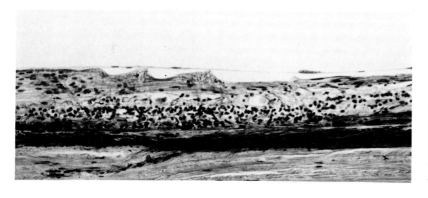

FIG. 8-14. Light micrograph, case 3. Nasal, parapapillary retina showing surface wrinkling of retina, single-layered epiretinal membrane drawing the inner retinal layers into crests with intervening troughs (hematoxylin-eosin, × 312).

Since autosomal dominant cone dystrophies may also have some rod dysfunction on ERG testing, it is important to establish whether the patient in question has a progressive pathologic process which is primarily like RP or a process similar to a cone dystrophy. There are many reports about cone-rod dystrophy, progressive cone-rod degeneration, progressive cone dystrophy, and so forth in the literature which actually discuss processes quite different from RP.

The easiest way to determine whether a patient with a cone-rod ERG degeneration pattern has RP or an RP-like process is to evaluate and follow the patient with serial visual fields; in many cases the diagnosis is obvious from the initial Goldmann field test. In most cone dystrophies, the peripheral visual field remains relatively stable and full, although central scotomata may be noted, while in the RP types, there is progressive peripheral visual field loss with ring scotomata (see Chapter 3). Both cone dystrophies and cone-rod degenerations may have a number of findings in common, so serial visual fields are very important for distinguishing these two entities; bull's-eye or atrophic macular lesions, peripheral

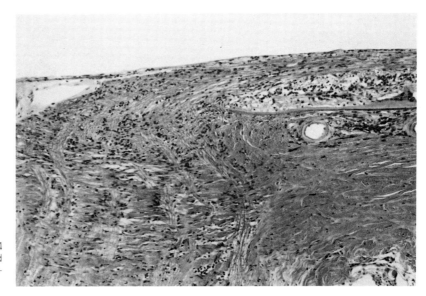

FIG. 8-15. Light micrograph, case 4 of ADRC. Temporal optic nervehead showing glial hyperplasia (hematoxylin-eosin, ×155).

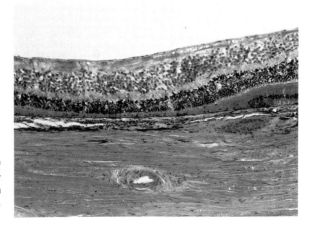

FIG. 8-16. Light micrograph, case 3 of ADRC. Macula of right eye showing abrupt loss of RPE, receptor cells, and outer limiting membrane with attenuation of choriocapillaris in atrophic area seen grossly (see Fig. 8-6B, hematoxylin-eosin, ×155).

pigmentary changes, and relatively good final rod thresholds may be seen both in cone dystrophy and cone-rod degeneration.

Occasionally, the picture is further confused by rare patients who demonstrate a type of "inverse" RP. While this term has been used in the literature for RP patients who have focal pigmentary or atrophic changes in the macular area, more commonly it refers to patients who have cone-rod degenerative patterns on the ERG and who may have bull's-eye or atrophic macular lesions with central scotomata which slowly enlarge.

COMPOSITE PICTURE

AD CONE-ROD DEGENERATION—RP TYPE

The average age of onset of symptoms was 22.2 years, with a mean duration of symptoms on the first visit of 10.5 years. Autosomal dominant cone-rod degeneration was found in 34 (5.6%) of 609 patients examined. The average refraction was $-4.13 +1.20 \times 79$ with a mean visual acuity of 20/40. The ERG was recordable in 6 of 11 patients, with an average final rod threshold of 1.25 log units of elevation in patients with recordable ERGs and 2.08 log units when non-

recordable. The cup-to-disc ratio was 0.24, and optic nervehead telangiectasia was present in 90%. Macular edema was present in 10%, macular hypofluorescence in 80%, macular window defect in 20%, paramacular window defect in 0%, and parapapillary edema in 10%.

One characteristic feature that separates the rod-cone degeneration patients from the cone-rod RP patients is that the latter are not night-blind until advanced stages of the disease; temporal optic atrophy, telangiectasia of the nervehead, and less pigmentary disruption of the retina are also commonly seen in this group as a whole. These features are well illustrated by the following pedigree (**Fig. 8-17**; Tables 8-2 and 8-3).

FAMILY ADRP-3[22]

Case 8 The propositus is a 55 year-old white man who was told of retinal abnormalities during an army physical examination at age 18, when he was diagnosed as having RP. The family history revealed three affected generations with four of seven children and two grandchildren with visual abnormalities **(Fig. 8-17).** The patient related that his visual acuity at the

---

TABLE 8-2

CLINICAL CHARACTERISTICS, DOMINANT CONE-ROD DEGENERATION

PATIENT	AGE	EYE	VISUAL ACUITY	GOLDMANN VISUAL FIELD (1–4)	COLOR VISION FARNSWORTH* ERROR SCORE/AXIS	FINAL ROD THRESHOLD (LOG UNITS)
Case 8	55	OD	10/200	barely detects	—	4.30
		OS	10/200	target centrally	—	
Case 9	33	OD	20/30	30°	214 early	0.20
		OS	20/30	15°	208 tritan	
Case 10	16	OD	20/30	15°	67 low dis	1.30
		OS	20/30	6°	149 crimination	
Case 11	8	OD	20/50	5°	not done	3.40
		OS	20/60	3°		

* Nagel Anomaloscope was normal in cases 2, 4, 5.
(Meyer K, Heckenlively JR, Spitznas M et al: Dominant retinitis pigmentosa: A clinicopathologic correlation. Ophthalmology 89:1418, 1982)

TABLE 8-3

ELECTROPHYSIOLOGICAL DATA, DOMINANT CONE-ROD DEGENERATION FAMILY

| PATIENT | EYE | ELECTRORETINOGRAM | | SAMP | SBIT | ELECTROOCULOGRAM DARK/LIGHT RATIO |
		Pamp	PBIT			
Case 8	OD	non-recordable				not done
	OS	non-recordable				
Case 9	OD	50 uv	36 ms	100 uv	60 ms	156%
	OS	20 uv	36 ms	70 uv	60 ms	148%
Case 10	OD	non-recordable				122%
	OS	non-recordable				135%
Case 11	OD	non-recordable				not done
	OS	non-recordable				

Pamp = photopic b-wave amplitude; PBIT = photopic b-wave implicit time; Samp = scotopic b-wave amplitude; SBIT = scotopic b-wave implicit time.

(Doc Ophthalmol Proc Ser 27:187, 1981)

time of diagnosis was 20/40. Severe visual problems were noted by age 35, and at age 43 he had bilateral cataracts removed.

Slit lamp and external examination were unremarkable with the exception of pigmented specks in the anterior vitreous space. Fundus examination revealed a pale optic nerve with flattening and atrophy of the temporal side of the disc **(Fig. 8-18***A&B***).** There were large areas of RPE loss, and the choroidal vessels were yellowish and appeared underperfused **(Fig.**

8-18*C***).** The retinal vessels were attenuated. Fluorescein angiography **(Fig. 8-18***D***)** demonstrated peripapillary loss of the RPE and choriocapillaris, with larger choroidal vessels remaining patent. There were multiple telangiectatic surface disc vessels temporally, some of which showed persistent fluorescence on late frames.

Case 9 The 33-year-old daughter of case 8 noticed some mild night blindness but reported no severe

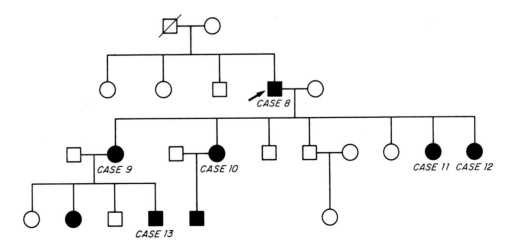

FIG. 8-17. Pedigree of ADRP-3, a three-generation family with autosomal dominant cone-rod degeneration.

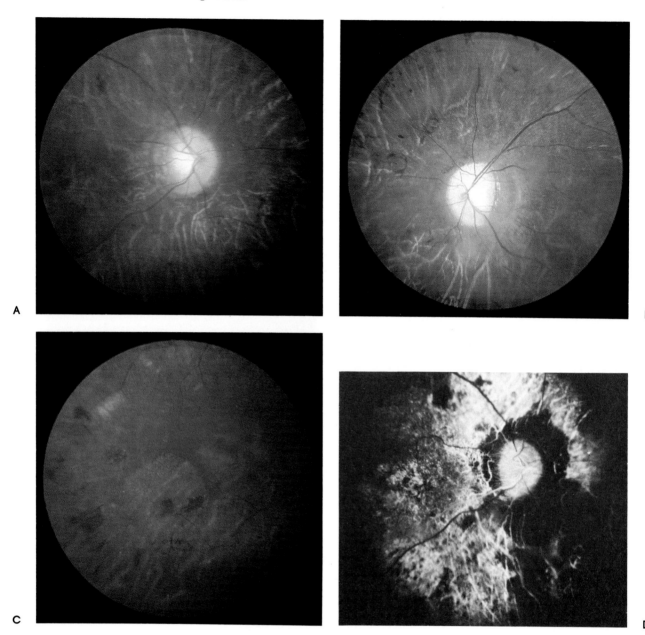

FIG. 8-18.   Case 8 with advanced autosomal dominant cone-rod degeneration demonstrating in the *(A)* right and *(B)* left eyes temporal flattening and atrophy of the disc, hypopigmentation and diffuse loss of RPE, pigmented deposits, and scattered white, elongated lesions of the nerve fiber layer; *(C)* posterior pole right, eye with atrophic macular changes with round pigmented lesions at the level of RPE and white lesions of the nerve fiber layer; *(D)* fluorescein angiogram showing patchy loss and granularity of RPE and choriocapillaris, disc temporal atrophy and telangiectasia, and macular degeneration.

problems functionally. Her medical history was negative. Biomicroscopy showed fine white deposits in the fetal nucleus. Fundus examination was remarkable for severe temporal disc tissue loss, with swelling of the nerve fiber layer overlying the disc **(Fig. 8-19**A**)**. Peripapillary atrophy was present, and on the nasal side of the disc the RPE was yellowish tan, giving a partial halo effect to the disc. The overall appearance of the fundus was a tigroid pattern from hypopigmentation of the RPE. Retinal vessels were not significantly attenuated. Fluorescein angiography

demonstrated severe temporal disc atrophy with telangiectasia **(Fig. 8-19**B**)**. Visual field and ERG test results were consistent with the diagnosis of RP (Tables 8-2 & 8-3).

Case 10 The 16-year-old daughter of the propositus (case 8) first noted visual field problems at age 12 and had no night vision problems. External and slit lamp examination were unremarkable. Indirect ophthalmoscopy revealed a tigroid blond fundus and a pink optic nerve which had severe temporal loss of

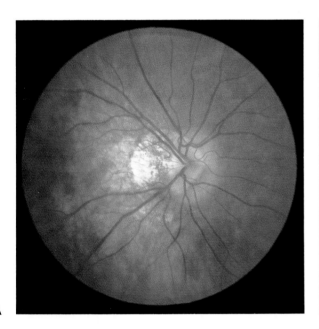

A

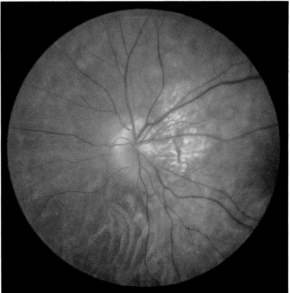

B

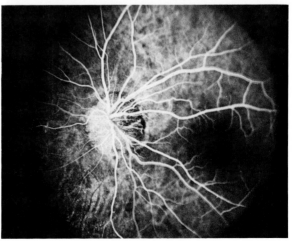

C

FIG. 8-19. Case 9, a 33-year-old woman with autosomal dominant cone-rod degeneration, with *(A)* generalized hypopigmented RPE, attenuation of vessels, hypoplastic disc with surrounding halo of peripapillary depigmented RPE in right eye, *(B)* severe temporal disc atrophy and disc swelling and telangiectasia in left eye. Peripheral retina was hypopigmented and had no pigmentary deposits in both eyes. *(C)* fluorescein angiography demonstrating disc telangiectasia and temporal atrophy, and generalized hypopigmented nature of RPE.

tissue **(Fig. 8-20**A**)**. The nerve fiber layer overlying the disc margin adjacent to the area of missing disc tissue was swollen. Fluorescein angiography demonstrated missing temporal disc tissue as well as telangiectasia of the disc vessels **(Fig. 8-20**B**)**. The patient's clinical and electrophysiologic test results are presented in Tables 8-2 and 8-3.

Case 11 The 8-year-old grandson of the propositus and son of case 9 is symptomatic from peripheral vision loss, often bumping into objects, and he also has mild difficulty in reading. His best corrected visual acuity was OD 20/50, OS 20/60. Slit lamp examination revealed fine deposits in the fetal nucleus of both eyes. Ophthalmoscopy demonstrated a tigroid fundus. The optic nerve was pink with flattening of the temporal side of the disc, and the nerve fiber layer was indistinct inferonasally **(Fig. 8-21)**. Disc telangiectasia was seen in both eyes.

FAMILY ADRP-4

Case 12 A 52-year-old woman noted visual acuity loss at age 45 and retrospectively feels that she had

visual field problems even as a child. The patient's mother had visual difficulties and never drove a car, and by history probably had the same problem. One of the patient's two daughters is affected (case 13 below). The medical history was noncontributory.

The visual acuity was 20/25 − in both eyes, and biomicroscopy revealed small posterior subcapsular opacities but no evidence of pigmented flecks in the anterior vitreous space. On funduscopy, the patient showed a blond fundus with minimal pigmentary changes in the equator region, some optic atrophy, moderate vessel attenuation, and telangiectasia of the temporal optic nervehead **(Fig. 8-22**A**)**. Fluorescein angiography highlighted the disc telangiectasia, with late frames showing leakage and staining over the telangiectatic areas **(Fig. 8-22**B**)**.

The ERG was nonrecordable, and the final rod threshold at 40 minutes was 2.7 log units elevated above normal. Goldmann visual field tests demonstrated baring of the blind spot and constriction **(Fig. 8-23**A**)**. The diagnosis of autosomal dominant cone-rod degeneration was made on the basis of three generations of affected individuals, supported by the

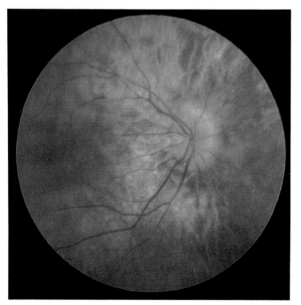

A

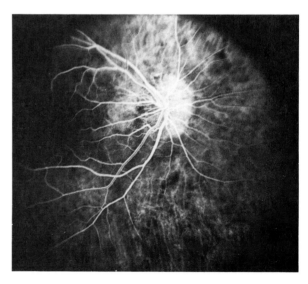

B

FIG. 8-20. Case 10, a 16-year-old woman with autosomal dominant cone-rod degeneration. *(A)* Vascular attenuation, hypopigmentation of the RPE, atrophy of temporal disc, and no pigmentary deposits were seen in the periphery (not shown). *(B)* Fluorescein angiography demonstrates disc telangiectasia and temporal atrophy or "tilted disc," and patchy loss of RPE and choriocapillaris. Nerve fiber layer swelling at disc margin was seen.

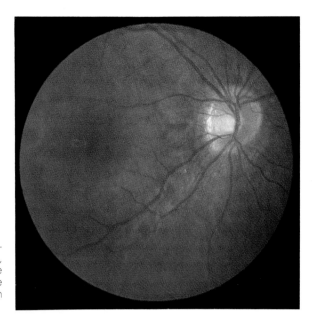

FIG. 8-21. Case 11, an 8-year-old boy with severe autosomal dominant cone-rod degeneration; fundus photograph, right eye, shows a thinning or hypopigmentation of RPE outside of posterior pole, a tilted disc or lack of temporal disc tissue and nerve fiber loss. Telangiectasia of discs was seen in both eyes. Peripheral retina showed early pigmentary deposition.

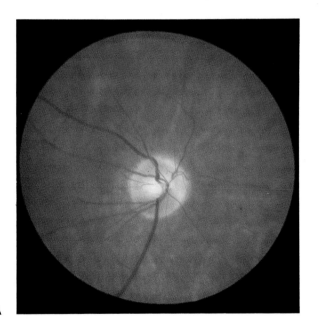

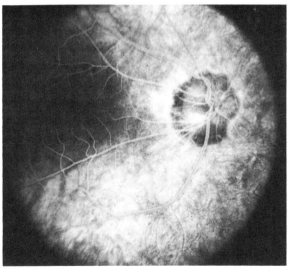

A

B

FIG. 8-22. Case 12, a 52-year-old woman with dominant cone-rod degeneration. *(A)* Fundus photograph showing mild optic nerve pallor, generalized hypopigmentation of RPE, vessel attenuation, and several scattered white lesions in the nerve fiber layer. *(B)* Fluorescein angiography demonstrates lack of pigment in the RPE outside the posterior pole and leakage of fluorescein from telangiectatic vessels on the disc.

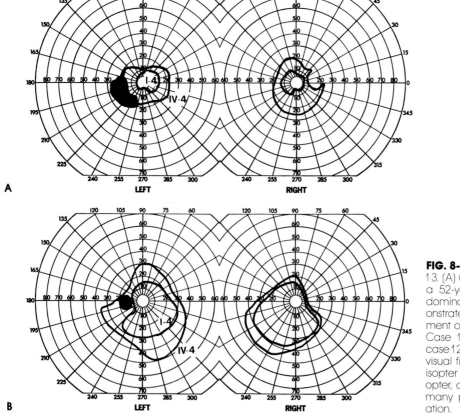

FIG. 8-23. Visual fields of cases 12 and 13. (A) Goldmann visual field of case 12, a 52-year-old woman with autosomal dominant cone-rod degeneration, demonstrated contracted fields, enlargement of the blind spot in the left eye. (B) Case 13, the 29-year-old daughter of case 12, also has moderately contracted visual fields with no temporal islands. I-4 isopter is nearly as sensitive as IV-4 isopter, a characteristic demonstrated by many patients with cone-rod degeneration.

fact that the daughter (case 13) had definite cone-rod ERG findings. However, the patient's relatively good final rod threshold in face of a small field and nonrecordable ERG and her temporal disc telangiectasia were evidence consistent with the diagnosis of cone-rod degeneration.

Case 13 The daugther of case 12 is a 29-year-old woman who had noted difficulty in entering darkened areas for at least 20 years but related no overt night blindness; she has had problems with side vision for 5 years. She reports light flashes all the time. The family history is consistent with autosomal dominant disease. Prior to the diagnosis of RP, the patient consulted several ophthalmologists who stated that she had retinal leakage OD and retinal spots not characteristic of RP.

The visual acuity was OD 20/25, OS 20/20. Biomicroscopy demonstrated clear lenses and fine pigment in the anterior vitreous space. There was a blond fundus with diffuse atrophy in equator regions but no

pigmentary deposition; vessel attenuation was apparent **(Fig. 8-24***A&B*).

On electroretinography, the scotopic amplitudes were slightly larger than the photopic (30 uV to 20uV), and the final rod threshold was within normal limits at 40 minutes. The Goldmann visual field tests showed moderately severe constriction **(Fig. 8-23***B*). Fluorescein angiography showed thinning and granularity of the RPE on early phases and marked retinal edema on late phases **(Fig. 8-24***C&D*).

There are a number of features distinguishing these patients from those with ADRC. Until advanced stages, these patients have little pigment deposition despite fairly severe disease (as evidenced by vessel attenuation or retinal atrophy in the equator and periphery and by their ERGs and visual fields).[21] These patients could thus be said to have what has been termed "retinitis pigmentosa sine pigmento," although this may not be the best term since many RP patients, including some with rod-cone degen-

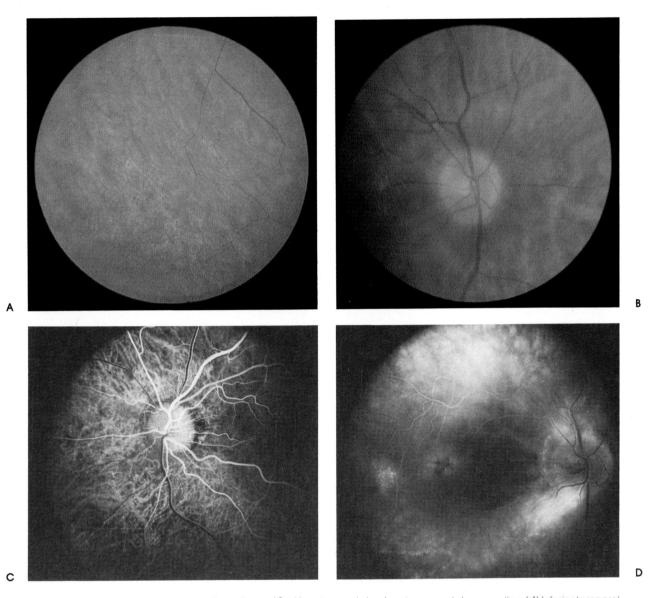

FIG. 8-24. Case 13, 29-year-old daughter of case 12 with autosomal dominant cone-rod degeneration. (*A*) Inferior temporal view of equator region demonstrates diffuse atrophy of RPE without pigment deposition. (*B*) Posterior pole shows vessel attenuation, a pink disc with small cup-to-disc ratio, and hypopigmentation of RPE. (*C*) Early phase of fluorescein angiogram shows hypopigmentation of RPE, patchy loss of choriocapillaris, and some granularity at level of RPE. (*D*) Late-phase view shows cystoid macular edema as well as diffuse edema in the vascular arcades.

eration, go through a stage in which the fundus is quite blond and there is no evidence of pigment deposition.

ADRC patients with visual fields more than 10° usually have normal or near-normal final rod thresholds which are not found in patients with ADRC who characteristically have childhood-onset night blindness. While telangiectasia is occasionally seen in ADRC, it is very common in the cone-rod degenerations as a group and was seen in all the above examples.

In contrasting members within families ADRP-2 and ADRP-3, there appears to be variable expressivity among members even though all individuals in a family can be assumed to have the same gene defect. Case 7 and case 11, many years younger than their mother and aunt, respectively (cases 6 and 5, and 9 and 10), were much more severely affected than the older generation.

SECTOR RP

In 1937, Bietti reported a case of RP in which the pigmentary retinopathy involved only the inferonasal quadrant of each eye. Since this first report a number of authors have reported this entity. While this degenerative pattern is most frequently found in the inferior nasal quadrants, the inferior temporal quadrant may also be involved. While all inheritance patterns have been noted in sector RP, the most common one is autosomal dominant.[23]

The most frequent complaint is night blindness, which may have a late onset. Visual field defects correspond to the areas of pigmentary retinopathy so that superior temporal or generalized superior defects are seen, particularly with smaller isopters. Some fields give the appearance of having a pseudoaltitudinal defect, as the superior field loss usually parallels the horizontal meridian. In prior years, a number of these patients undoubtedly had evaluations for pituitary adenoma. Omphroy reported an unusual pedigree of sector RP with chronic angle-closure glaucoma in which field defects and fluorescein angiographic changes are well documented.[24]

Some patients may have elevated final rod thresholds in areas of intact retina, while other patients may have normal final rod thresholds in uninvolved areas.[25] The visual acuity is generally normal in most patients. Most patients remain relatively stable, although progression is occasionally found, and in families the severity of the disease has been found to be age-dependent.[26]

The regionalized nature of the pigmentary retinopathy is quite striking, since there is usually a sharp demarcation line between intact RPE and inferior atrophied areas (**Fig. 8-25**). In many cases retinal vessels will suddenly attenuate as they reach the atrophied retinal areas.

Most patients have a subnormal ERG; Berson found reduced amplitudes but normal implicit times in three patients with sector RP.[27] He contrasted this finding with typical early RP in which diffuse disease resulted in delayed cone and rod implicit times.

AUTOSOMAL DOMINANT LEBER'S AMAUROSIS CONGENITA

Dominant Leber's amaurosis congenita is rarely mentioned in the literature; Sorsby reported one pedigree[28] and François had three pedigrees[29] which

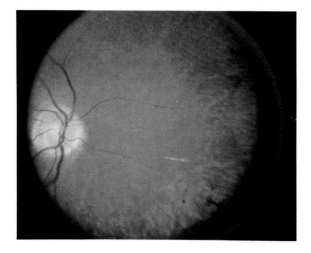

FIG. 8-25. Sector RP. Fundus photograph, left eye, a 49-year-old woman with autosomal dominant sector RP showing demarcation between abnormal- and normal- appearing RPE in the nasal equator region.

he stated had clinical manifestations similar to those of the typical autosomal recessive form.

At UCLA we have seen one six-generation pedigree, ADRP-5 (**Fig. 8-26;** Table 8-4) in which the family experiences a severe progressive retinal degeneration that begins in infancy. Some patients develop a roving nystagmus before the first year of life with severe vision loss, while others have a mild nystagmus and visual field loss similar to early-onset RP. All members have progressed to light-perception level of vision by age 30. Four generations (severely affected patients) have attended state schools for the blind from first or second grade because of severe visual impairment. The macular bull's-eye lesions (**Fig. 8-27A&B**) along with the better than usual final rod threshold in case 1 suggest that this family may have some type of aggressive cone-rod dystrophy. Whether this is the same entity reported by François and Sorbsy is not known.

DIFFERENTIAL DIAGNOSIS

In addition to the four main types of primary RP covered above, there are a number of autosomal dominant inherited disorders that may have a pigmented retinopathy (although not necessarily progressive visual field loss); these include Charcot-Marie-Tooth disease, familial exudative vitreoretinopathy, Flynn-Aird syndrome, myotonic dystrophy, olivopontocerebellar atrophy, Paget's disease, Pierre-Marie syndrome, snowflake vitreoretinal degeneration, Stickler syndrome, Wagner's disease, and Waardenburg's syndrome. A summary of the features of these disorders can be found in Table 13-5.

Another main type of autosomal dominant retinal dystrophy that possibly could be confused with RP consists of the autosomal dominant cone dystrophies. These patients have distinctive features differing from RP, including atrophic macular lesions (by

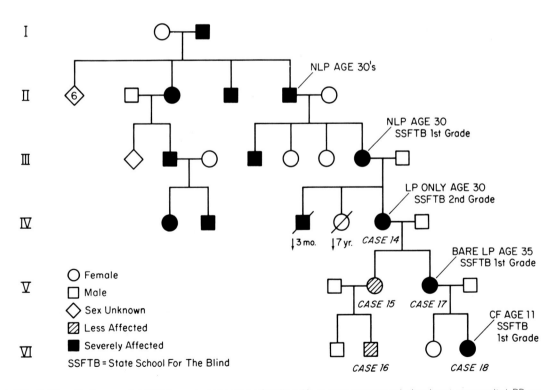

FIG. 8-26. Pedigree of ADRP-5, a six-generation family with a rare autosomal dominant congenital RP or Leber's amaurosis. Both typical and juvenile Leber's amaurosis congenita are inherited in an autosomal recessive fashion, and ADRP-5 can be assumed to have a different gene from typical forms of Leber's amaurosis.

TABLE 8-4

CLINICAL CHARACTERISTICS OF FAMILY ADRP-5 WITH AUTOSOMAL DOMINANT CONGENITAL RETINITIS PIGMENTOSA

	CASE 14	CASE 15	CASE 16	CASE 17	CASE 18
Age at time of examination	52	30	11.5	35	11
Age at onset	Birth	Birth	Birth	Birth	Birth
Visual acuity Bare LP Bare LP	20/200 20/100	20/200 20/60	NLP Bare LP	CF 3′ CF 3′	
Visual fields OD OS	None None	IV–4 10° IV–4 15°	1–4 20° 1–4 20°	None None	Temporal islands O.U.
ERG OU	NR	NR	NR	NR	NR
Final rod threshold OD OS	Can't do	4.4 4.4	20° 2.3 30° 4.0	Can't do	4.0 4.0
Refraction or retinoscopy OD OS	− 3.00 − 3.50	− 4.75 + 1.75 × 85 − 2.50 + 1.00 × 75	+ .75 + 1.00 × 105, + .50 + .75 × 75	− 1.75 + 1.00 × 135 − 1.25	+ 3.50 + 2.00 × 105 + 4.75 + 2.00 × 75
Nystagmus	Mild	Yes	Mild	Yes	Yes
Fundus changes	Bull's-eye macular, severe RPE atrophy	Bull's-eye macular, mild RPE bull's-eye alterations	Mild RPE changes	Bull's-eye macular, moderate RPE alterations	Bull's-eye macular, mild RPE alterations

Age is expressed in years, visual fields were performed by Goldmann perimetry, and final rod thresholds are expressed in log units of elevation after 40 minutes of dark adaptation; NR = nonrecordable ERG.

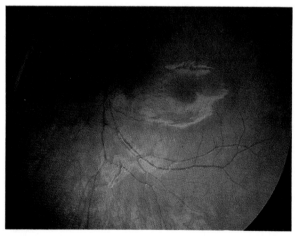
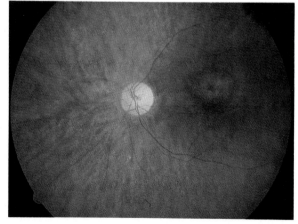

A

B

FIG. 8-27. Fundus photographs from family members of ADRP-5. *(A)* Case 16, an 11-year-old boy who was noted to have visual problems from birth, has no sign of RPE pigmentary changes in the equatorial and peripheral retina while the posterior pole shows early bull's-eye maculopathy. *(B)* Case 15, the 30-year-old mother of case 16, demonstrates optic atrophy, severe retinal vessel attenuation, no RPE pigmentary changes, and a bull's-eye maculopathy.

midadult life), full peripheral visual fields, monophasic dark adaptation curves with relatively normal final rod thresholds, and extinguished photopic ERGs in the face of normal to relatively normal scotopic (rod) ERGs.[30]

Advanced cases of Sorby's pseudoinflammatory dystrophy, an autosomal dominant disorder, may look like sector RP, choroidal sclerosis, or typical RP.

REFERENCES

1. Vannas S, Setälä M: On atypical night blindness. Acta Ophthalmol 36:849–89, 1958
2. Heckenlively JR, Yoser S: Autosomal dominant Leber's amaurosis congenita: A report of a six generation pedigree (submitted)
3. Boughman JA, Conneally PM, Nance WE: Population genetic studies of retinitis pigmentosa. Am J Hum Genet 32:223–235, 1980
4. Marmor MF: Visual loss in retinitis pigmentosa. Am J Ophthalmol 89:692–698, 1980
5. Jay B: Hereditary aspects of pigmentary retinopathy. Trans Ophthalmol Soc UK 92:173–178, 1972
6. Fishman GA: Retinitis pigmentosa: Visual loss. Arch Ophthalmol 96:1185–1188, 1978
7. Pruett RC: Retinitis pigmentosa: Clinical observations and correlations. Trans Am Ophthalmol Soc 81:693–735, 1983
8. Fishman GA, Maggiano JM, Fishman M: Foveal lesions seen in retinitis pigmentosa. Arch Ophthalmol 95:1993–1996, 1977
9. Heckenlively J, Friederich R, Farson C et al: Retinitis pigmentosa in the Navajo. Metab Pediatr Syst Ophthalmol 5:201–206, 1981
10. Arden GB, Carter RM, Hogg CR et al: Rod and cone activity in patients with dominantly inherited retinitis pigmentosa: Comparisons between psychophysical and electroretinographic measurements. Br J Ophthalmol 67:405–418, 1983
11. Berson EL, Sandberg MA, Rosner B et al: Natural course of retinitis pigmentosa over a three-year interval. Am J Ophthalmol 99:240–251, 1985
12. Marmor MF: The electroretinogram in retinitis pigmentosa. Arch Ophthalmol 97:1300–1304, 1979
13. Berson EL, Gouras P, Gunkel RD: Rod responses in retinitis pigmentosa, dominantly inherited. Arch Ophthalmol 80:58–67, 1968
14. Berson EL, Goldstein EB: Recovery of the human early receptor potential during dark adaptation in hereditary retinal disease. Vision Res 10:219–226, 1970
15. Berson EL, Simonoff EA: Dominant retinitis pigmentosa with reduced penetrance. Arch Ophthalmol 97:1266–1291, 1979
16. Massof RW, Finkelstein D: Two forms of autosomal dominant primary retinitis pigmentosa. Doc Ophthalmol 51:289–346, 1981
17. Lyness AL, Ernst W, Quinlan MP et al: A clinical, psychophysical, and electroretinographic survey of patients with autosomal dominant retinitis pigmentosa. Br J Ophthalmol 69:326–339, 1985
18. Meyer KT, Heckenlively JR, Spitznas M et al: Dominant retinitis pigmentosa: A clinicopathologic correlation. Ophthalmology 89:1414–1424, 1982
19. Hansen RI, Friedman AH, Gartner S et al: The association of retinitis pigmentosa with preretinal macular gliosis. Br J Ophthalmol 61:597–600, 1977
20. Foos RY: Surface wrinkling retinopathy. In Freeman HM, Hirose T, Schepens CL (eds): Vitreous Surgery and Advances in Fundus Diagnosis and Treatment, pp 23–83. New York, Appleton-Century-Crofts, 1977
21. Heckenlively JR, Martin DA, Rosales TO: Telangiectasia and optic atrophy in cone-rod degenerations. Arch Ophthalmol 99:1983–1991, 1981
22. Heckenlively JR, Rosales T, Martin D: Optic nerve changes in dominant cone-rod dystrophy. Doc Ophthalmol 27:183–192, 1981
23. Hellner KA, Rickers J: Familiary bilateral segmental retinopathia pigmentosa. Ophthalmologica 166:327–341, 1973
24. Omphroy CA: Sector retinitis pigmentosa and chronic angle-closure glaucoma: A new association. Ophthalmologica 189:12–20, 1984
25. Krill AE, Archer D, Martin D: Sector retinitis pigmentosa. Am J Ophthalmology 69:977–987, 1970
26. Krill AE: Incomplete rod-cone degenerations. In Krill AE, Archer D (eds): Krill's Hereditary Retinal and Choroidal Diseases, p 616. Harper & Row, Hagerstown, 1977
27. Berson EL, Howard J: Temporal aspects of the electroretinogram in sector retinitis pigmentosa. Arch Ophthalmol 86:653–665, 1971
28. Sorsby A, Williams CE: Retinal aplasia as a clinical entity. Br Med J 30:293–297, 1960
29. François J, de Rouck A: Degenerescence tapeto-retienne-congenitale de Leber. 18 Cong Ass Pediat Langue Fr. Geneva, 1961. Cited in Franceschetti A, François J, Babel J (eds): Chorioretinal Heredodegenerations, p 316. Charles C Thomas, Springfield, IL, 1974
30. Berson EL, Gouras P, Gunkel RD: Progressive cone degeneration, dominantly inherited. Arch Ophthalmol 80:77–83, 1968

9

Autosomal Recessive Retinitis Pigmentosa

JOHN R. HECKENLIVELY

There are a number of types of ocular-only autosomal recessive (AR) retinitis pigmentosa (RP); these include AR rod-cone, cone-rod, retinitis punctata albescens, preserved para-arteriolar retinal pigment epithelium, Goldmann-Favre disease, and three forms of congenital RP (Leber's congenital amaurosis). It is important to *not* automatically term cases of *simplex* (isolated) or *multiplex* RP as autosomal recessive RP. While many of these cases undoubtedly are autosomal recessive, some of them will be found to have other modes of inheritance. These issues are discussed more fully in Chapters 2 and 11; congenital RP is reviewed in Chapter 7.

There are a number of RP syndromes inherited in the autosomal recessive fashion in which other organ systems are affected; the more common ones include Usher's syndrome, Bardet-Biedl syndrome, Refsum's disease, Batten's disease(s), mucopolysaccharidoses I, IS, and III, Pierre-Marie syndrome, and Saldino-Mainzer syndrome. These entities are reviewed in Chapter 12.

The frequency of autosomal recessive RP has been variously reported to be 14% to 19%,[1-3] with an estimated rate in the population of 6.40/100,000.[4] Higher frequencies occasionally are reported but usually are the result of combining simplex and multiplex cases with those patients who have more definitive family histories (see Pedigree Analysis, Chapter 2). One exception to this is in the Navajo, in which 56.5% of RP patients (or 1/3000 of the population) have the autosomal recessive form. All patients have similar fundus appearance (**Fig. 9-1**) with multiple focal thinning of the retinal pigment epithelium (RPE) in early stages; this progresses to a generalized atrophy, giving an overall gray, granular appearance, with minimal pigmentary deposition. Patients have an early onset of night blindness and visual acuity impairment by the early twenties.[5] It is not known whether the Navajo AR RP is the same genetic disease or differs from AR RP in other populations.

Since the concept of the basic clinical differences between RP patients with rod-cone and cone-rod degeneration is fully covered in other sections, it

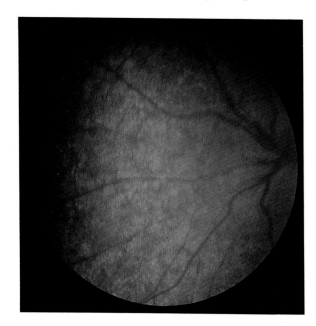

FIG. 9-1. Fundus photograph, 14-year-old Navajo woman with autosomal recessive RP; most AR RP Navajo patients demonstrated diffuse RPE atrophy, starting as multiple focal areas of dropout. The choriocapillaris and retinal vessels were less affected than might be expected.[5]

will not be repeated here. Both types of degenerative patterns are seen with autosomal recessive inheritance. While patients with cone-rod degeneration tend to have less pigmentary change with optic nervehead telangiectasia and temporal atrophy, these changes are not exclusive.

COMPOSITE PICTURE

AR ROD-CONE AND CONE-ROD DEGENERATION

AR ROD-CONE The average age of onset of symptoms was 16.1 years, with the mean age of diagnosis of 31.2 years. The electroretinogram (ERG) was recordable in 29% of patients, and the mean final rod threshold after 40 minutes of dark adaptation was 4.6 log units of elevation above normal. The mean visual acuity was 20/50 with a mean refraction of −1.82 +1.17 ×93. On average, 49% had posterior subcapsular cataracts. On fluorescein angiography, no patients had macular edema or paramacular window defect, 60% macular hypofluoresence, 20% macular window defect and vascular arcade edema, 30% parapapillary edema, 70% optic nervehead telangiectasia, and 50% temporal optic atrophy. The frequency of AR RC at UCLA was 3.9% (excluding simplex RC).

AR CONE-ROD The average age of onset of symptoms was 12.8 years, with the duration of the disease on the first visit of 8.2 years. The ERG was recordable on the first visit in 83% of patients, and the mean final rod threshold after 40 minutes of dark adaptation was 0.5 log units above normal baseline. The mean refraction was −3.25 +1.56 ×92 with a mean visual acuity of 20/50. On the fluorescein angiogram, no patients had macular edema, 63% had macular hypofluorescence, 50% macular window defect, 38% parapapillary edema, 78% temporal optic nervehead atrophy, and 88% disk telangiectasia. The average size of the visual field was 25° with a pseudoaltitudinal-like defect seen in 37% of eyes. The frequency of AR CR at UCLA was 2.0% (excluding simplex CR).

Two types of AR RP have unique fundus alterations which help to identify them as separate types of RP; these are preserved para-arteriolar RPE (PPRPE) and retinitis punctata albescens.

PRESERVED PARA-ARTERIOLAR RETINAL PIGMENT EPITHELIAL RP

PPRPE is an aggressive childhood-onset form of RP first reported by Heckenlively; it is inherited in the autosomal recessive fashion.[6] In areas where there is diffuse atrophy of the retina, a relative preservation

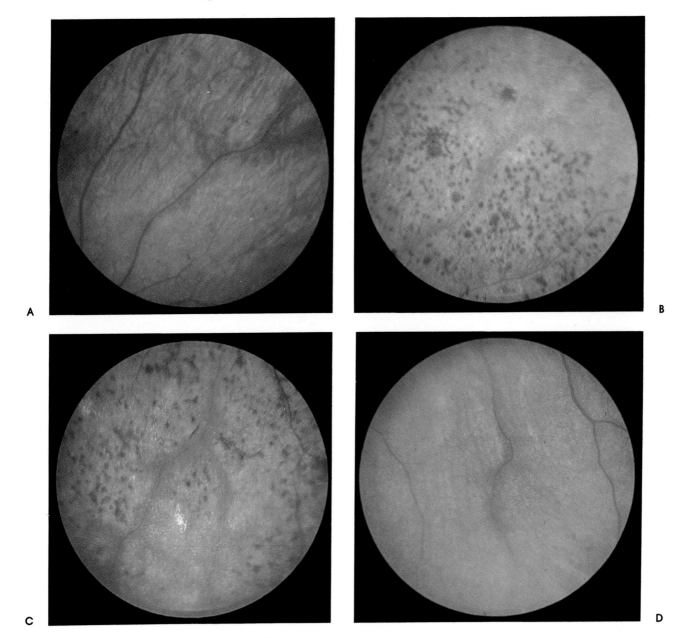

FIG. 9-2.   Preserved para-arteriolar RPE (PPRPE) RP. *(A)* A 9-year-old boy, case 1, Table 9-1 and 9-2, with PPRPE pattern under retinal arteriole superior temporal, left eye. *(B,C)* A 33-year-old woman, case 2, whose parents were first cousins with areas of RPE preservation inferior nasally in the left eye, and in the inferior equatorial region, right eye. *(D)* A 15-year-old boy, case 5, with no family history of RP, who demonstrated preservation under all retinal arterioles of anterior equatorial regions. Over time, some areas of preservation have been lost.

of the RPE can be seen underneath and adjacent to the retinal arterioles, with most of the patients demonstrating the pattern in the equatorial or anterior retina (**Fig. 9-2A–D**). The RPE preservation is best described as a relative retardation of the RP process, as several patients seen at UCLA have had documented loss in areas of previous RPE preservation. Fluorescein angiography may enhance the PPRPE pattern (**Fig. 9-3A–D**). The few PPRPE patients who have been identified to date are all hypermetropic, while most RP patients are myopic. The clinical and electrophysiologic features of the disease are presented in Tables 9-1 and 9-2.

Six patients have been seen at UCLA with this condition. In all cases the pattern was consistent with autosomal recessive inheritance. Visual acuity was affected early in contrast to the typical RP pattern of macular preservation, and many of the patients had disc drusen (**Fig. 9-4**). Patients with PPRPE also tend to have retinal vessels that are less attenuated than in many forms of RP, with patent vasculature into the peripheral retina, often through areas of pigmentary deposits (**Fig. 9-2B&C**).

The PPRPE pattern is uncommon, and its frequency is less than 1% of the RP population. The pattern should be sought especially in RP patients who are hypermetropic, since it appears to be a specific type of RP. Currently, the reason for the relative preservation under retinal arterioles is not known; one hypothesis is that there is a permeable factor that diffuses to the level of the RPE from the retinal arteriole and retards the RP process.

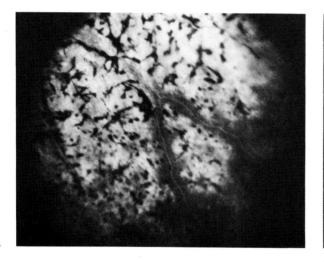

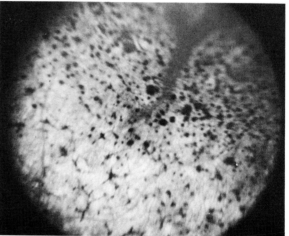

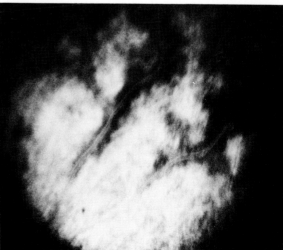

FIG. 9-3. Fluorescein angiograms of PPRPE RP. *(A)* Inferior temporal and *(B)* superior temporal anterior equatorial views of late venous phase, case 2, demonstrating preserved areas of RPE under and adjacent to retinal arterioles; *(C)* superior nasal view of PPRPE in case 5.

TABLE 9-1

SUMMARY OF CLINICAL FINDINGS IN SIX PATIENTS WITH PPRPE

CASE	AGE	AGE OF ONSET (YRS.)	INHERITANCE PATTERN	EYE	VISUAL ACUITY	REFRACTION
1	9	6	Simplex	OD OS	20/30 20/40	+6.00+1.00 × 75 +6.00+1.00 × 105
2	33	5	Parents 1st cousins	OD OS	CF 4/200	+3.00+.75 × 120 +2.50
3	18	8	Maternal aunt blind	OD OS	20/60 20/50	+2.00+2.25 × 90 +1.50+2.75 × 95
4	65	35	RP in sister, maternal GGM	OD OS	20/200 20/400	+3.75 +2.75
5	15	3	Simplex	OD OS	20/300 20/400	+3.00+.75 × 90 +2.50+.75 × 90
6	25	3	Parents 1st cousins	OD OS	HM HM	+4.00+1.25 × 90 +3.75+.75 × 90

CF = counting fingers; HM = hand motion; GGM = great grandmother

TABLE 9-2

ELECTROPHYSIOLOGICAL/PSYCHOPHYSICAL EVALUATION OF SIX PATIENTS WITH PPRPE

CASE	DARK ADAPTATION ROD THRESHOLD	ERG FINDINGS	GOLDMANN VISUAL FIELDS (IV–4 ISOPTER)
1	4.6 log unit*	rod-cone degeneration	OD 30° OS 15°
2	4.2 log units*	nonrecordable	OD–peripheral OS 3° islands OU
3	3.2 log units*	nonrecordable	OD 3° OS 3°
4	5.0 log units*	nonrecordable	OD 5° OS 4°
5	3.2 log units*	nonrecordable	OD 7° peripheral OS 7° islands OU
6	2.4 log units*	nonrecordable	OD–small temporal island OS–eccentric large temporal field

*Final rod threshold after 40 minutes of dark adaptation using a 2° target.

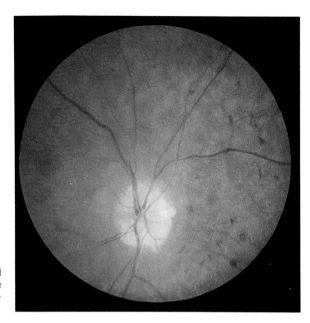

FIG. 9-4. Optic nervehead drusen in case 2, a 33-year-old woman with PPRPE. Most of the PPRPE RP patients had some fine yellow-golden crystals or deposits in their optic nerveheads.

Retinitis Punctata Albescens

DON S. ELLIS
JOHN R. HECKENLIVELY

Retinitis punctata albescens (RPA), an autosomal recessive progressive retinal degeneration, was first reported by Mooren in 1882.[7] RPA is distinguished from other forms of RP primarily by a fundus appearance characterized by numerous punctate whitish-yellow spots, often fanning out from the posterior pole in a radial pattern (**Fig.** 9-5). The spots are most numerous in the equatorial region and usually spare the macula. While these lesions have been observed to remain unchanged over many years, there is a concurrent diffuse degeneration of the RPE which begins peripherally and progresses toward the macula (**Fig.** 9-6). Advanced cases of RPA may reveal pigment deposition and bone spicule formation, especially in the anterior equatorial and peripheral retina. Atrophic disc changes and arteriolar attenuation are often present.

There may be some variation from the classic description of punctate lesions which are unchanged over long periods. Cases have been reported in which the punctate lesions have decreased or completely disappeared with time.[8]

An atypical case was reported by us in which the fundus revealed numerous confluent yellow spots of irregular shape distributed in a radial pattern with a perimacular ring and another ring in the midperiphery (**Fig.** 9-7*A&B*)[9]; in this patient the spots were found to disappear as the disease and functional abnormalities progressed (**Fig.** 9-7*C*). The progression of subretinal deposits often does not correlate with the progression of retinal dysfunction. It is not clear whether these different patterns represent unique entities or the variable expression of one disease.

CASE STUDIES

CASE 7

A 59-year-old woman was seen on referral in April 1975 for evaluation of retinal spots. There was a history of night blindness since the age of 7. There was no known family history of similar eye disease or consan-

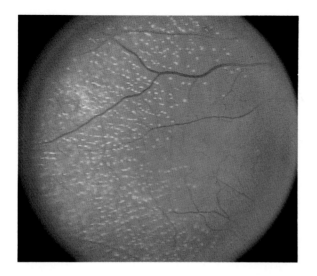

FIG. 9-5. Retinitis punctata albescens. A 59-year-old woman, case 7, demonstrating a radial pattern of punctate spots temporal to the macula, right eye, which on stereoscopic examination were at the level of the RPE.

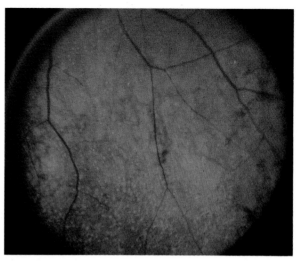

FIG. 9-6. Retinitis punctata albescens. Case 7, inferior nasal equatorial retina, right eye showing pigmentary deposits and diffuse RPE atrophy.

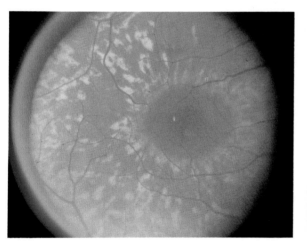

A

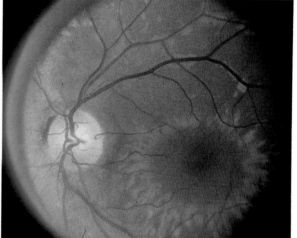

B

FIG. 9-7. Atypical retinitis punctata albescens. Case 8, age 55, with atypical spots or deposits at the level of the RPE, *(A)* right eye and *(B)* left eye. The spots are confluent, in a radial pattern, with two concentric rings. *(C)* Eight years later, at age 63, the same area in the left eye shows loss of the confluent spots, RPE atrophy with baring of large choroidal vessels, and pigment deposition.

C

guinity. The disease did not worsen during two pregnancies. External and slit lamp examinations were within normal limits.

On initial examination, the visual acuity was 20/25 in both eyes. The ERG was nonrecordable in both eyes, and dark-adaptation testing with a 5° object showed a final rod threshold elevation of 3.2 log units at 40 minutes. In June 1976, Goldmann visual field measured with the IV-4 isopter was 40° in both eyes.

Funduscopic examination revealed numerous punctate whitish-yellow spots, about the diameter of a second-order arteriole, which appeared by stereoscopic examination to be deep to the retinal vessels. Distribution was in a radial pattern throughout the fundus of both eyes. The spots were most numerous in the periphery where there was obvious degeneration of the RPE **(Fig. 9-5)**. Pigment clumping was beginning in the nasal periphery. The macula and peripapillary area were free of spots, but the peripapillary area showed signs of atrophic change.

The fluorescein angiogram was essentially normal; there was some mottling of the RPE, and the yellow spots were mainly hypofluorescent, although a few spots were hyperfluorescent. A few areas of the retina without obvious spots also had focal hyperfluorescence and hypofluorescence.

In February 1979, the visual acuity was 20/20 in both eyes. The photopic, scotopic, and bright flash dark-adapted ERG was nonrecordable, and dark adaptation testing demonstrated a 4.2-log unit elevation of the final rod threshold at 40 minutes. There was marked progression of the Goldmann visual fields, with the IV-4 isopter decreasing to 20° in both eyes and an increase in the size of the blind spot.

Funduscopy revealed greater pigment clumping, more dense in the periphery where bone spicule formation could be seen **(Fig. 9-6)**. The number, size, color, and position of the spots remained unchanged, although they appeared less intense owing to the surrounding diffuse RPE atrophy.

CASE 8

A 63-year-old woman was first seen at UCLA in May 1973 for evaluation of night blindness of 3 years' duration. There was no known family history of similar eye disease or consanguinity. The visual acuity was 20/20 in both eyes. The dark-adapted bright flash ERG was barely recordable, with only a 20-to-30-microvolt b-wave amplitude in both eyes. Dark adaptation testing using a 2° test object showed a 2.2-log unit elevation of the final rod threshold at 40 minutes of dark adaptation. Goldmann visual fields with IV-4 isopter were 10° to 15° with ring scotomata in both eyes.

Funduscopic examination revealed numerous confluent yellow spots of irregular shape that appeared to be deep to the retinal vessels by stereoscopic examination. They were distributed in a radial pattern with a perimacular ring and another ring in the midperiphery **(Fig. 7A)**. The spots were most numerous in the posterior pole surrounding the macula. A sharp border of the inner ring separated the uninvolved macula **(Fig. 9-7A&B)**.

The patient was followed for 9 years, during which time further progression of the disease was demonstrated. By September 1979, the ERG was completely nonrecordable. Dark adaptation testing using a 10° test object showed a 4.1-log unit elevation of the final rod threshold. Goldmann visual field measured with the IV-4 isopter decreased to 2° for both eyes. Visual acuity was 20/30 for both eyes.

Three years later the patient's visual acuity had decreased to 20/60 in the right eye and light perception in the left eye. Funduscopy showed that the subretinal deposits were almost completely gone, while there was further progression of RPE atrophy except for some macular sparing **(Fig. 9-7C)**. Pigment clumping was noted in the midperiphery and periphery. The arterioles were attenuated, most severely in areas of RPE loss.

Lauber first described RPA as an autosomal recessive trait in 1910,[10] and most cases are consistent with this inheritance pattern. RPA has been reported to occur in families in which some members demonstrated RP without the spots characteristic of RPA. Rare examples of this have been reported in autosomal dominant forms[11] and in autosomal recessive pedigrees of RP.[12–14]

The symptoms and electrophysiologic abnormalities of RPA are the same as those of other rod-cone degenerations. Symptoms include progressive loss of the visual fields, night blindness, decreased visual acuity, color vision impairment, and photophobia. In early stages of RPA, the scotopic ERG is more severely abnormal than the photopic ERG. In advanced stages, the photopic, scotopic, and flicker ERG responses become severely abnormal and often nonrecordable, and the final rod threshold for dark adaptation testing becomes greatly elevated. On the basis of these abnormalities, RPA is classified as a type of RP.

Fluorescein angiography reveals the progression of abnormalities typical of the rod-cone degenerations. In advanced stages, there are window defects with hyperfluorescence and increased visualization of the choroidal circulation due to RPE atrophy; arteriolar attenuation is usually seen. In addition, the subretinal spots characteristic of RPA may have corresponding hypofluorescence or hyperfluorescence (sometimes with central hypofluorescence) in the mid-late venous phase. The former changes are due to blockage of fluorescence. The later changes are indicative of dye leakage and are not consistent with window defects due to RPE atrophy.

The spots in RPA are at the level of the RPE, deep to the retinal vessels, and should not be confused with punctate depigmentation of the RPE commonly seen in many types of advanced RP. In these RP cases, there is a degeneration of the RPE in the equatorial regions which is diffusely and focally depigmented. Many patients with RP have fine scattered drusen which may appear similar to patterns seen in RPA. Initially, drusen begin as small punctate lesions in the posterior pole, and over many years they may increase in number and become confluent.

DIFFERENTIAL DIAGNOSIS

RPA and fundus albipunctatus (FA), which in the past has been referred to as the stationary form of RPA by many authors including Krill,[15] should be considered two distinct entities. Work by Carr[16] and Marmor[17] suggests that RPA is a progressive degeneration that permanently damages the RPE and photoreceptors, while FA is a stationary disorder of visual pigment kinetics with transitory loss of night vision. The cases of RPA reported as intermediate forms are probably examples of slowly progressive RPA. Alternatively, these are cases of fundus albipunctatus in which full regeneration of visual pigments has not yet occurred, and the visual thresholds are elevated and ERG tracings abnormal.

There has been confusion between RPA and FA in the past; RPA and FA were first separated in 1910 by Lauber,[5] who suggested, as have others since,[18-20]

that there may be intermediate forms of the disease. A wide range of abnormalities have been reported in ERG and dark adaptation testing in FA.[18,21] This may be one of the reasons for the earlier confusion between RPA and FA.

The fundus appearance of FA is very similar to that of RPA, but it lacks the RPE degeneration, pigment deposition, and progression to severe functional abnormalities. FA has a better prognosis, since night blindness is usually the only symptom.

In FA, the ERG and dark adaptation testing have been reported to be within normal limits after a prolonged adaptation to the dark from one-half[13] to more than 3 hours.[11,16] This is a fundamental difference from RPA in which night blindness does not show improvement on dark adaptation. In FA, the scotopic and flicker fusion ERG responses and dark adaptation testing show mild abnormalities that are characteristic of congenital stationary night blindness.[22] In RPA, the severely abnormal ERG and dark adaptation test results (which do not improve with dark adaptation), the progressive visual field loss, and the RPE atrophy along with pigment deposition indicate a diffuse process of tapetoretinal degeneration that clearly distinguishes RPA from FA.

Fundus flavimaculatus may demonstrate a funduscopic appearance somewhat similar to RPA, as in case 9-2 (**Fig. 9-8A&B**). Fundus flavimaculatus is characterized by numerous yellow flecks in the posterior fundus, which may regress with time. However, unlike RPA, central vision loss is usually the only complaint, and macular involvement has been reported in up to 90% of cases.[10] Although areas of atrophic RPE and subnormal ERG and dark adaptation test results are sometimes present,[23] the severe electrophysiologic abnormalities characteristic of the rod-cone degenerations are not seen. Fluorescein angiography may reveal paramacular and midperipheral degeneration of the RPE,[10] and a diffuse generalized hypofluorescence called the "dark choroid effect" is frequently present.[24]

Neuroretinitis may present a funduscopic picture similar to an atypical appearance of RPA (case 9-2, **Fig. 9-7A&B**). Although peripheral field loss may be associated with neuroretinitis, many factors easily distinguish this disease from the hereditary pigmentary degenerations. In neuroretinitis, vision loss is

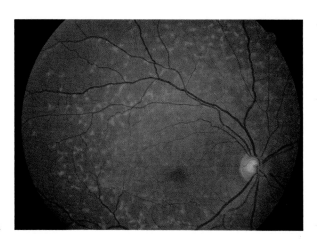 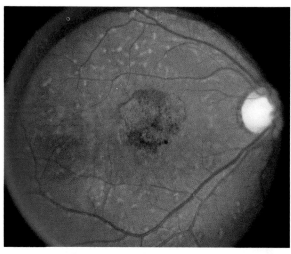

FIG. 9-8. Fundus flavimaculatus *(A)* without macular involvement and *(B)* with macular degeneration. On occasion, cases of fundus flavimaculatus can appear very similar to RPA on fundus examination, but electrophysiological testing will clearly differentiate the two entities.

usually unilateral, of sudden onset, seen more often in younger patients, and possibly associated with pain. The prognosis is good even with massive disc edema and hemorrhages. Degeneration of the RPE, pigment deposition, and a chronic progressive course are not characteristic of neuroretinitis.[25]

Fundus xerophthalmicus and other vitamin A deficiency states,[26] and abetalipoproteinemia[27] may present with a fundus appearance of numerous discrete white spots resembling RPA or FA (**Fig. 9-9**). Dark adaptation testing is abnormal in both of these conditions. Systemic manifestations of vitamin A deficiency distinguish it from RPA. Abetalipoproteinemia may show degenerative changes of the RP type, including ERG abnormalities, peripheral visual field loss, pigment deposition, and bone spicule formation.[21] Patients with these diseases have a history of late onset of night blindness, and the family history for night blindness is negative. Many of these patients have a reversal of symptoms, but not of pigment deposition, on vitamin A therapy.[20,21]

Other systemic conditions may cause fundus changes that resemble RPA or FA. Fundus lesions of calcium oxalate deposits in oxalosis[28] and crystal deposits in cystinosis[29] have been reported. Cases of pancreatitis[30] and hereditary nephropathies[31] have also demonstrated yellow punctate or fleck-like le-

sions in the fundus. In addition, yellow fleck-like lesions in the fundus were reported in a case of embolization of the choroidal circulation.[32] Other conditions which can cause scattered retinal spots include macular degeneration with cholesterol deposits, *peau d' orange* spots of pseudoxanthoma

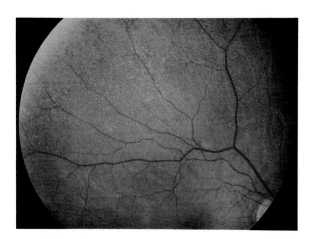

FIG. 9-9. Vitamin A deficiency mimicking the retinal findings of retinitis punctata albescens or fundus albipunctatus; a 53-year-old woman with documented vitamin A deficiency from complications secondary to a large intestine resection necessitated by Crohn's disease. Her barely recordable ERG and night vision became normal on parenteral vitamin A and E therapy.

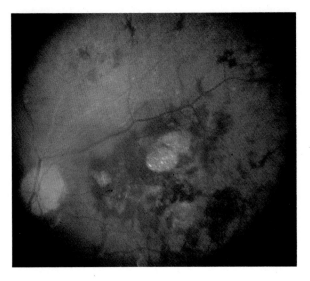 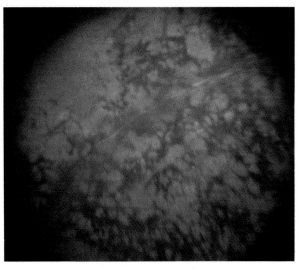

A   B

FIG. 9-10. Goldmann-Favre disease; a 32-year-old woman from a consanguineous marriage, who had poor vision from childhood. Fundus photographs show *(A)* severe macular atrophy and pigmentation from degeneration of previous macular cysts, as well as diffuse retinal atrophy and vessel attenuation, posterior pole, left eye; *(B)* peripheral view demonstrates epiretinal membrane over pigmented area.

elasticum, vitelliruptive macular degeneration (Best's disease) with multiple lesions confined to the arcades, the lacunae of Aicardi syndrome, the carrier state for X-linked albinism, punched-out lesions of presumed histoplasmosis syndrome, and scattered lesions of "birdshot retinochoroiditis." The associated features of these diseases are quite distinct from the inherited retinal dystrophies.

It is important to recognize patterns that may signify separate entities, since it is becoming increasingly evident that RP is a collection of many different diseases with common findings. However, the relationship of RPA to the other rod-cone degenerations remains unclear. To date, no histologic and biochemical studies delineating pathophysiologic mechanisms have been performed on eyes with RPA. The classification of RPA is based primarily on the funduscopic appearance and the electrophysiological differentiation from FA.

GOLDMANN-FAVRE DISEASE

Goldmann-Favre disease is a distinctive autosomal recessive vitreoretinal dystrophy characterized by peripheral and macular retinoschisis, chorioretinal atrophy, vitreous degeneration and veils, and epiretinal membranes (**Fig. 9-10**).[33] Coarse microcystic macular changes, cataracts and night blindness, and a progressive course are typical findings. The ERG is nonrecordable early in the disease, and visual fields and dark adaptation study results are similar to those of typical RP.

Advanced stages of the disease may appear similar to congenital RP with macular colobomata as the macular cysts degenerate and the tissue atrophies, although the uneven perimacular pigmentation, as well as the peripheral veils and epiretinal membranes help to differentiate patients with Goldmann-Favre disease.

REFERENCES

1. Berson EL, Rosner B, Simonoff E: Risk factors for genetic typing and detection in retinitis pigmentosa. Am J Ophthalmol 89:763-775, 1980
2. Boughman JA, Fishman GA: A genetic analysis of retinitis pigmentosa. Br J Ophthalmol 67:449–454, 1983
3. Fishman GA: Retinitis pigmentosa: Genetic percentages. Arch Ophthalmol 96:822–826, 1978
4. Bunker CH, Berson EL, Bromley WC et al: Prevalence of retinitis pigmentosa in Maine. Am J Ophthalmol 97:357–365, 1984

5. Heckenlively JR, Friederich R, Farson C et al: Retinitis pigmentosa in the Navajo. Metab Pediatr Syst Ophthalmol 5:201–206, 1981
6. Heckenlively JR: Preserved para-arteriole retinal pigment epithelium (PPRPE) in retinitis pigmentosa. Br J Ophthalmol 66:26–30, 1982
7. Mooren A: Fünf lustren ophthalmologischer wirksamkeit, pp 216–229. Wiesbaden, Bergmann, 1882
8. François J: The differential diagnosis of tapetoretinal degenerations. Arch Ophthalmol 59:86–120, 1958
9. Ellis D, Heckenlively J: Retinitis punctata albescens. Fundus appearance and functional abnormalities. Retina 3:27–31, 1983
10. Lauber H: Die sogenaunte Retinitis punctata albescens. Klin Monatsbl Augenhenkd 48:133–148, 1910
11. Vannas S, Setala M: On atypical night blindness. Acta Ophthalmol 36:849–859, 1958
12. Merin S, Auerbach, E: Retinitis pigmentosa. Surv Ophthalmol 20:303–346, 1976
13. Franceschetti A, François J, Babel J: Chorioretinal Heredodegenerations, pp 222–250. Springfield, IL, Charles C Thomas, 1974
14. Galindez-Iglesias: Retinitis punctata albescens. Am J Ophthalmol 37:436–438, 1954
15. Krill AE: Hereditary Retinal and Choiroidal Diseases, vol II, pp 739–824. Hagerstown, Harper & Row, 1977
16. Carr RE, Ripps H, Siegel IM: Visual pigment kinetics and adaptation in fundus albipunctatus. Doc Ophthalmologica Proc Ser 4:193–204, 1974
17. Marmor MF: Dystrophies of the retinal pigment epithelium. In Zinn KM, Marmor MF (eds): The Retinal Pigment Epithelium, pp 424–453. Cambridge, Harvard University Press, 1979
18. Smith BF, Ripps HA, Goodman G: Retinitis punctata albescens. A functional and diagnostic evaluation. Arch Ophthalmol 61:93–101, 1959
19. Nettleship E: A note on the progress of some cases of retinitis pigmentosa and of retinitis punctata albescens. Roy Lond Ophthalmol Hosp Rep 19:123, 1941
20. Tamai A, Setogawa T, Kandori F: Electroretinographic studies on retinitis punctata albescens. Am J Ophthalmol 62:125–131, 1966
21. Marmor MF: Defining fundus albipunctatus. Doc Ophthalmologica Proc Ser 13:227–234, 1977
22. Carr RE: Congenital stationary night blindness. Trans Am Ophthalmol Soc 72:448–487, 1974
23. Klien BA, Krill AE: Fundus flavimaculatus. Clinical, functional and histopathological observations. Am J Ophthamol 64:3–23, 1967
24. Eagle RC, Lucier AC, Bernardino VB et al: Retinal pigment epithelial abnormalities in fundus flavimaculatus. Opthalmology 87:1189–1200, 1980
25. Fish G, Grey R, Seyhmi KS et al: The dark choroid in posterior retinal dystrophies. Br J Ophthalmol 65:359–363, 1981
26. Glaser JS: Topical diagnosis: Prechiasmal visual pathways. In Duane TD, Jaeger E (eds): Clinical Ophthalmology, vol 2, pp 23–24. New York, Harper & Row 1986,
27. Levy NS, Toskes PP: Fundus albipunctatus and vitamin A deficiency. Am J Ophthalmol 78:926–929, 1974
28. Gouras P, Carr RE, Gunkel RD: Retinitis pigmentosa in abetalipoproteinemia: Effects of vitamin A. Invest Ophthalmol 10:784–793, 1971
29. Bullock J, Albert DM: Flecked retina appearance secondary to oxalate crystals from methoxyflurane anesthesia. Arch Ophthalmol 93:26–31, 1976
30. Sanderson PO, Kuwabara T, Stark WJ et al: Cystinosis: A clinical histologic and ultrastructure study. Arch Ophthalmol 91:270–274, 1974
31. Peterson WS, Albert DM: Fundus changes in the hereditary nephropathies. Trans Am Acad Ophthalmol Otolaryngol 78:762–771, 1974
32. Ellis DS, Heckenlively JR, Martin CL et al: Leber's congenital amaurosis associated with familial juvenile nephronophthisis and cone-shaped epiphyses of the hands (the Saldino-Mainzer syndrome). Am J Ophthalmol 97:233–239, 1984
33. Byers B: Blindness secondary to steroid injections into the nasal turbinates. Arch Ophthalmol 97:79–80, 1979
34. Favre M: A propos de deux cas de degenerescence hyaloideo-retinienne. Ophthalmologica 135:604–609, 1958 97:233-239, l984.

10

X-linked Recessive Retinitis Pigmentosa (X-linked Pigmentary Retinopathies)

ALAN C. BIRD
JOHN R. HECKENLIVELY

Numerous surveys comparing the sex distribution of patients with retinitis pigmentosa (RP) have demonstrated a male preponderance.[1,2] In 1908, Nettleship reported that of 1381 affected individuals 61.21% were male and 38.8% were female. Nettleship concluded that there was a greater susceptibility of men to suffer RP.[3] These statistics were reconfirmed by Sorsby in 1966, when he found that 59.5% of the population of England and Wales registered as blind or partially sighted because of RP and allied disorders were male.[4]

RP occurs in males at a higher frequency because of the unique features of X-linked recessive inheritance in which males who are hemizygotic for the condition are affected, while most females carriers usually have minimal or no features of the disease.

DIAGNOSIS OF X-LINKED INHERITANCE

X-linked recessive inheritance can be identified in pedigree analysis when only males are severely affected by the disease and when there is no evidence of male-to-male transmission. In a large pedigree, X-linked disease is easily identified; this inheritance is suggested if a maternal uncle or grandfather has RP with the mother having no or minimal symptoms. (The characteristics of the mendelian X-linked recessive pattern are reviewed more fully in Chapter 2.)

Because males have only one X chromosome, they may be said to be hemizygous for any X-linked disease, while female carriers of X-linked diseases have two X chromosomes, one with and one without the RP gene, and are said to be heterozygous for the condition. However, female carriers of RP may show signs of the disease, which is probably determined by the degree of lyonization present (see Chapter 2 for details of lyonization.)

The identified frequency of X-linked recessive RP varies with the country in which the survey is performed (Table 10-1).

The highest reported frequency of X-linked recessive RP is in the United Kingdom, where at least 20% of presenting RP patients have X-linked recessive inheritance.[5,10,11] Of these, 15.76% were identi-

TABLE 10-1

INCIDENCE OF X-LINKED RP

AUTHOR	PERCENT XL-RP	COUNTRY
Jay[5]	22.3%	United Kingdom
Fishman[6]	7.0%	United States
Voipio[7]	4.5%	Finland
Francois[8]	4.0%	Europe
Ammann[9]	1.0%	Switzerland

fied clinically, while the remaining 6.6% were determined by segregation analysis. The higher incidence in the U.K. is not the result of inbreeding as is commonly suggested, but it is likely that the gene has been present in the population for many generations, probably dating to times when the population of Great Britain was small. Nettleship in 1907 found a 55% to 45% ratio of males to females in his survey of patients with RP from across Europe,[3] suggesting that X-linked disease may be more prevalent in other European countries than is thought.

Because all affected males' daughters will carry the gene, and on the average half the sons of a carrier will inherit the RP gene, the potential for increasingly large numbers of affected individuals to develop with subsequent generations is easily seen. Pedigrees with affected individuals have been found dating back to the early 1700s.

Patients with X-linked RP have been assumed to have the same disease process as the result of a single gene defect. The evidence for this assumption is incomplete, and when RP pedigrees with X-linked inheritance are carefully reviewed, there are numerous important differences which may be the result of variable expressivity, allelic genetic defects, or even different gene loci. Frequently, reports on X-linked RP do not carefully define the characteristics of visual loss, so it is hard to tell whether different reports concern the same or different diseases. However, linkage studies using restriction fragment length polymorphisms continue to suggest that the gene locus for X-linked RP is in the region of Xp11

on the short arm of the X chromosome, and only one gene locus has been found to date.[12–14] Whether the actual gene defect is one or more than one remains to be determined.

CLINICAL HETEROGENEITY

As an example of the diversity of findings in X-linked RP, we looked at more than 25 hemizygotic males from 11 pedigrees and found that, when electroretinograms (ERGs) were recordable, some patients had cone-rod ERG patterns, while other members had rod-cone patterns on the ERG (Family XL-10-1, cases 1–5).

The issue is further complicated by potential confusion caused by other X-linked recessive diseases; unless careful family and clinical studies are performed, patients with juvenile retinoschisis, choroideremia, blue cone monochromatism, and X-linked recessive cone-rod dystrophy may be mistakenly diagnosed as having typical X-linked RP (see differential diagnosis discussion, this chapter).

CLINICAL PICTURE OF X-LINKED RP (HEMIZYGOTES)

Bird studied 23 families, in which 42 males were affected.[10] Details of visual loss were obtained about affected relatives in a further 69 cases. Early studies suggested less variation in the severity of the disease from one family to another, but more recent studies of several large pedigrees demonstrated variation of expressivity between cousins, or between affected uncles and nephews in the same pedigree, all of whom presumably have the same gene defect. The visual loss was found to be severe in nearly all males; night blindness was reported early in the first decade of life in all affected males, and symptoms referable to visual field loss were reported within the second decade. Unlike many forms of RP, central vision loss is found earlier in the disease, with difficulty in reading noted as early as age 20, and count finger to hand motion level of vision in many patients by age 35. By the midforties to fifties, no light perception is common (**Fig. 10-1**). Exceptions to this severe loss are recorded, with some patients maintaining good visual acuity into the fifth decade of life.

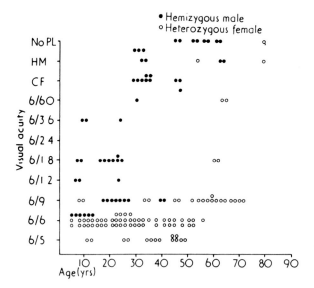

FIG. 10-1. Best visual acuity of each eye in hemizygous males and heterozygous females, by age, in X-linked RP (Bird AC: Br Ophthalmol 59:191, 1975)

Early Hemizygotic RP Changes

The earliest detectable change in young boys is an increased granularity or pigmentation of the anterior equatorial RPE (**Fig. 10-2A**). Pigment migration into the neuroretina may be minimal (**Fig. 10-2B**), and most patients have a blond fundus appearance. Retinal vascular attenuation may be seen, and temporal optic atrophy is common.

The diagnosis is usually made quite early (e.g., by age 4) in families in which the relevance of symptoms is well known, while it may not be detected in some cases until the middle teenage years in families who have no immediate affected members and who are not seeking signs of the disease.

The most common symptom is night blindness, manifested by the child crying in dimly lighted areas or grabbing onto a parent's hand when walking in a darkened area. Early visual field loss may manifest itself as stumbling over objects at ground level while walking.

The ERG may demonstrate a cone-rod or a rod-cone pattern and becomes nonrecordable by adulthood. Visual fields show contraction, which is accentuated with smaller isopters. Superior depression and ring scotomata may be present.

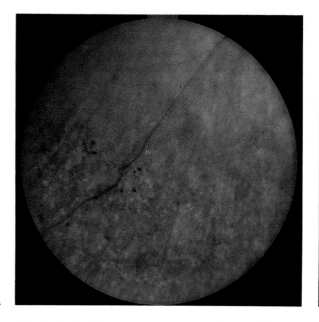
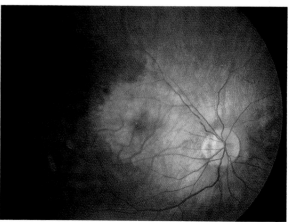

A   B

FIG. 10-2. Early funduscopic changes in X-linked RP. (A) An 11-year-old boy with equatorial granularity and early pigment deposits. (B) A 9-year-old boy with a visual acuity of OD 20/70, OS 20/100 and myopic changes of the posterior pole, mild granularity of equatorial region with no pigment deposits. This latter pattern is relatively common in X-linked RP.

Second Decade

By the beginning of the second decade, obvious RPE changes are seen in the equatorial region, with discernible pigment deposits. The posterior pole may also show disruption and focal areas of atrophy of the RPE, which may be more pronounced in cases that are more myopic. The retinal vasculature is attenuated. By the second decade, most patients have increased visual difficulties in bright light (e.g., sunlight).

Slit lamp examination reveals clear lenses, but pigmented flecks or cells can be seen in the anterior vitreous space, and the vitreous appears syneretic.

By the midteens, visual field loss is noticeable, and the visual acuity may be as low as 6/36. Patients retain adequate central vision to complete normal schooling.

Third Decade

In their twenties, hemizygotic RP patients show a marked loss of visual acuity, a phenomenon that usually occurs later in the course of the disease in most other types of primary RP. The visual field becomes considerably contracted, with a 10°-to-15° central field and a temporal island that often is connected centrally by a small isthmus (see Fig. 3-9B). Severe retinal vessel attentuation is seen, and pigment deposits occur in the posterior pole in addition to heavy deposits nasally and equatorially. Optic nervehead waxy pallor and posterior subcapsular cataracts may develop. Careful evaluation of the future visual potential should be given prior to extraction of the cataract, particularly in view of the macular damage often found in hemizygotic RP patients. Guidelines for cataract extraction in RP patients can be found in Chapter 6.

Fourth Decade

By the end of the fourth decade, most males have advanced stages of the disease with hand motion to light perception level of vision. At this stage, some patients develop nystagmus and consequently oscillopsia, which is often disturbing to the patient. Severe atrophy of the RPE is present, with areas of hyperpigmentation or pigment clumps and other areas showing no clinical evidence of RPE. Choroidal atrophy may occur, and it is sometimes profound,[15] but fluorescein angiography reveals a patchy loss rather than the confluent scalloped loss of choriocapillaris seen in choroideremia.

COMPOSITE PICTURE

X-LINKED RP (Hemizygotes)

The frequency of X-linked RP in the UCLA RP Registry is 5.5%; the average age of patients examined was 34 years. The mean age of onset of symptoms was 5.5 years. The average refractive error was $-5.75 +1.60 \times 120$. The mean final rod threshold was elevated 4.2 log units above normal. Recordable ERGs, when obtainable, tended to occur more frequently in patients with cone-rod patterns.

Fundus examination revealed that 22% had macular staphylomata, 55% had paramacular atrophy, and 33% had macular degeneration. The mean cup-to-disc ratio was 0.21. Fluorescein angiographic parameters showed the following occurrences: macular edema, 13%; macular hypofluorescence, 63%; macular window defect, 13%; temporal optic atrophy, 75%; optic nervehead telangiectasia, 75%. Approximately 40% of presenting X-linked RP patients had posterior subcapsular cataracts; this appeared to be age-related, with about 80% of patients over 30 years of age having at least 1- to 2-mm posterior subcapsular cataracts.

X-LINKED RECESSIVE RP CARRIERS (HETEROZYGOTES)

Carriers of X-linked recessive RP are both diagnostically challenging and scientifically interesting, since they may show absolutely no evidence of the disease, or in some cases they may appear to have RP. This variation is believed to be due to the degree of lyonization of normal genes in contrast to that of RP genes. It is commonly reported by heterozygotes that once visual loss begins, it may be rapid and follow a time course similar to that experienced by hemizygotes, the difference being that it starts much later in life in the affected carriers.

Prior to linkage studies demonstrating only one locus for X-linked RP, it had been hypothesized, on the basis of variability seen in heterozygotes, that there was more than one gene involved in transmitting the disease. At one time this variability led some investigators to hypothesize that there were dominant, intermediate, and recessive subdivisions of X-linked RP.

However, severely affected heterozygotes are found in all large pedigrees, which implies that a subdivision on the basis of severity of disease in heterozygotes is not justified.[16] While it has not been proven that the variable expressivity in heterozygotes relates to the degree of lyonization, the clinical findings are explained by lyonization.

The carrier status may be diagnosed on genetic grounds alone when a female has an affected son in a pedigree which clearly demonstrates X-linked inheritance. In addition, any daughter of an affected male will also be a carrier for the X-linked RP gene. In both these situations, the term obligate carrier is used. Every heterozygote has a 50% chance of passing the RP gene to offspring, male or female, so daughters of heterozygotes are at a 50% risk to be X-linked carriers.

Until recently the carrier state was determined by pedigree analysis and by examination of females at risk for fundus carrier signs. Fortunately, X chromosome recombinant DNA probes can now detect specific DNA fragments from white blood cell nuclei, and the location of the X-linked RP gene has been mapped to the proximal portion of the short arm of the X chromosome. Evaluating these restriction fragment length polymorphisms within pedigrees will allow, in some X-linked families, the possibility of predicting inheritance of the RP gene in males or females by blood or cell studies. Prenatal diagnosis may be possible in selected cases.

Clinical Studies of Carriers

Clinical and electrophysiological evaluations of 61 proven, presumed, and possible carriers from 23 families with X-linked RP were performed by Bird.[10] Of 61 females seen, 19 were obligate and 15 presumed heterozygotes, since all had evidence of fundus disease. Of 23 possible heterozygotes, 14 had evidence of fundus disease and 9 were normal.

In mildly affected carriers, fundus changes consisted of irregularity of pigmentation in the RPE in localized areas with or without associated migration of pigment into the retina. In the least severe cases, the changes were largely in the pre-equatorial fundus. Fluorescein angiography proved helpful in confirming the loss of pigment epithelium in affected areas (**Fig. 10-3**).

In more severe cases, widespread abnormalities were seen, which in some were restricted to a single sector or hemisphere and sometimes resembled sector RP (**Fig. 10-4A&B**).[17] While the most severe disease was seen in older carriers, two of five in the second decade and two of nine in the third decade of life had more extensive changes than simple peripheral RPE atrophy. Profound and localized atrophy of the choroid was seen in the peripheral fundus in some older cases. In one family, glistening white reflexes were seen in the midperipheral fundus of

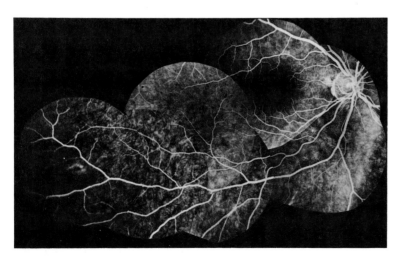

FIG. 10-3. Fluorescein angiogram of a 28-year-old asymptomatic female carrier with an affected brother; her visual acuity was 20/20 in each eye, and the visual fields were normal. The equatorial RPE appeared mottled, and the periphery of the right fundus showed a small atrophic patch with migration of pigmented cells into the retina. Abnormal function was confirmed by estimation of retinal rhodopsin concentration, which was reduced by 40%. (Bird AC: Trans Am Acad Ophthalmol Otolaryngol 77:649, 1973)

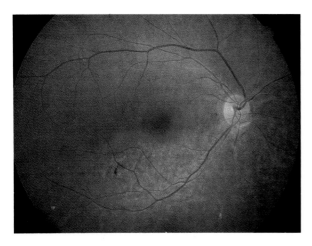
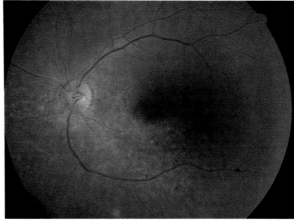

A   B

FIG. 10-4. Carrier of X-linked RP with fundus findings resembling sector RP; nasal and inferior retina are particularly affected.

some heterozygotes, but these were not seen in all carriers.

As early as 1914, Diem reported abnormal fundus reflexes in females heterozygous for X-linked RP.[18] In subsequent years, abnormal fundus reflexes were reported in different genetic forms of RP and were referred to as "tapetal reflexes."[19]

Falls and Cotterman found that this abnormal tapetal reflex was the most common expression of the heterozygous state in their family, and others have emphasized the importance of this ophthalmoscopic sign.[20-22] Similarly, Fishman found that 52% of his obligate carriers had tapetal reflexes.[23] Schappert-Kimmijser identified the tapetal reflex in one family out of eight and concluded that while this sign might be useful at the time of presentation, no conclusions could be drawn when the reflex could not be identified.[24]

In our experience, the tapetal reflex is most easily seen with direct ophthalmoscopy in the temporal paramacular region (**Fig. 10-5***A&B*) in heterozygous women in their second and third decade of life.

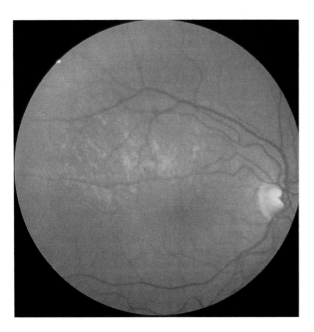
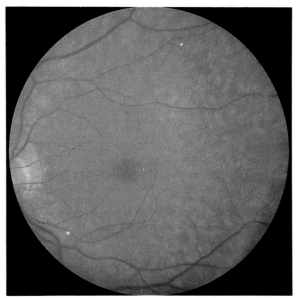

A   B

FIG. 10-5. Tapetal reflex, X-linked RP. (A) A 52-year-old woman with an affected son. (B) A 36-year-old woman whose father had X-linked RP.

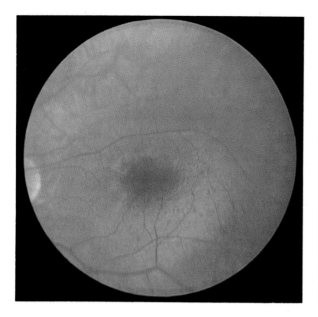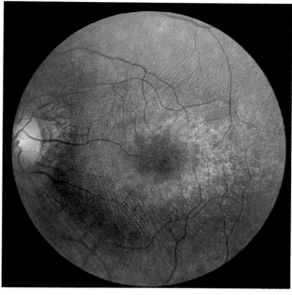

A   B

FIG. 10-6. Tapetal-like reflex from young males with X-linked RP. (A) A 14-year-old boy with X-linked RP showing tapetal-like reflex from paramacular region. His visual acuity was 20/50. (B) A 25-year-old X-linked male with paramacular tapetal-like changes and surface wrinkling retinopathy. The visual field was 10° with the IV-4 target, final rod threshold 4.8 log units elevated, and visual acuity 20/30–

Young hemizygotes (males) also may have tapetal-like reflexes in the paramacular region (**Fig. 10-6A&B**). Gieser, Fishman, and Cunha-Vaz have published examples of the tapetal reflex.[25] Ricci reported that this reflex may not be seen after exposure to light and will reappear after a period of darkness, terming this the *phenomne de mizuo* inverse.[26]

Visual field loss was found in 35 of 36 heterozygotes tested and corresponded to visual fundus abnormalities. The loss consisted most commonly of irregular peripheral and midzone changes, sectoral loss, or even marked contraction in more severe cases. The most severe loss has been seen in older women, although two heterozygotes in the second and two in the third decades of life were symptomatic and had significant visual field loss.

Dark adaptation was abnormal in 32 of 37 heterozygotes tested, ranging from 0.3 to 2.5 with a mean of 0.5 log units of elevation of the final rod threshold above the high normal value (0.5).

Electro-oculography was within normal limits in 15 of 42 tested, even in cases in which fundus abnormalities, field loss, and abnormal dark adaptation was identified.

ERG b-wave amplitudes were abnormal in 11 of 42 tested, but did not add diagnostically to the evaluation, since all of these cases had easily recognizable fundus changes, field loss, and abnormal dark adaptation.

Further ERG studies in 36 women, aged between 11 and 78 years, found that abnormalities to blue scotopic and white light flicker ranged from 30% to 75% of patients.[27] By contrast, Berson reported a 96% abnormal photopic implicit time using an averaged flicker technique.[28] Fishman reported that 86% of his 46 hemizygote patients had reductions in ERG amplitudes.[23] In addition, seven carriers had appreciable asymmetry in ERG amplitude reduction between the two eyes; five had asymmetric fundus pigmentary changes.

The early receptor potential (ERP) was evaluated by Berson and Goldstein in an affected boy and two heterozygotes.[16] Using a bright flash, the ERP measures the electrical signal generated by the outer segments during bleaching, and the amplitude of the response depends on visual pigment concentration, receptor function and number, and orientation of the pigment molecules within the receptor. They reported that the affected boy's ERP was less than 20% of normal, while the heterozygotes had a 50% reduction in ERP amplitude, even though their rod and cone function was normal on ERG and psychophysical testing.

Hyman and Weale measured rhodopsin levels in six carriers of X-linked RP with reflectometry. All of these patients had normal ERGs, while three of the six had abnormal electro-oculograms, and two of the six had abnormal dark adaptations.[29] Fundus reflectometry, however, showed that all six of the heterozygotes had rhodopsin levels well below normal values. The authors suggested that the ability to identify heterozygous females in a family with X-linked RP is greatly facilitated by estimation of retinal rhodopsin concentration.

Vitreous fluorophotometry, in a small series with four X-linked carriers, demonstrated abnormal blood–retinal barriers in all cases, with the most leakage occurring in the case which had the only abnormal ERG.[25]

Histopathological studies by Szamier and coworkers in a 24-year-old male with X-linked RP who died of cancer showed that central foveal cones were reduced in number by about 50% and had intact though distorted outer segments (Fig. 4-11).[30] Rods were absent in the center and midperiphery, cones had shortened inner segments and no organized outer segments from the para-fovea to midperiphery,

and in the far periphery cones and rods both had normal inner segments and slightly short outer segments (Fig. 4-4). The RPE contained abnormally large numbers of melanolysosomes and few free melanin granules from the fovea through the midperiphery, and few melanolysosomes and many free melanin granules in the far periphery (see Chapter 4).

Psychophysical testing by Massof and Finkelstein in two patients with X-linked RP, aged 16 and 28, correlated well with the histopathology found by Szamier and associates and may be representative of the overall disease process.[31] Using blue-green and red stimuli to measure rod and cone sensitivity thresholds, respectively, they found that the cones of these two patients were mediating detection of both stimuli in the central 10°, that there was a ring scotoma in the midperiphery, and rods mediated detection of the stimuli in the far periphery. They felt that their test results were in agreement with those of Szamier and colleagues.

CASE EXAMPLES

FAMILY XL-1

Case 1 A 14-year-old male (**Fig. 10-7**, Pedigree V-24) gave a history of night blindness for as long as he can remember. He first noted visual field difficulties at

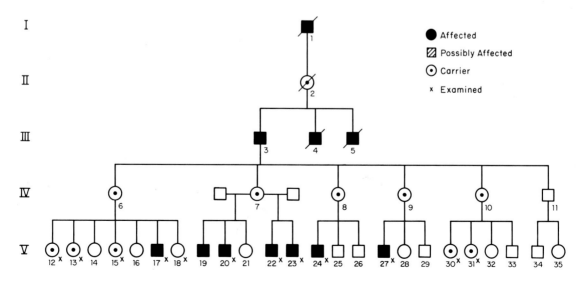

FIG. 10-7. Pedigree, X-linked RP: five-generation family with 11 males known to be affected.

the age of 7 and has noted visual acuity problems from early childhood. The medical history is noncontributory. Family history demonstrates an X-linked inheritance pattern, with 11 males affected in five generations.

On examination with myopic correction, his visual acuity was 20/40 OU. Fundus examination revealed pigmentary deposits in the equatorial region, disc pallor with temporal atrophy, vessel narrowing, and mild retinal and choroidal atrophy **(Fig. 10-8A&B)**.

Visual fields demonstrated **(Fig. 10-9)** nearly complete ring scotomata with large temporal islands connecting to the central field by an isthmus of intact field (similar to that seen in Fig. 3-2).

Electroretinographic testing showed a barely recordable cone ERG while the rod tracing was well formed with reduced amplitudes (cone-rod pattern). Psychophysical testing showed residual rod function.

Case 2 (Fig. 10-7, Pedigree V-20) The 23-year-old first cousin of cases 1 and 5 and half brother of cases 3 and 4 noted the onset of night blindness at the age of 13 years, but he was not able to identify a date of onset for his visual field loss. His visual acuity was OD 20/40, OS 20/60. Goldmann visual fields were re-stricted to central islands with an inferior peripheral island circumscribing 12 clock hours in each eye **(Fig. 10-10)**. Biomicroscopy showed clear lenses, but there were pigmented flecks in his anterior vitreous space. Fundus examination revealed a blond tigroid fundus with bone spicules in equatorial regions, vessel attenuation, and optic nerve pallor **(Fig. 10-11A&B)**. His ERG was nonrecordable under all test conditions, but psychophysical testing showed residual rod function.

Case 3 A 19-year-old man **(Fig. 10-7,** Pedigree V-22) first noted the onset of night blindness at age 10. His visual acuity with myopic correction was 20/30 OU; Goldmann visual field tests in the right eye show a central 18° area with a ring scotoma and an inferior peripheral island for 12 clock hours, while the left eye has a central area connected to a 5-clock-hour peripheral island by an isthmus **(Fig. 10-12)**. Biomicroscopic examination revealed pigmented flecks in the anterior vitreous space and clear lenses. Funduscopy showed diffuse retinal atrophy and some pigment deposits **(Fig. 10-13)**. The ERG was abnormal under all testing conditions, with the rods showing a greater reduction in amplitude (rod-cone pattern). Scotopic

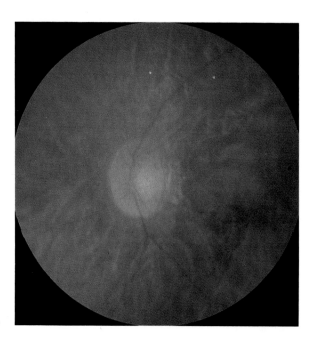
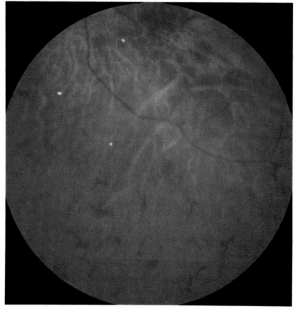

A   B

FIG. 10-8. Case 10-1, a 24-year-old man with X-linked RP who had night blindness from infancy and visual field loss from age 7, 20/50 vision OU, and a cone-rod pattern on his ERG showing (A) blond fundus, pale discs with temporal atrophy, vessel narrowing, and (B) pigment deposits in equatorial region.

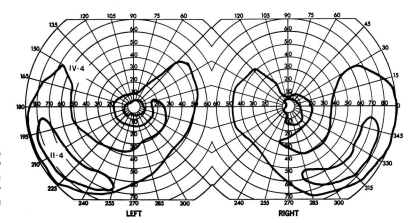

FIG. 10-9. Goldmann visual field, case 1, a 14-year-old boy with X-linked RP demonstrating a partial ring scotoma and a peripheral island connected by an isthmus to his central field in both eyes.

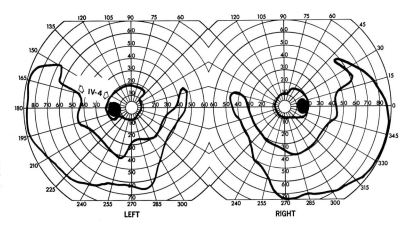

FIG. 10-10. Goldmann visual field, case 2, a 23-year-old man with X-linked RP demonstrating small central fields and complete ring scotomata, with large inferior peripheral islands.

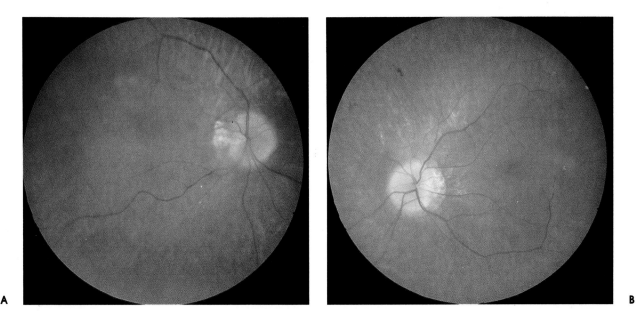

FIG. 10-11. Fundus photographs, case 10-2, a 23-year-old male with X-linked RP and nonrecordable ERG: (A) right eye and (B) left eye show diffuse retinal pigment epithelial atrophy outside of posterior pole with some pigment deposits. Discs are pale with temporal portion missing.

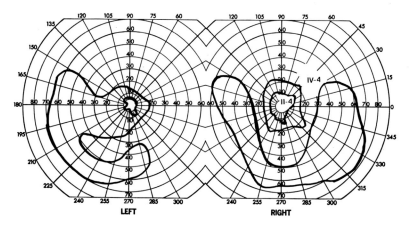

FIG. 10-12. Goldmann visual field, case 3, a 19-year-old man with X-linked RP demonstrating a full-ring scotoma in the right eye and a partial one in the left eye in which the central island of vision is connected to his peripheral island by a large isthmus.

static perimetry demonstrated less rod function than in cases 2 and 4 (i.e., the patient's rod threshold sensitivity was elevated).

Case 4 (Fig. 7, Pedigree V-23**)** A 17-year-old man, brother of 3, was first noted to have night blindness by age 1, but he has noted no visual field problems. His visual acuity was OD 20/40, OS 20/60 with myopic correction. The ERG was abnormal, with the cones showing greater amplitudes than the rods (rod-cone pattern). Fundus examination revealed a blond fundus with diffuse retinal atrophy in the equatorial re-

gions with early bone spicule formation. There was some retinal vessel attenuation **(Fig. 10-14).**

Case 5 (Fig. 10-7, Pedigree V-27**)** The 20-year-old first cousin of the above cases was found to be night blind before age 1 and noted visual field loss at age 6. His visual acuity was OD 20/20, OS 20/40. The ERG was abnormal, with the cones showing a greater reduction in amplitude than the rods (cone-rod pattern). Psychophysical testing showed good residual rod function. Fundus examination showed a blond fundus with paramacular retinal atrophy, vessel attenuation,

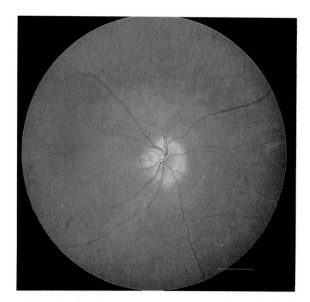

FIG. 10-13. Fundus photograph, case 3. The right eye demonstrates diffuse retinal atrophy and vascular attenuation; there appears to be some nerve fiber layer swelling at disc margin.

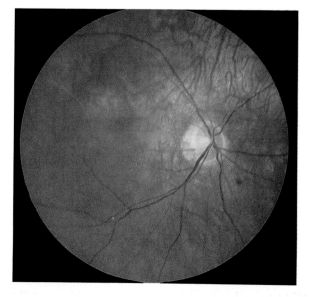

FIG. 10-14. Fundus photograph, case 4. The right eye shows a blond fundus with some attenuation of the vasculature, with thinning of nasal paramacular and peripapillary RPE. There were no pigment deposits in the periphery.

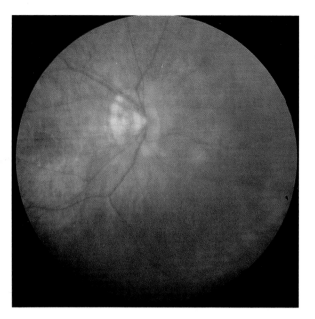 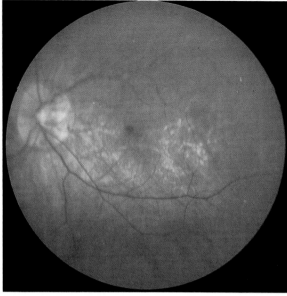

A   B

FIG. 10-15. Fundus photographs, case 5, a 20-year-old man with X-linked RP. (A) The right eye and (B) left eye reveal a blond myopic fundus with diffuse retinal atrophy in the paramacular area.

and severely "tilted" discs with no temporal disc tissue apparent **(Fig. 10-15A&B).**

CARRIER EXAMPLES

Case 6 (Fig. 10-7, Pedigree V-13**)** The 27-year-old female first cousin of the above cases complained of night blindness for as long as she could remember. She had not noticed any changes in her visual field, although her Goldmann visual field test showed a nasal step in the left eye and a general superior field suppression. The patient reported light sensitivity. She had −8.00 diopters of myopia, and her best cor-

rected visual acuity was 20/25 OU. Biomicroscopy demonstrated some pigmented flecks in the anterior vitreous space. Indirect ophthalmoscopy revealed an appearance consistent with high myopia with some generalized RPE mottling in the equatorial regions and some atrophy in the paramacular region in the posterior pole.

Case 7 (Fig. 10-7, Pedigree V-12**)** This 31-year-old sister of case 10-6 was asymptomatic and had vision of 20/15 in each eye. Goldmann visual field showed mild constriction of the II-4 isopter in both eyes with a nasal step in the left eye **(Fig. 10-16).** Fundis exami-

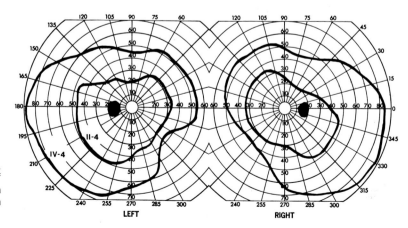

FIG. 10.16. Goldmann visual field, case 7, a 31-year-old female carrier of X-linked RP, showing some constriction with the II-4 isopter and a nasal step in the left eye.

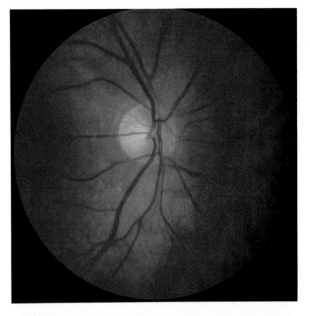
A

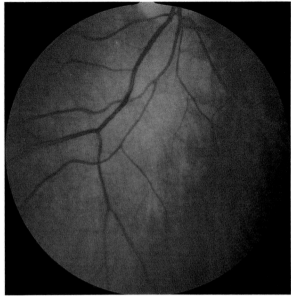
B

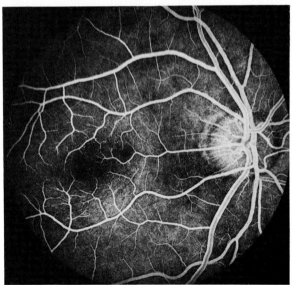
C

FIG. 10-17. (*A*) Fundus photograph of optic nerve and posterior pole and (*B*) inferior to nervehead, demonstrating thinning and atrophy of RPE of case 7, but overall the fundus appearance was relatively normal. Disc telangiectasia was seen on direct ophthalmoscopy and confirmed on (*C*) fluorescein angiography; this mid-transit phase view shows marked telangiectasia of the temporal optic nervehead as well as capillaries in the macular region.

nation showed some RPE thinning or atrophy **(Fig. 10-17 *A&B*)**, while there was marked disc telangiectasia which was confirmed on fluorescein angiography **(Fig. 10-17 *C*)**.

Case 8 (Fig. 10-7, Pedigree V-15) The 22-year-old sister of cases 6 and 7 had no visual complaints and had uncorrected visual acuity of 20/15 in each eye. Goldmann visual fields showed some superior field suppression and mild constriction on fields **(Fig.**

10-18). Fundus examination revealed some RPE atrophy and fine pigmentation in the equitorial regions which was even more obvious, though subtle on fluorescein angiography **(Fig. 10-19 *A&B*)**.

Differential Diagnosis

When a pedigree with an X-linked pattern of inheritance is found in a patient with a retinal problem,

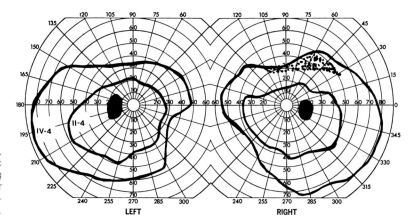

FIG. 10-18. Goldmann visual field, case 8, in a 22-year-old asymptomatic female carrier of X-linked RP, showing enlarged blind spots, mild superior depression, nasal steps, and mild constriction with the II-4 isopter in both eyes.

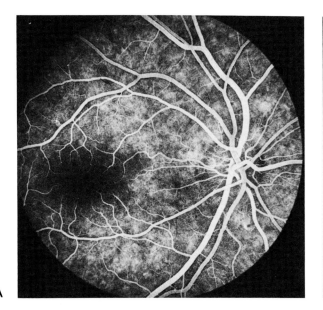 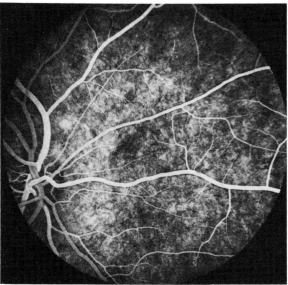

FIG 10-19. Fluorescein angiogram, case 8, demonstrating (*A*) right eye posterior pole RPE mottling and mild disc telangiectasia (*B*) Area nasal to disc shows multiple hyperpigmented granules with difuse mottling at the level of the RPE.

there are a number of possible diseases that must be carefully considered (Table 10-2).

Juvenile Retinoschisis. In its early and middle stages, juvenile retinoschisis is easily distinguished from X-linked RP, since patients have microcystic-like changes of the macular region but less than half have obvious equatorial or peripheral retinal schisis. Many patients present with a vitreous hemorrhage when the schisis process breaks a retinal vessel. Interestingly, some older patients with juvenile retinoschisis may present with severe visual loss and

TABLE 10-2

(NON-RP) X-LINKED RECESSIVE RETINAL DISORDERS

1. Juvenile retinoschisis
2. Blue cone monochromatism*
3. X-linked late-onset cone dystrophy with tapetal reflex and Mizuo-Nakamura effect
4. Cone-rod dystrophy (rare)
5. Protanopia, deutanopia*
6. X-linked congenital stationary night blindness*

* Stationary problems

pigmentary retinopathy[32] (**Fig. 11-7A&B**); with an X-linked pedigree, these patients may be assumed incorrectly to have X-linked RP. In some of these patients, remnant vitreal retinal blood vessels may be observed. Examination of younger affected members will ensure that the correct diagnosis is made.

Blue Cone Monochromatism.   Blue cone monchromatism is a rare X-linked recessive cone disorder characterized by males who present with a history of poor vision from birth, a visual acuity of 20/60 to 20/200, nystagmus, and relatively full visual fields. Except for severe temporal optic atrophy, no obvious fundus disturbance is seen, although older patients may have mild macular atrophy. The ERG demonstrates a nonrecordable photopic ERG and a normal to near-normal rod ERG. Carriers may show loss of the cone portion of the dark-adapted bright red stimulus waveform.

X-linked Cone-Rod Dystrophy.   X-linked cone-rod dystrophy is a rare disorder, and patients present with decreased central vision, may have a bull's-eye lesion in the macula, a fine nystagmus, and no or very little pigmentary change in the fundus until advanced stages of the disease. The visual field loss is slower than in X-linked RP, and the ERG shows a cone-rod pattern if the ERG is recordable, which is often the case, unlike X-linked RP in which the ERG is severely affected early in the disease.

Congenital Stationary Night Blindness.   X-linked congenital stationary night blindness is characterized by high myopia, tilted or misshapened optic nerveheads, normal visual field and fundus consistent with myopia, and moderately severe night blindness. The ERG demonstrates a photopic ERG which has normal to subnormal amplitudes and a rod ERG which is barely recordable to nonrecordable. The oscillatory potentials are missing in these patients.[33] Sharpe and colleagues recently demonstrated that these patients have residual rod function.[34]

Color Blindness.   Protonopia and deutanopia are congenital forms of X-linked recessive color blindness, which are generally considered benign disorders, since persons with these entities have normal visual acuities and fields and no evidence of pathological sequelae.

Choroideremia.   Choroideremia (below) is a progressive form of retinal degeneration that can be classified under the broad umbrella of peripheral retinal receptor dystrophy or RP (note definitions, Chapter 1). Patients with early choroideremia may not be distinguishable clinically from those with early X-linked RP, since fine pigmentary or granular changes can be seen in the peripheral retina of each disorder (**Figs. 10-2A&B and 10-20A–C**). Examining other affected members in the family or following the patient over time will clarify which disorder is occurring.

Choroideremia

JOHN R. HECKENLIVELY
ALAN C. BIRD

Choroideremia, an X-linked recessive disease, is characterized by diffuse progressive degeneration of the retinal pigment epithelium (RPE) and choriocapillaris. The degeneration is first manifest in the equatorial region as mottled areas of pigmentation, which progresses to scalloped areas of confluent loss of RPE and choriocapillaris with preservation of larger choroidal vessels. The fluorescein angiographic changes are even more marked, with the scalloped areas of missing choriocapillaris appearing quite hypofluorescent next to brightly hyperfluorescent patent choriocapillaris.

Choroideremia meets all the standard definitions of retinitis pigmentosa (RP) except for the fundus appearance. Patients are night blind from an early age, with progressive visual field loss leading to tunnel vision; when the electroretinogram (ERG) can be recorded, a rod-cone degenerative pattern is seen. Inheritance is well established to be X-linked recessive. This group of patients has been considered to be separate from RP patients because of their distinctive retinal changes. Since most RP patients

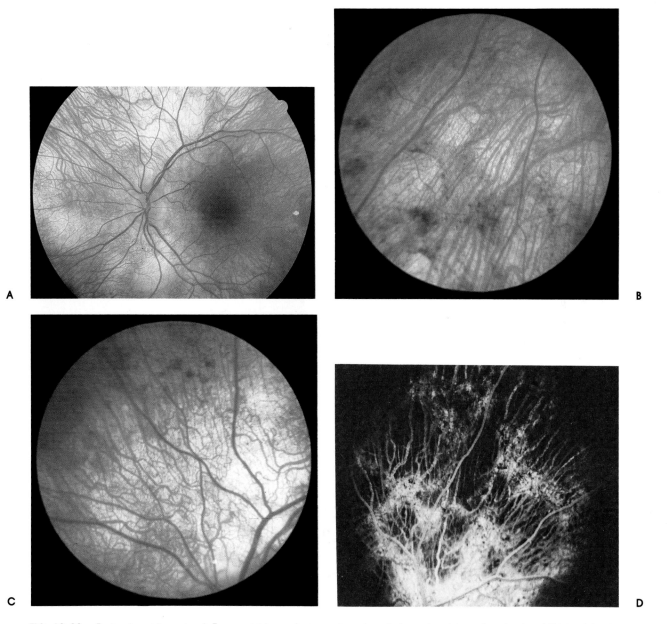

FIG. 10-20. Early choroideremia. A 7-year-old boy whose maternal uncle has choroideremia, who has (A) blond fundus with (B,C) peripheral granularity and fine pigmentary deposits; (D) fluorescein angiogram demonstrates patchy loss of RPE and choriocapillaris area superior temporal *A*.

present with similar clinical features, researchers have been eager to focus on those retinal degenerative changes that make choroideremia distinctive. Now that RP is accepted as a term referring to a number of different disorders, it is reasonable to consider choroideremia as a single nosological entity within the group of diseases causing widespread degeneration of the outer retina.

HISTORICAL REVIEW

Choroideremia was first identified as an entity separate from "typical" RP in 1871 by Mauthner,[35] who reported two male patients with pigmentary changes in the fundus, night blindness, and constricted visual fields. However, he noted features different from typical RP: atrophy of the choroid, normal retinal vessels, and absence of optic atrophy. Noting a similarity to choroidal coloboma, he described his cases as having "choroideremia." Subsequent reports in 1920 by Zorn,[36] who found six cases in three generations and in 1938 by Schutzbach,[37] who reported 13 cases in four generations, established the X-linked recessive nature of choroideremia.

Establishing the hereditary pattern was not without some confusion, for as earlier cases were seen, the distinctive scalloped pattern of tissue loss was noticed and confused with gyrate atrophy, which is inherited in an autosomal recessive fashion. However, in 1942, Goedbloed[38] and Waardenberg[39] independently suggested a sex-linked pattern of inheritance for the condition; this was confirmed in 1948 by McCulloch,[40] who presented 86 cases of choroideremia in two families, one with more than 600 members. McCulloch demonstrated that the disease follows mendelian inheritance patterns and that females may have a "benign" form of the disease.

There has been speculation that X-linked choroidal sclerosis[41] may be a different entity; however, there is little evidence to support the view that this is not just another name given to families with choroideremia.

The finding of elevated plasma ornithine levels in association with gyrate atrophy by Kirsten Takki in 1971,[42] as well as a second article[43] in which she reported that choroideremia patients had normal ornithine levels, gave a definitive method for separating gyrate atrophy from choroideremia in cases in which the inheritance pattern is not clear.

CLINICAL FINDINGS IN CHOROIDEREMIA

HEMIZYGOTE (MALES)

Young patients in the preschool years may experience night blindness, but visual field loss usually is not found until the teenage years. The early funduscopic appearance is a generalized loss of the RPE, resulting in a blond fundus. Areas of fine granular subretinal pigment deposits are seen in the anterior and midequatorial regions (**Fig. 10-20A–C**). Fluorescein angiography shows a hypofluorescent macula, and possibly localized patchy loss of RPE and choriocapillaris equatorial regions (**Fig. 10-20D**).

After a time, multifocal areas of RPE loss with concurrent underlying choriocapillaris atrophy in a scalloped pattern (**Fig. 10-21**) become more widespread and slowly progress over years to a generalized confluent loss, which for a time spares the macula, leaving an island of tissue (**Fig. 10-22**), occasionally areas nasal to the disc, and frequently the most anterior retina. As the RPE and choriocapillaris atrophy, uveal pigment is also lost, which results in variable pigmentation in areas of degeneration. Eventually, after many years, the macula succumbs to the disease. The UCLA RP Registry has several choroideremia patients in their fifties who have tiny 3° to 4° fields and 20/30 visual acuity; however, the Registry also has several patients in their thirties with as severe findings, so there is a spectrum of disease expression.

The fluorescein angiographic findings are the hallmark of the disease. The scalloped areas of RPE atrophy with choriocapillaris loss are hypofluorescent except for the prominent hyperfluorescent larger choroidal vessels that cross the area of missing tissue. The remaining RPE is granular appearing and hyperfluorescent; the edge of the remaining RPE and choriocapillaris usually is stained on later frames of the angiogram.

Visual fields early in the disease reveal multiple

scotomatous areas corresponding to the scalloped tissue loss seen on funduscopy. As the disease progresses, ring scotomata usually develop, and typical RP-type visual field loss is seen with preserved central fields and often temporal islands of vision (Fig. 3-3A–C). The anterior retina often has preserved function.*

The ERGs of patients with choroideremia are usually nonrecordable or, if recordable, are abnormal with a rod-cone pattern of degeneration. Sieving reviewed the ERG findings in 47 hemizygotic and 26 heterozygotic cases. He found that rod responses were markedly reduced while cone responses, even if in the normal range, have increased implicit

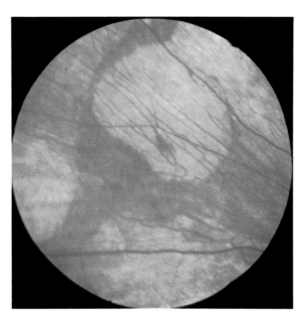

FIG. 10-21. Early choroderemia. A 19-year-old man with scalloped loss of RPE in equatorial regions.

---

*This late preservation of anterior retinal function in many patients may complicate a choroideremia victim's disability examination. The 360° remnant of anterior retina detects the target, giving the impression of a full field while the gigantic ring scotoma may not be found by the examiner. Other types of RP may also demonstrate this finding on visual field examination.

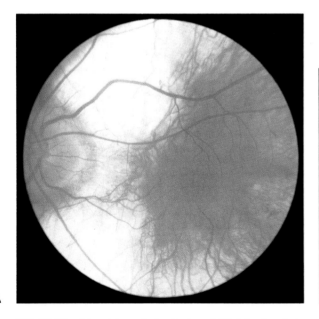

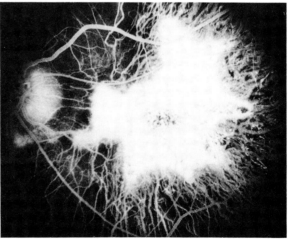

A   B

FIG. 10-22. Choroideremia fundus type I. (A) A fundus photograph, left eye of a 27-year-old man, demonstrating preservation of the RPE in the macula while there is generalized loss of retinal and uveal tissue outside the macula. (B) A fluorescein angiogram of the same area showing patency of the choriocapillaris in macular region while extramacular regions show loss of RPE and choriocapillaris and preservation of larger choroidal vessels.

times.[44] The ERG responses in the female carriers of choroideremia were mainly normal.

COMPOSITE PICTURE

CHOROIDEREMIA (Hemizygote Male)

Choroideremia patients represent approximately 6% of RP patients seen at UCLA. The average age for patients with choroideremia was 31 years, with, on average, a 21-year history of symptoms of night blindness and visual field loss. The mean visual acuity was 20/30, while the visual field with the IV-4 target averaged 24°, and ring scotomata and enlarged blind spots were common. Posterior subcapsular cataracts occurred, on average, in 31% of patients. The average refraction was $-3.53 +.076 \times 97$.

The ERG was recordable only in children in a rod-cone pattern. The mean final rod threshold was 4.1 log units of elevation.

On funduscopy, patients have pink discs with a cup-to-disc ratio of 0.21 (normal, 0.35), and near normal-sized retinal vessels. Temporal optic atrophy, defined as missing tissue, was seen in 29% of patients and nerve fiber alterations in 47% (some patients had such blond fundi that it was impossible to discern). Analysis of fluorescein angiography in 25 patients showed temporal optic atrophy (missing tissue) in 29%, optic nervehead telangiectasia in 50%, macular edema in 0%, parapapillary edema in 8%, vascular arcade edema in 15%, macular window defect in 21%, and paramacular window defect in 0%. All patients demonstrated on fluorescein angiography the characteristic scalloped loss of RPE and choriocapillaris in the equatorial and anterior retinal regions, leaving islands of intact macular tissue.

Three fundus appearances have been identified in patients with choroideremia. All patients have had pedigrees consistent with X-linked recessive inheritance, and the variability seen in fundus appearance can be regarded as variable expressivity of a single gene defect. Note that these patients have pink optic discs and minimally attenuated retinal vessels, even with advanced disease. Similar observations were demonstrated by Kustjens in his thesis on choroid-

eremia and gyrate atrophy[45]; he illustrated fundus changes with color fundus photographs but did not further characterize the various appearances in the disease.

Fundus Appearance I

Patients with fundus appearance I usually have fair complexions in general, although some patients have darker hair. On funduscopy, these patients have loss of the RPE and choroidal pigmentation, leaving only bare sclera and larger choroidal vessels (**Figs. 10-21, 10-22A**). Fluorescein angiography reveals confluent loss of choriocapillaris, with only larger choroidal vessels remaining patent (**Fig. 10-23B**).

Fundus Appearance II

Patients with fundus appearance II usually have more skin pigmentation, and if caucasian may have origins from the Mediterranean region or may have had an ancestor with more pigmentation (e.g., American Indian). There is a complete loss of RPE in affected areas, with partial loss of uveal pigmentation (**Fig. 10-23A&C**). The fluorescein angiogram pattern is identical to appearance I (**Fig. 10-23B&D**). About half of the patients followed at UCLA have this fundus appearance.

Fundus Appearance III

Three patients from two famlies have been seen at UCLA with fundus appearance type III. One pedigree was clearly X-linked recessive, but because the overall fundus appearance was a pink-orange with patches of black pigmentation throughout (**Fig. 10-24A–C**), the diagnosis was initially thought to be X-linked RP. However, the fluorescein angiogram clearly revealed the same characteristic pattern of confluent scalloped choriocapillaris loss seen in choroideremia (**Fig. 10-24D&E**).

Patients with fundus appearance III have loss of the RPE with only subtle loss of choroidal pigmentation. Subretinal pigment clumps may be seen.

HETEROZYGOTES FOR CHOROIDEREMIA (CARRIERS)

The carrier status for choroideremia is probably the easiest to detect among the various X-linked reces-

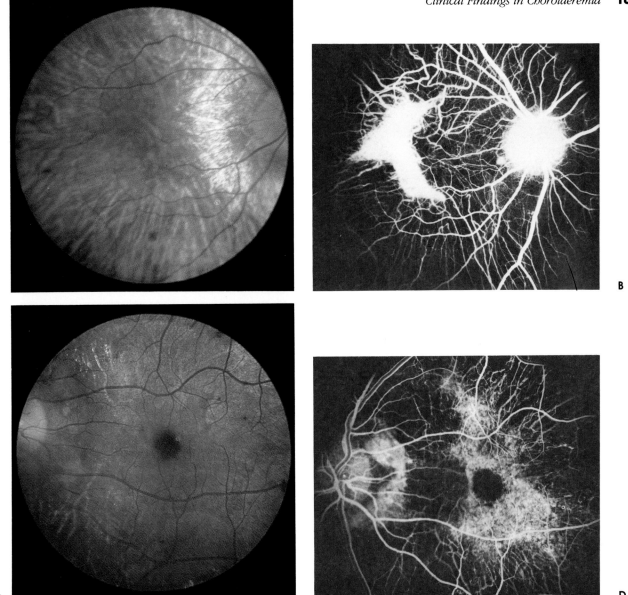

FIG. 10-23. Choroideremia fundus type II. (A) A fundus photograph, right eye, showing posterior pole of 28-year-old man with a small island of RPE in the macula. (B) A fluorescein angiogram of the same area shows patent choriocapillaris only in the area of intact RPE with preservation of larger choroidal vessels. (C) A fundus photograph, left eye of a 22-year-old Japanese man with obvious macular island of preserved RPE. (D) Fluorescein angiography confirms presence of choriocapillaris in the macula but also shows a parapapillary area of patent choriocapillaris, whereas on funduscopy, the RPE appears to be missing.

sive ophthalmologic diseases. In fact, many choroideremia carriers with the most marked fundus changes are referred with the diagnosis of RP but on testing generally are found to have normal ERGs and visual fields. Other carriers may have more subtle changes, with lightly scattered pigment deposits that

might be considered a normal variant except for the family history of choroideremia. The fundus changes appear to be age-related such that as carriers age they may show areas of retinal degeneration, which occasionally may be quite marked, with functional loss.

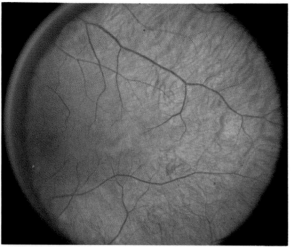

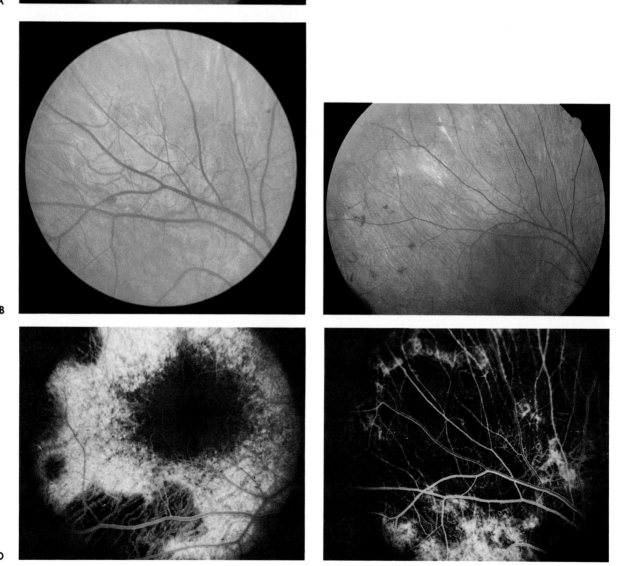

FIG. 10-24. Choroideremia fundus type III. (A–C) Fundus photographs of a 44-year-old man with subtle loss of choriocapillaris and RPE. Initially, because of the large clumps of pigment and the X-linked pedigree, it was thought that he had X-linked RP. (D,E) Fluorescein angiography, right eye, of the inferior and superior posterior pole and equatorial region, showing scalloped confluent loss of choriocapillaris, a pattern characteristic of choroideremia.

The clinical findings in the choroideremia carrier state are usually found because an affected male has been seen and female members of the family are examined to confirm the diagnosis or to answer, for genetic counseling reasons, which female members of the family are at risk for bearing affected offspring. A few carriers, mainly in later years, will have symptoms of night blindness, photophobia, and occasionally visual field loss. In looking at a dozen obligate carriers at UCLA, we found that there was a bimodal distribution for refractive error, with half the carriers showing marked hypermetropia averaging +3.10, while the others averaged plano. No correlation was seen between the amount of refractive error and the ERG or other clinical findings. Further studies may clarify the significance of the bimodal refractive error distribution.

Electrophysiological and psychophysical testing in a dozen obligate carriers was performed at UCLA. Patients' ages ranged from 23 to 71, with a mean of 45 years. Final rod thresholds mean value at 40 minutes was 0.56 log units elevated, which is a borderline abnormal value (normal is 0.0–0.3). However, two patients were more severely affected, with an elevation of the final rod threshold of 1.2 and 2.0 log units, respectively. Mean electro-oculogram values (light peak to dark trough) in five carriers were 213% (normal). Color vision was normal.

Asymmetry of normal values between eyes was common for all tests, which is unusual, since most patients typically have symmetrical test values between eyes.

The electroretinographic findings were particularly interesting because most carriers, even ones with marked fundus changes, had normal records when compared with age-matched normal controls. Two older carriers with obvious degenerative changes had subnormal ERG values.

Funduscopy revealed variable findings. The more severely affected carriers demonstrated focal areas of RPE loss (**Fig. 10-25***A*) and/or extensive subretinal granular pigment deposits (**Fig. 10-25***B&C*). Affected carriers have been reported.[46,47] A few carriers have minimal pigmentary changes (**Fig. 10-25***D*); these changes are often enhanced by the use of fluorescein angiography (**Fig. 10-25***E*).

Many carriers of choroideremia have other subtle changes which include nerve fiber layer dropout[48] and telangiectasia of the optic nervehead.

ORIGIN OF CHOROIDEREMIA

For many years it was assumed that the primary defect in choroideremia was vascular in origin, affecting primarily the choriocapillaris. However, there is increasing evidence that the basic defect is in the RPE. Krill in his text[49] reported histology for a carrier in which the abnormality was alternating areas of RPE atrophy and pigment clumping, with the retina and choroid otherwise appearing normal. A summary of three histopathologic cases can be found in Chapter 4.

Clinically, there are indications that the defect lies in the RPE; carriers clearly have their pigmentary granular changes in the RPE layer. In one 22-year-old Japanese man with choroideremia followed at UCLA, there was clear evidence that his RPE was showing depigmentation prior to the choriocapillaris atrophy (**Fig. 10-23***C&D*). Whatever process is affecting the RPE cells, it clearly involves Bruch's membrane, since the choriocapillaris atrophies soon after the RPE is lost.

Further evidence of an RPE abnormality was shown in a biochemical study from a 19-year-old man with choroideremia which revealed a reduction in interphotoreceptor retinoid-binding protein and cyclic AMP several-fold higher in the RPE-choroid complex of the affected eye compared with the control.[50]

OTHER OUTER RETINAL DYSTROPHIES WITH CHOROIDAL ATROPHY

Ayazi studied a three-generation family with "choroideremia," obesity, and congenital deafness; those affected were male, while carriers were asymptomatic, with normal ERGs but with peripapillary atrophy and pigmentary stippling.[51]

Van Den Bosch described a syndrome of choroideremia, mental deficiency, acrokeratosis verruciformis, anhidrosis, and skeletal deformity in a three-generation Dutch pedigree.[52]

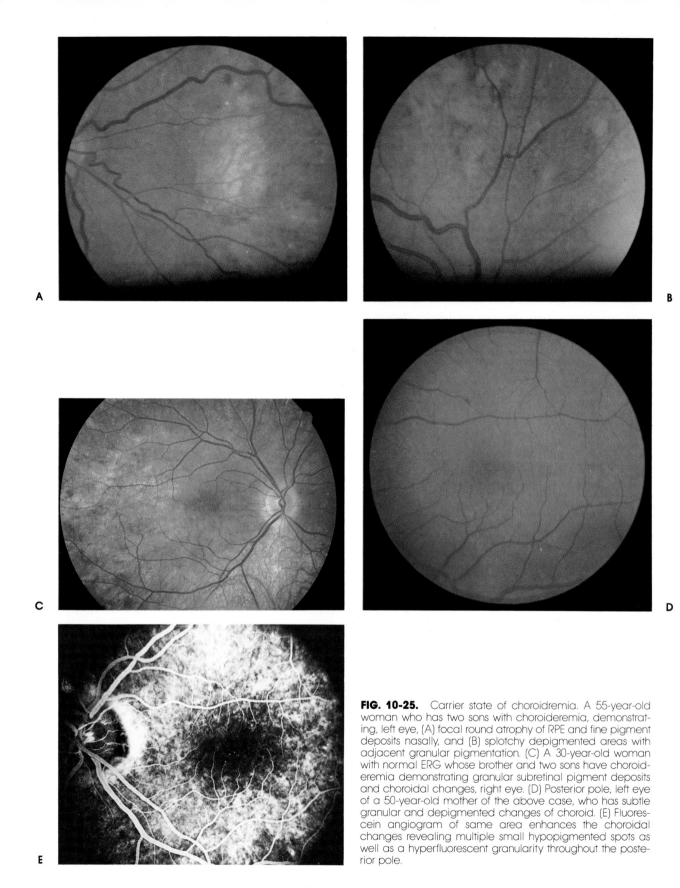

FIG. 10-25. Carrier state of choroidremia. A 55-year-old woman who has two sons with choroideremia, demonstrating, left eye, (A) focal round atrophy of RPE and fine pigment deposits nasally, and (B) splotchy depigmented areas with adjacent granular pigmentation. (C) A 30-year-old woman with normal ERG whose brother and two sons have choroideremia demonstrating granular subretinal pigment deposits and choroidal changes, right eye. (D) Posterior pole, left eye of a 50-year-old mother of the above case, who has subtle granular and depigmented changes of choroid. (E) Fluorescein angiogram of same area enhances the choroidal changes revealing multiple small hypopigmented spots as well as a hyperfluorescent granularity throughout the posterior pole.

DIFFERENTIAL DIAGNOSIS

The disease most similar to choroideremia is gyrate atrophy, which is covered in detail in Chapter 12. The major diagnostic difference is the inheritance pattern, with choroideremia patients being X-linked and gyrate atrophy patients having autosomal recessive inheritance. In addition, gyrate atrophy patients' RPE is hyperpigmented, while choroideremia patients tend to have a generalized depigmentation of the RPE. While both groups of patients tend to be myopic, gyrate atrophy patients tend to high myopia and are more likely to develop significant cataracts at an earlier age. A plasma ornithine or skin fibroblasts for ornithine aminotransferase activity will answer the question of whether gyrate atrophy is present.

Patients with Bietti's crystalline retinal dystrophy may exhibit a scalloped confluent loss of RPE in the paramacular posterior pole, and the fluorescein angiographic pattern in this area looks like that seen in choroideremia, but the crystalline deposits

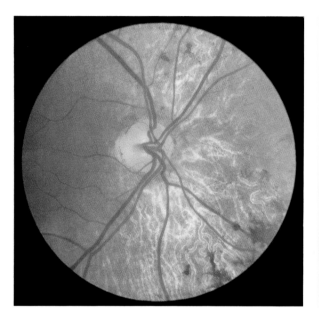

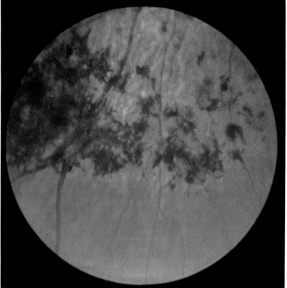

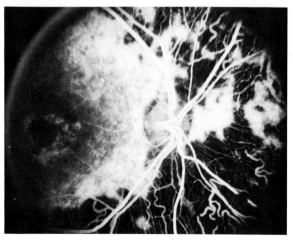

FIG. 10-26. Pericentral RP resembling choroideremia in a 72-year-old man. (A,B) Fundus photographs reveal pigmentary deposits and loss of RPE in equatorial regions. (C) Fluorescein angiography confirms confluent loss of choriocapillaris in posterior equatorial region only.

throughout the retina (and sometimes limbal cornea), the lack of equatorial involvement in the RPE–choriocapillaris atrophy, and the lack of an X-linked inheritance pattern are clear clues that choroideremia is not present.[53] Other diseases in which a scalloped loss of RPE and choriocapillaris may be seen include mitochondrial myopathy[54] and chorioretinopathy and pituitary dysfunction (CPD) syndrome.[55] Mellaril retinal toxicity may also demonstrate a nummular loss of RPE and choriocapillaris.[56]

Occasionally, patients with severe myopia will present with a scalloped loss of the RPE under the vascular arcades into the equatorial region[57]; no inheritance pattern has been established in these patients, and the progression is quite different from that of choroideremia patients. The onset of myopic retinal degeneration occurs in late adulthood, and there is usually a history of progressive myopia.

Rare RP patients of all inheritance patterns can demonstrate severe equatorial RPE and choriocapillaris atrophy which looks similar to the changes seen in choroideremia, but RPE is preserved in the posterior pole and anterior retina. One such patient is presented below:

CASE STUDY

This 71-year-old man first noted difficulty driving at night in his thirties, but had few peripheral vision problems until his forties. He reported typhoid fever at age 14, but there was no family history of ocular disorders. On examination, his visual acuity was OD 20/30-, OS 20/40 with mild nuclear sclerosis. Fundus examination revealed marked RPE and choroidal atrophy in the midperiphery with bone spicule deposits, parafoveal RPE atrophy, and preservation of the posterior pole and anterior retina RPE **(Fig. 10-26A&B)**. Fluorescein angiography of the posterior pole showed a pattern of RPE and choriocapillaris loss very similiar to that seen in choroideremia **(Fig. 10-26C)**. However, the negative family history and intact anterior to midequatorial retina with no scalloped loss of tissue, particularly at age 71, rule out the diagnosis of choroideremia in this patient.

REFERENCES

1. Usher CH: Bowman's lecture on a few hereditary eye affections. Trans Ophthalmol Soc UK 55:164–245, 1935
2. Kjerrumgaard E: Retinitis pigmentosa with special reference to otologic, neurologic and endocrine complications. Acta Opthalmol (Kbh) 26:55–65, 1948
3. Nettleship E: On retinitis pigmentosa and allied diseases. Roy Lond Ophthalmol Hosp Rep 17:333–426, 1908
4. Sorsby A: The incidence and causes of blindness in England and Wales 1948–1962. Reports on Public Health and Medical Subjects, no. 114, HMSO, London
5. Jay M: On the heredity of retinitis pigmentosa. Br J Ophthalmol 66:405–416, 1982
6. Fishman GA: Retinitis pigmentosa. Genetic percentages. Arch Ophthalmol 96:822–826, 1978
7. Voipio H, Gripenberg U, Raitta C et al: Retinitis pigmentosa; a preliminary report. Hereditas (Lund) 52:247, 1964
8. François J: Chorioretinal heredodegeneration. Proc Roy Soc Med 54:1109–1118, 1961
9. Ammann F, Klein D, Franceschetti A: Genetic and epidemiological investigations of pigmentary degeneration of the retina and allied disorders in Switzerland. J Neurol Sci 2:183–196, 1965
10. Jay B: Hereditary aspects of pigmentary retinopathy. Trans Ophthalmol Soc UK 92:173–178, 1972
11. Bird AC: X-linked retinitis pigmentosa. Br J Ophthalmol 59:177–199, 1975
12. Bhattacharya SS, Wright AF, Clayton JF et al: Close genetic linkage between X-linked retinitis pigmentosa and a restriction fragment length polymorphism identified by recombinant DNA probe L1.28. Nature 309:253–255, 1984
13. Mukai S, Dryja TP, Bruns GAP et al: Linkage between the X-linked retinitis pigmentosa locus and the L1.28 locus. Am J Ophthalmol 100:225–229, 1985
14. Nussbaum RL, Lewis RA, Lesko JG et al: Mapping X-linked ophthalmic diseases: II. Linkage relationship of X-linked retinitis pigmentosa to X chromosomal short arm markers. Hum Genet 70:45–50, 1985
15. Sorsby A, Savory M: Choroidal sclerosis: A possible intermediate sex-linked form. Br J Ophthalmol 40:90–95, 1956
16. Berson EL, Goldstein EB. The early receptor potential in sex-linked retinitis pigmentosa. Invest Ophthalmol Vis Sci 9:58–63, 1970
17. Krill AE: Observations of carriers of X-chromosomal-linked chorioretinal degenerations. Am J Ophthalmol 64:1029–1040, 1967
18. Diem M: Retinitis punctata albescens et pigmentosa. Klin Monatsbl Augenheilkd 53:371–379, 1914
19. Mann I: Developmental abnormalities of the eye, Fig 105. London, Cambridge University Press, 1937
20. Falls HF, Cotterman CW: Choroido-retinal degeneration. A sex-linked form in which heterozygous women exhibit a tapetal-like retinal reflex. Arch Ophthalmol 40:685–703, 1948
21. Goodman G, Ripps H, Siegel IM: Sex-linked ocular disorders: Trait expressivity in males and carrier females. Arch Ophthalmol 73:387–398, 1965
22. Krill AE: X-chromosomal-linked diseases affecting the eye: Status of the heterozygote female. Trans Am Ophthalmol Soc 67:535–608, 1969
23. Fishman GA, Weinberg AB, McMahon TT: X-linked recessive retinitis pigmentosa: Clinical characteristics of carriers. Arch Ophthalmol 104:1329–1335, 1986

24. Schappert-Kimmijser J: Les Dégénérescences tapéto-rétiniennes du type X chromosomal aux Pays-Bas. Bull Soc Fran Ophtal 76:122–129, 1963
25. Gieser DK, Fishman GA, Cunha-Vaz J: X-linked recessive retinitis pigmentosa and vitreous fluorophotometry. Arch Ophthalmol 93:307–310, 1980
26. Ricci A, Ammann F, Franceschetti A: Reflet taptoderversible (phnomenomne de Mizuno inverse) chez desconductrices de rtinopathie pigmentaire rcessive lie au sexe. Bull Soc Fran Ophtal 76:31, 1963
27. Arden GB, Carter RM, Hogg CR et al: A modified ERG technique and the results obtained in X-linked retinitis pigmentosa. Br J Ophthalmol 67:419–430, 1983
28. Berson EL, Rosen JB, Siminoff EA: Electroretinographic testing as an aid in detection of carriers of X-chromosome-linked retinitis pigmentosa. Am J Ophthalmol 87:460–468, 1979
29. Hyman VN, Weale RA: Rhodopsin density and visual threshold in retinitis pigmentosa. Am J Ophthalmol 75:822–832, 1973
30. Szamier RB, Berson EL, Klein R et al: Sex-linked retinitis pigmentosa: Ultrastructure of photoreceptors and pigment epithelium. Invest Ophthalmol Vis Sci 18:145–160, 1979
31. Massof RW, Finkelstein D: Vision threshold profiles in X-linked retinitis pigmentosa. Invest Ophthalmol Vis Sci 18:426–429, 1979
32. Tanino T, Katsumi O, Hirose T: Electrophysiological similarities between the eyes with x-linked recessive retinoschisis. Doc Ophthalmol 60:149–148, 1985
33. Heckenlively JR, Martin DA, Rosenbaum AL: Loss of electroretinographic oscillatory potentials, optic atrophy, and dysplasia in congenital stationary night blindness. Am J Ophthalmol 96:526–534, 1983
34. Sharpe D, Arden G, Bird AC et al: X-linked congenital stationary night blindness. (submitted)
35. Mauthner L: Ein Fall von Choroideremia. Berd Naturw Med Ver Innsbruck 2:191, 1871
36. Zorn B: Ueber familiare atypische Pigment degeneration der Netzhaut (totale Aderhautatrophie). Graefes Arch Ophthalmol 101:1–13, 1920
37. Schutzbach M: Uber erbliche Aderhaut-Netzhauterkrankung. Graefes Arch Ophthalmol 138:315–331, 1938
38. Goedbloed J: Mode of inheritance of choroideremia. Ophthalmologica 104:308, 1942
39. Waardenburg PJ: Choroideremie als Erbmerkmal. Acta Ophthalmol 20:235, 1942
40. McCulloch C, McCulloch RJP: A hereditary and clinical study of choroideremia. Trans Am Acad Ophthalmol Otolaryngol 542:160–190, 1948
41. Shapiro I, Gorlin RJ: X-linked choroidal sclerosis: A stage of choroideremia. Minn Med 57:259–262, 1974
42. Takki K: Gyrate atrophy of the choroid and retina associated with hyperornithinemia. Br J Ophthalmol 58:3–23, 1974
43. Takki K: Differential diagnosis between the primary total choroidal vascular atrophies. Br J Ophthalmol 58:24–35, 1974
44. Sieving PA, Niffennegger JH, Berson, EL: Electroretinographic findings in selected pedigrees with choroideremia. Am J Ophthalmol 101:361–367, 1986
45. Kurstejens JH: Choroideremia and gyrate atrophy of the choroid and retina. Doc Ophthalmol l9(suppl):1–122, 1965
46. Harris GS, Miller JR: Choroideremia. Visual defects in a heterozygote. Arch Ophthalmol 80:423–429, 1968
47. Fraser GR, Friedmann AI: Choroideremia in a female. Br Med J 2:732, 1968
48. Newman N, Stone R, Heckenlively JR: NFL defects in outer retinal disease. (submitted)
49. Krill AE: Hereditary Retinal and Choroidal Diseases, vol II, p 1036. Harper & Row, Hagerstown, l977
50 Rodrigues MM, Ballintine EJ, Wiggert BN et al: Choroideremia: A clinical, electron microscopic, and biochemical report. Ophthalmology 91:873–883, 1984
51. Ayazi S: Choroideremia, obesity, and congenital deafness. Am J Ophthalmol 92:63–69, 1981
52. van den Bosch J: A new syndrome in three generations of a Dutch family. Ophthalmologica 137:422–423, 1959
53. Welch RB: Bietti's tapetoretinal degeneration with marginal corneal dystrophy: Crystalline retinopathy. Trans Am Ophthalmol Soc 75:164–179, 1977
54. Unpublished data, ACB
55. Judisch GF, Lowry RB, Hanson JW et al: Chorioretinopathy and pituitary dysfunction. The CPD syndrome. Arch Ophthalmol 99:253–256, 1981
56. Meredith TA, Aaberg TM, Willerson WD: Progressive chorioretinopathy after receiving thioridazine. Arch Ophthalmol 96:1172–1176, 1978
57. Heckenlively J: Possible syndrome of high myopia with retinal degeneration, cataract, manic depression, and elevated aminio acids. Metab Pediatr Syst Ophthalmol 4:155–160, 1980

11

Simplex Retinitis Pigmentosa (Nonhereditary Pigmentary Retinopathies)

JOHN R. HECKENLIVELY

Isolated retinitis pigmentosa (RP) cases or patients whose inheritance is poorly defined are the largest "type" of RP seen by most ophthalmologists. It can be presumed that some cases represent acquired disease while others are hereditary with no family history of RP known. The frequency of simplex or multiplex cases has been reported to range from 18% to 58% with several large studies reporting about 39%.[1-4] At UCLA, simplex and multiplex cases on one survey constituted 42% of 609 patients (see Table 2-6).

When there is only one (isolated) affected member in a family, the term *simplex* is employed; if more than one sibling is affected and no other family member outside of the sibship is known to have RP, then the term *multiplex* is used. The rationale for the use of these terms and a discussion of simplex and multiplex RP can be found in Chapter 2.

In classifying the types of RP, Mendelian inheritance pattern plays an important role. The inheritance of most simplex/multiplex cases cannot be ascertained unless there is a highly characteristic finding

such as choroideremia or congenital RP with macular colobomata. Each case has to be judged on its own merits.

COMPOSITE PICTURE

SIMPLEX ROD-CONE DEGENERATION*

The average age of onset of symptoms was 17.7 years, with a duration of 14.2 years before the diagnosis of RP was made. The mean visual acuity was 20/40 with a mean refractive error of $-2.71 +1.14 \times 96$. Various types of cataracts were seen: anterior subcapsular, 2%; nuclear sclerotic, 12%; and posterior subcapsular, 39%. The electroretinogram (ERG) was recordable in 27 of 64, while the mean final rod threshold after 40 minutes of dark adaptation was 4.02 log units above normal. The average visual field with the IV-4 isopter was 10° on initial presentation. Fundus photography or fluorescein angiography revealed the following: macular edema, 16%; macular window defect, 24%; paramacular window defect,

1%; parapapillary edema, 27%; nerve fiber alterations, 47%; vascular arcade edema, 39%; optic nervehead telangiectasia, 50%; temporal optic atrophy, 50%; and macular hypofluorescence, 61%.

SIMPLEX CONE-ROD DEGENERATION (RP TYPE)*

The average age of onset of symptoms was 26.5 years and the average age for diagnoses was 40.6 years. The mean visual acuity was 20/30 with a mean refraction of −4.09 +1.52 ×97. The ERG was recordable in 19 of 26 cases, with a mean final rod threshold of 2.3 log units above normal at 12° above fixation. Most patients did not have subjective night blindness although many noticed problems with dark adaptation. The mean size of the visual field with a IV-4 isopter was 20.5°. On fundus photography or fluorescein angiography, the following parameters were found: macular edema, 15%; macular hypofluorescence, 69%; macular window defect, 15%; paramacular window defect, 0%; parapapillary edema, I5%; vascular arcade edema, 27%; optic nervehead telangiectasia, 54%; and temporal optic atrophy, 58%.

---

*These data are presented with some reservation, since simplex RP is a mixture of RP types; however, there are still distinguishing features which eventually may allow for a more definitive diagnosis in these patients.

PIGMENTED PARAVENOUS RETINOCHOROIDAL ATROPHY (PPRCA)

One type of pigmentary retinopathy, pigmented paravenous retinochoroidal atrophy (PPRCA), to date generally has been found to occur without an inheritance pattern. Both progressive and nonprogressive forms have been reported, and thus PPRCA will be considered in this chapter as one identifiable type of simplex pigmentary retinopathy. It should be noted that most forms of simplex/multiplex RP are not cases of PPRCA (Table 2-6).

There are two exceptions in the literature in which patients with the PPRCA pattern have been found to have other affected family members. Skalka reported a father and son,[5] and Traboulsi reported a mother and three of her children with the PPRCA pattern.[6] It was suggested that Skalka's cases could have represented Wagner's disease,[7,8] an autosomal dominant disorder, while Traboulsi's cases could be examples of pseudodominance or autosomal dominant inheritance. These two familial examples are still the exception to the rule.

PPRCA is a degenerative pattern with paravenous localization of retinal pigment epithelial degeneration and pigment deposition. The cause and pathophysiologic mechanisms of this condition are not known, but to date no definite hereditary form of this disease has been clearly demonstrated. The one slight exception to this statement is in Stickler syndrome in which some patients have a PPRCA pattern in localized areas of the retina, while other areas are free of the pattern. At UCLA and the Berman-Gund laboratory in about 40 cases, no hereditary PPRCA has been found to date.[9,10] In fact, both research centers have seen the same PPRCA patient who has an identical twin free of retinal disease, while the affected patient has a diffuse pigmentary retinopathy in one eye and a definite PPRCA pattern in the other (**Fig. 11-1A&B**). The PPRCA pattern has been seen in a well-documented case of measles retinopathy (**Fig. 11-2**), a further indication of a nonhereditary etiology for these cases.[11]

PPRCA was first reported by Brown as retinochoroiditis radiata[12] and has been described under a variety of names, including paravenous retinal degeneration, parvenous retinochoroidal atrophy, and congenital pigmentation of the retina.[13] Many cases of helicoid peripapillary chorioretinal degeneration have marked paravenous atrophy (**Fig. 11-3A&B**) and may be what other researchers would term PPRCA.[14] There are reports that this entity is stationary and geographic in nature[15,16] and other reports that it is progressive.[17,18] Many researchers prefer to give the PPRCA diagnosis only to the stationary type. One of the reasons that PPRCA is so poorly understood is that it is relatively rare, with about five dozen cases reported in the world literature.

Some cases are asymptomatic and are picked up on fundus examination. These cases tend to be nonprogressive, but in all cases, serial visual fields must

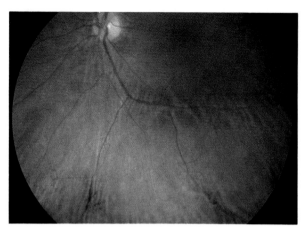

A

B

FIG. 11-1. Monocular pigmented paravenous retinochoroidal atrophy in a 28-year-old woman whose identical twin is completely normal. *(A)* Right eye, nasal retina shows heavy bone spicule-like pigmentary pattern, while *(B)* left eye demonstrates mild paravenous pigmentation.

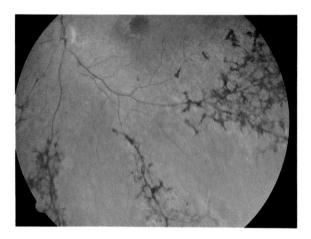

FIG. 11-2. Pigmented paravenous retinochoroidal atrophy pattern of degeneration in a woman who had a well-documented case of rubeola retinopathy in childhood.[11]

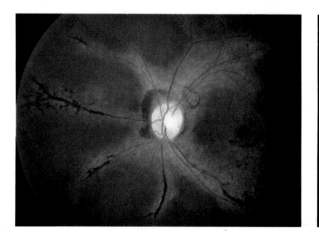
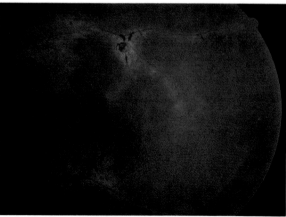

A

B

FIG. 11-3. Helicoid peripapillary and pigmented paravenous retinochoroidal atrophy degeneration in a 26-year-old woman with cone-rod degeneration. *(A)* Posterior pole, left eye, shows retinal degeneration under vascular arcades and peripapillary area which extends *(B)* into equatorial regions under retinal veins.

be performed over many years before it can be assumed that the disorder is the stationary variety. Some cases have rod-cone and others cone-rod patterns on the ERG. On visual field testing, some patients-have enlarged blind spots, ring scotomata, radially oriented scotomata corresponding to the paravenous atrophic areas, and peripheral constriction. The final rod threshold is quite elevated in most patients, and even retinal areas which are free of obvious disease show elevations of the final rod threshold.

Some cases have demonstrated asymmetry between eyes, which is characteristic of inflammatory insults to the retina rather than a hereditary disease.

PSEUDORETINITIS PIGMENTOSA

There are a number of disorders that may have a pigmentary retinopathy or mimic RP but are not called RP because another diagnosis is known to be present. Carr has classified the forms of pseudoretinitis pigmentosa into idiopathic, acquired, and hereditary forms.[19]

IDIOPATHIC PSEUDORETINITIS PIGMENTOSA

The idiopathic types of pseudoretinitis pigmentosa include pigmented paravenous retinochoroidal atrophy, birdshot retinochoroidal atrophy, pericentral RP, reticular degeneration of the elderly, advanced cases of Harada's disease, and some cases in which there is residual retinal damage from toxemia of pregnancy or resolution of an exudative retinal detachment.

Acquired forms of pseudoretinitis pigmentosa may be the result of ocular infection, drug toxicity, or trauma. The most common known infectious forms are leutic chorioretinitis and measles retinopathy. The former tends to be progressive, while the latter may be stationary.

LEUTIC CHORIORETINITIS

Whenever a patient with a pigmentary retinopathy presents with no family history, and particularly if there is asymmetric involvement on the visual field

or ERG, an FTA-ABS blood test is needed to rule out syphilitic chorioretinitis. Some patients who are inadequately treated for central nervous system involvement or who may have been given antibiotics for other reasons, may clear their VDRL, but the retina may continue to show degeneration. The FTA-ABS test usually remains positive in these cases, and it is the dignositic test of choice for leutic chorioretinitis. Some patients have a history of recurrent or chronic uveitis.

Congenital syphilis frequently has a diffuse salt-and-pepper pigmentary degenerative pattern (**Fig. 11-4**) with severely attenuated visual fields. Some patients with acquired leutic chorioretinitis may have a fundus appearance similar to choroidal sclerosis with scattered bone spicules and yellow, apparently nonperfused choroidal vessels (**Fig. 11-5***A&B*), but often have asymmetric visual fields.[20] A few patients with leutic chorioretinitis have a fundus appearance that looks like typical RP, but there is no family history.

Other inflammatory or infectious disorders that occasionally result in a pigmentary retinopathy

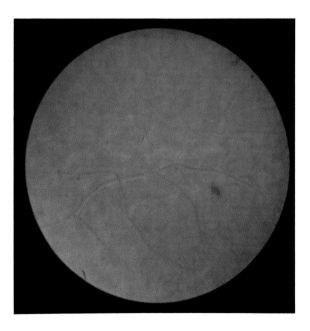

FIG. 11-4. Congenital syphilis. A 45-year-old woman with 12° fields with a large target and 20/60 visual acuity in both eyes. Fundus photograph shows diffuse retinal atrophy with granularity to the retinal pigment epithelium.

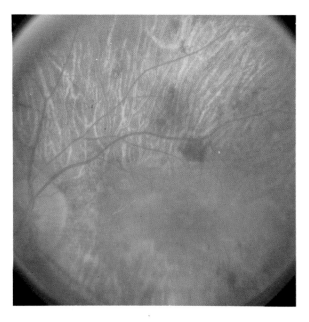

A

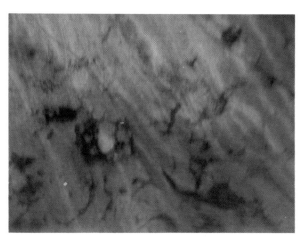

B

FIG. 11-5. Acquired syphilitic chorioretinitis. A 67-year-old woman who recalled that her former husband had been treated for syphilis 20 years previously. Her visual acuity was OD light perception, OS 20/50 + 2. The visual fields were asymmetric, OD none, OS 35° with the III-4 isopter. Fundus photographs: *(A)* Left eye, showing RPE atrophy and apparent choroidal sclerosis outside the macular area where the RPE is preserved. The patient's fluorescein angiogram, however, showed that the choroidal vessels were patent. *(B)* Right eye, equatorial view demonstrating bone spicule-like pigment deposition similar to that of RP.

which may mimic retinitis pigmentosa include measles retinopathy, disseminated choroiditis, chorioretinitis, serpiginous or geographic atrophy. Many of these conditions have asymmetric involvement, which is a clue to the nongenetic nature of the illness.

Patients with rubella retinopathy commonly have scattered pigmentary deposits, but more often subretinal clumps or salt-and-pepper pigmentation (**Fig. 11-6A–E**).[21] On occasion, the pigmentation may be bone spicule-like, and the retinal vessel caliber tends to be more normal. Some patients will present with full or partial deafness, and Usher's syndrome will be in the differential diagnosis until the patient has been followed for a period of years with visual fields to document the lack of progression of the disorder. Often, however, the patient is aware of the diagnosis since there are other manifestations or sequelae of rubella, or the mother was known to have the disease during pregnancy.

Obenour performed ERGs in 30 eyes with rubella retinopathy unassociated with other ocular defects and found that the ERGs were normal in 28 and borderline in the other 2.[22] Berson has emphasized that patients with chorioretinal scars may have decreased photopic and scotopic ERG amplitudes but that the implicit times are normal.[23] Certainly, in stable or nonprogressive chorioretinal disease (usually following a single insult) this is true. A careful study, however, in a large population of pseudoretinitis pigmentosa patients might find a few exceptions to this rule.

DRUG TOXICITIES

A few drugs dispensed for systemic disease may have an associated retinal toxicity in susceptible individuals resulting in a pigmentary retinopathy. The most common ones include chloroquine, hydroxychloroquine, thioridazine (Mellaril), stelazine, chlorpromazine, Indomethacin, and Tomoxifen.[24–26]

Chloroquine and its derivatives, originally prescribed for malaria, are among the most frequently encountered class of drugs with the potential for retinal toxicity, since they are often used for chronic treatment of collagen vascular disease and arthritis.

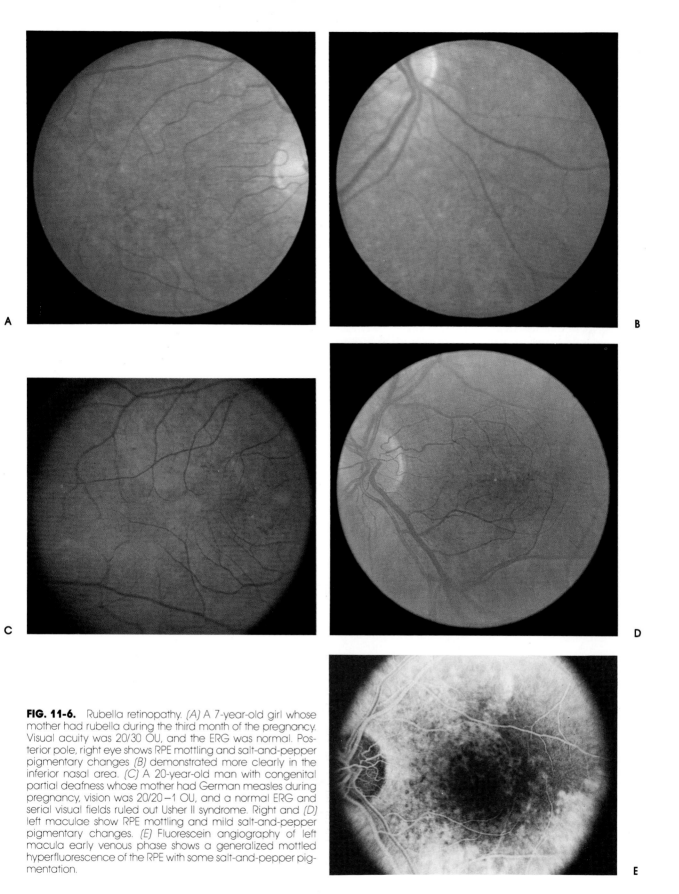

FIG. 11-6. Rubella retinopathy. *(A)* A 7-year-old girl whose mother had rubella during the third month of the pregnancy. Visual acuity was 20/30 OU, and the ERG was normal. Posterior pole, right eye shows RPE mottling and salt-and-pepper pigmentary changes *(B)* demonstrated more clearly in the inferior nasal area. *(C)* A 20-year-old man with congenital partial deafness whose mother had German measles during pregnancy, vision was 20/20−1 OU, and a normal ERG and serial visual fields ruled out Usher II syndrome. Right and *(D)* left maculae show RPE mottling and mild salt-and-pepper pigmentary changes. *(E)* Fluorescein angiography of left macula early venous phase shows a generalized mottled hyperfluorescence of the RPE with some salt-and-pepper pigmentation.

While most patients show no retinal toxicity, a few develop mottled retinal pigment epithelial areas and bull's-eye macular lesions which may progress to atrophic macular scars similar to advanced fundus flavimaculatus with central involvement. A rare patient will develop a pigmented retinopathy.[27] Studies have suggested a relationship between accumulated drug (total dose) and occurrence of retinopathy.[28] Krill reported that the ERG was normal to subnormal in early to intermediate stages of chloroquine retinopathy, and was abnormal in advanced cases.[29]

With the advent of use of hydroxychloroquine, the incidence of retinal toxicity has decreased. Increased awareness and prophylactic testing also have helped to better regulate dosage to avoid retinal toxicity. The retinal degeneration produced by chloroquine is usually reversible if diagnosed in its early stages. Clinically, the most common method of following patients for retinal toxicity is examining for loss of the foveal reflex or increased granularity of the RPE of the macula.[30] At UCLA we have followed large numbers of patients on chloroquine and have found that early retinal toxicity (in a reversible stage) is easily identified by serial testing using a combination of the electro-oculogram and the Farnsworth 100-hue color vision test. One distinct drawback in using these two tests is that their use on a long-term basis is relatively expensive and time-consuming.[31]

In a few patients, thioridazine and stelazine have been found to be associated with diffuse damage and discrete nummular loss of choriocapillaris and RPE.[32,33] Because lower doses are now commonly used, cases of retinal toxicity from thioridazine are infrequent, and prophylactic testing is not usually done nor known to be effective in this group of patients.

Chlorpromazine-related toxicity has been reported in the cornea, lens, and retina and is proportional to total drug given. Retinal toxicity manifests as a granular or salt-and-pepper change in the RPE. Retinal function often remains good despite extensive retinal pigmentary changes.[34,35]

HEREDITARY FORMS OF PSEUDORETINITIS PIGMENTOSA

There are several hereditary retinal diseases that, at times, closely resemble RP. Some of the most striking

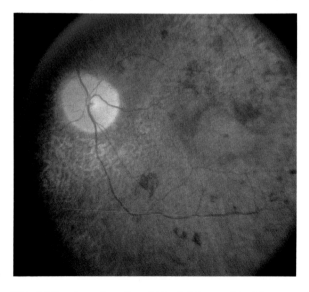

A

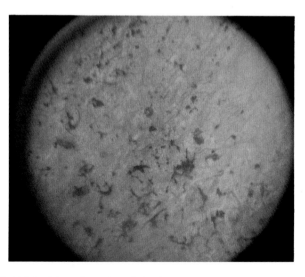

B

FIG. 11-7. Juvenile retinoschisis. A 54-year-old white man with X-linked juvenile retinoschisis demonstrated a pigmentary retinopathy similar to RP. Because of a definite X-linked recessive pedigree, the initial diagnosis was incorrectly thought to be X-linked RP, but examination of the patient's grandsons showed typical changes of juvenile retinoschisis. The visual acuity was OD light perception, OS 20/200. *(A)* Left eye shows a diffuse retinal atrophy, pigmentary deposits, and paramacular RPE preservation; *(B)* right eye, equatorial view with pigmentary bone spicule-like deposition.

are advanced cases of juvenile retinoschisis. These male patients may present with strong X-linked recessive pedigrees, night blindness, a pigmentary retinopathy, and a long history of visual dysfunction (**Fig. 11-7A&B**). The correct diagnosis is established by examining other younger affected male members in the family in whom macular and peripheral schisis changes should be apparent.[36]

Reticular dystrophy of the RPE may be inherited in the autosomal recessive or dominant fashion and has a characteristic "fishnet" pigment clumping at the level of the RPE.[37,38] In the dominant form, the ERG is reported to be normal, while the EOG and dark adaptation are usually abnormal in affected individuals.

Severe cases of senile reticular degeneration (not known to be related to reticular dystrophy) can present like a mild form of RP; patients are mildly night-blind and have slightly constricted visual fields, and their ERGs are subnormal (**Fig. 11-8**). Since all are elderly, there is no reason for the patient to be seriously concerned about the RP-like findings, since the disease does not seriously threaten the peripheral visual function. Macular degeneration, however, occurs more often in reticular degeneration patients than in elderly patients free of peripheral changes.

There are a number of autosomal dominant vitreoretinal degenerations, including Wagner's disease, Stickler syndrome, snowflake vitreoretinal degeneration, and familial exudative vitreoretinopathy, all of which can have a pigmentary retinopathy, particularly in more advanced stages.

Patients with severe fundus flavimaculatus rarely may have pigment clumps scattered throughout the equatorial region, usually have atrophy of the retina in the macula (often of the entire posterior pole), and may have residual flecks next to atrophic edges of the posterior pole. Fluorescein angiography may show the dark choroid sign.

Patients with stationary night blindness may present with a strong history of nyctalopia, but investigation with visual field tests, funduscopy, and electrophysiological studies will sort out most initially; a few stationary night blindness patients may have findings that leave the diagnosis in question, and may have to be followed for signs of progression over 5 or even 10 years to permanently settle the

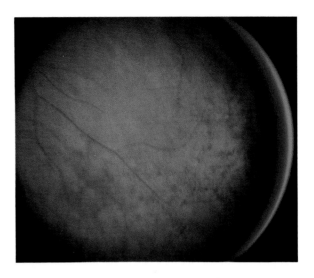

FIG. 11-8. Reticular degeneration. An 86-year-old man with bilateral atrophic macular degeneration and extensive "fishnet" shaped pigmentary deposits in the peripheral retina. The ERG and visual fields were subnormal for the patient's age-group.

issue, although they seldom have retinal pigment epithelial changes of consequence.

One form of congenital stationary night blindness, fundus albipunctatus, may be confused with retinitis punctata albescens; visual field and electrophysiological testing will differentiate these two entities, both of which have tiny whitish yellow flecks or dots scattered in a radial pattern from the posterior pole. Fundus albipunctatus patients have normal visual fields, and after prolonged dark adaptation, their scotopic ERG returns to normal values, while retinitis punctata albescens patients have constricted visual fields and ERGs that do not improve with dark adaptation (see Chapter 9).

Finally, a rare patient with advanced cone degeneration may present with peripheral pigmentary deposits or even bone spicules, but the family history, visual fields, and ERG should differentiate most of these patients.

UNIOCULAR RETINITIS PIGMENTOSA

While there have been a number of reports of uniocular RP, this entity has never been demonstrated in hereditary forms, and thus the term "uniocular

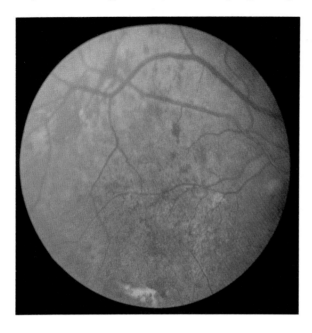

FIG. 11-9. Uniocular pigmentary retinopathy, right eye, in a 32-year-old man who had retinal detachment repair 7 years previously.

pigmentary retinopathy" would be preferred. Occasionally, a patient may have asymmetric ocular involvement from inflammatory disease with an initial presentation of a uniocular pigmentary retinopathy in which the second eye shows pigmentary changes after a number of years. The most common causes of unilateral pigmentary retinopathy have proven to be blunt trauma,[39,40] parasitic infection, retained foreign bodies, resolved exudative or rhegematogenous retinal detachments (**Fig. 11-9**), choroidal or retinal vascular occlusions, or chorioretinitis. Hereditary retinal diseases are symmetric in presentation, and when this rule is broken, other causes should be carefully evaluated.

REFERENCES

1. Boughman JA, Caldwell RJ: Genetic and clinical characterization of a survey population with retinitis pigmentosa. Prog Clin Biol Res pp 147–166, 1982
2. Jay B: Hereditary aspects of pigmentary retinopathy. Trans Ophthalmol Soc UK 92:173–178, 1972
3. Voipio H, Gripenberg V, Raitta C et al: Retinitis pigmentosa; a preliminary report. Hereditas 52:247, 1964
4. Fishman GA: Retinitis pigmentosa: Genetic percentages. Arch Ophthalmol 96:822–826, 1978
5. Skalka HW: Hereditary pigmented paravenous retinochoroidal atrophy. Am J Ophthalmol 87:286–291, 1979
6. Traboulsi E, Maumenee IH: Arch Ophthalmol 104:1636–1640, 1986
7. Cotlier E: Pigmented retinochoroidal atrophy, cases of Wagner's disease? (letter to editor) Am J Ophthalmol 88:134–135, 1979
8. Heckenlively J: Hereditary pigmented paravenous retinochoroidal atrophy. (letter to editor) Am J Ophthalmol 88:136, 1979
9. Berson E: Personal communication, June, l984
10. Heckenlively JR, Kokame GT: Pigmented paravenous retinochoroidal atrophy; clinical and electrophysiological findings. Doc Ophthalmol Proc Ser 40:235–241, 1985
11. Foxman SG, Heckenlively JR, Sinclair SH: Rubeola reti-

nopathy and pigmented paravenous retinochoroidalatrophy. Am J Ophthalmol 99:605–606, 1985
12. Brown TH: Retino-choroiditis radiata. Br J Ophthalmol 21:645–648, 1937
13. Krill AE: Incomplete rod-cone degenerations. In Krill AE, Archer D (eds): Krill's Hereditary Retinal and Choroidal Diseases, p 625. Hagerstown, Harper & Row, l977
14. Franceschetti A: A curious affection of the fundusoculi: Helicoid peripapillary chorioretinal degeneration. It's relation to pigmentary paravenous chorioretinaldegeneration. Doc Ophthalmol 16:81–110, 1962
15. Noble KG, Carr RE: Pigmented paravenous chorioretinal atrophy. Am J Ophthalmol 96:338–344, 1983
16. Chisholm IA, Dudgeon J: Pigmented paravenous retinochoroidal atrophy. Br J Ophthalmol 57:584–587, 1973
17. Pearlman JT, Heckenlively JR, Bastek JV: Progressive nature of pigmented paravenous retinochoroidal atrophy. Am J Ophthalmol 85:215–217, 1978
18. François J, DeRouck A: Paravenous pigmentary retinopathy. Doc Ophthalmol Proc Ser 10:281–289, 1976
19. Carr RE: Primary retinal degenerations. In Duane T, Jaeger E (eds): Clinical Ophthalmology. Philadelphia, JB Lippincott, 1984
20. Heckenlively JR: Secondary retinitis pigmentosa (syphilis).

Doc Ophthalmol Proc Ser 13:245–255, 1976

21. Metz HS, Harkey ME: Pigmentary retinopathy following maternal measles (Morbilli) infection. Am J Ophthalmol 66:1107–1110, 1968
22. Obenour LC: The electroretinogram in rubella retinopathy. Int Ophthalmol Clin 12:105–110, 1972
23. Berson EL: Electroretinographic testing as an aid in determining visual prognosis in families with hereditary retinal degenerations. In Pruett RC, Regan CDJ (eds): Retina Congress, pp 41–53. New York, Appleton-Century-Crofts, 1974
24. Burns CA: Indomethacin, reduced retinal sensitivity and corneal deposits. Am J Ophthalmol 66:825–835, 1968
25. Henkes HE, van Lith GHM, Canta LR: Indomethacin retinopathy. Am J Ophthalmol 73:846–856, 1972
26. Carr RE, Siegel IM: Retinal function in patients treated with indomethacin. Am J Ophthalmol 75:302–306, 1973
27. Brinkley JR, Dubois EL, Ryan RJ: Long-term course of chloroquine retinopathy after cessation of medication. Am J Ophthalmol 88:1–11, 1979
28. Nylander ULF: Ocular damage in chloroquine therapy. Acta Ophthalmol 44:335–348, 1965
29. Krill AE, Potts AM, Johanson CE: Chloroquine retinopathy. Investigation of discrepancy between dark adaptation and electroretinographic findings in advanced stages. Am J Ophthalmol 71:530–543, 1971
30. Carr RE, Henkind P, Rothfield N et al: Ocular toxicity of antimalarial drugs. Am J Ophthalmol 66:738–744, 1968
31. Infante R, Martin DA, Heckenlively JR. Hydroxychloroquine and retinal toxicity. Doc Ophthalmol Proc Ser 37:121–126, 1983
32. Cameron ME, Lawrence JM, Olrich JG: Thioridazine (Melleril) retinopathy. Br J Ophthalmol 56:131–134, 1972
33. Meredith TA, Aaberg TM, Willerson WD: Progressive chorioretinopathy after receiving thioridazine. Arch Ophthalmol 96:1172–1176, 1978
34. Siddal JR: The ocular toxic findings with prolonged and high dosage chlorpromazine intake. Arch Ophthalmol 74:460–464, 1965
35. Mathalone MBR: Eye and skin changes in psychiatric patients treated with chlorpromazine. Br J Ophthalmol 51:86–93, 1967
36. Tanino T, Katsumi O, Hirose T: Electrophysiological similarities between two eyes with X-linked recessive retinoschisis. Doc Ophthalmol 60:149–161, 1985
37. Sjogren H: Dystrophia reticularis laminae pigmentosae retinae. Acta Ophthalmol 28:279–295, 1950
38. Kingham JD, Fenzl RE, Willerson D et al: Reticular dystrophy of the retinal pigment epithelium; clinical and electrophysiologic study of three generations. Arch Ophthalmol 96:1177–1184, 1978
39. Cogan DG: Pseudoretinitis pigmentosa. Arch Ophthalmol 81:45–53, 1969
40. Bastek JV, Foos RY, Heckenlively J: Traumatic pigmentary retinopathy. Am J Ophthalmol 92:621–624, 1981

12

Gyrate Atrophy of the Choroid and Retina

RICHARD G. WELEBER
NANCY G. KENNAWAY

Gyrate atrophy of the choroid and retina is one of several disorders related to retinitis pigmentosa (RP) which are genetically determined and which produce slow deterioration of the retina (and choroid) with loss of retinal function and eventual blindness. Of the 80 to 100 disorders allied with RP, the biochemical defect is understood to the degree that rational treatment protocols have been proposed and tested in only three—abetalipoproteinemia, Refsum's disease, and gyrate atrophy. The diagnosis of gyrate atrophy can be suspected to a high degree of confidence on clinical grounds. However, measurement of serum or plasma amino acids to determine whether ornithine levels are high will establish the diagnosis with certainty. Although the precise pathophysiology of the disorder has yet to be worked out, the underlying enzyme deficiency is known. Heterogeneity exists even within the clinical picture of gyrate atrophy. Some forms are responsive and others nonresponsive to vitamin B_6 therapy. Uncommon but clinically similar disorders may demonstrate neither hyperornithinemia nor deficiency for the enzyme known to be abnormal in classic gyrate atrophy. It is for these reasons that considerable space will be devoted to this newly rediscovered, important metabolic disorder.

HISTORY

Gyrate atrophy of the choroid and retina is a progressive dystrophy that was first described almost 100 years ago.[10,16,27] More than 100 patients have been reported in the world's literature or are known to the authors.* The inheritance pattern is autosomal recessive.[3,69,72] Within the first decade of life, circular areas of total vascular choroidal atrophy appear in the mid- and far periphery of the fundus (Fig. 12-1).[33,69,74] These areas slowly enlarge, eventually coalescing to produce a jagged, serrated, or "gyrate" border between atrophic choroid and retina anter-

Supported in part by funding from the National RP Foundation Fighting Blindness, Baltimore, MD.

*References 1,7,12,14,23,33,34,45,53,69,71,74,81,86,88,90

iorly and more intact retina and choroid posteriorly (**Figs. 12-2 to 12-6**). The regions of atrophy are associated with absolute scotomata on visual fields. As the atrophy progresses posteriorly, the visual field constricts, eventually producing legal blindness, usually by midlife.

Simmell and Takki first reported the consistent association of hyperornithinemia with gyrate atrophy in 1973.[63] In 1974, Takki described the ophthalmic findings in 15 Finnish patients with gyrate atrophy and hyperornithinemia.[69] In 1960, François and associates, had reported elevated excretion of an amino acid, initially thought to be lysine, in the urine of a patient with gyrate atrophy and Adler's anomaly.[15] Later evaluation of this patient in 1979 revealed that the abnormal amino acid was, indeed, ornithine.[14] The magnitude of the elevation of serum or plasma ornithine varies in gyrate atrophy from 10- to 20-fold over normal (51 patients averaged 916 μM; 22 controls, 75 $\pm$ 5 μM).[63,69,78] Cerebrospinal fluid and aqueous humor levels of ornithine are similarly elevated.[69,78] Plasma, cerebrospinal fluid and aqueous humor lysine and glutamate, and plasma glutamine are all lower than normal in gyrate atrophy.[2,7,46,69,73,75,86,90] Urine excretion of ornithine, arginine, and lysine are all high.[78] In her original paper, Takki alluded to the preliminary finding of deficient levels of ornithine ketoacid aminotransferase, also called ornithine-δ-aminotransferase (OAT), in liver biopsy. However, Sengers and co-workers in 1976 presented the first data to document this enzyme deficiency.[56] Others have confirmed deficiency of OAT in cultured fibroblasts[36,47,57] and lymphocytes.[35,77]

Because OAT was known to be an enzyme that uses pyridoxal phosphate as a cofactor, several investigators have tried oral administration of vitamin B_6 to patients with gyrate atrophy in an attempt to alleviate the metabolic defect. Vitamin B_6 responsiveness has been determined in gyrate atrophy either in vivo, as manifested by approximately 50% lowering of serum ornithine and normalization of serum lysine levels with oral supplements of the vitamin, or in vitro, as manifested by an increase of residual enzyme activity in cultured fibroblasts when assayed at high concentrations of pyridoxal phosphate. Six patients, none of Finnish extraction, have

been reported to show vitamin B_6 responsiveness by one or both of the above described measures.[8,20,37,57,68,85,86,88] None of 22 reported Finnish cases have responded to vitamin B_6.[73] Somatic cell hybridization studies have failed to show complementation among vitamin B_6-responsive and nonresponsive forms of gyrate atrophy.[59,89] Thus these two forms, at least for the patients studied, appear to represent different allelic mutants of the same gene. Recently, the gene for human OAT has been localized to chromosome 10.[48] The mRNA for human ornithine aminotransferase has been cloned and the sequence for human OAT cDNA has been determined.[26]

CLINICAL FINDINGS

Gyrate atrophy begins in early childhood as slowly enlarging circular or irregular but discrete areas of total vascular choroidal atrophy in the mid- to far peripheral fundus (**Fig. 12-1**).[33,69] The retina adjacent to the areas of atrophy usually has a hyperpigmented, often maroon, discoloration (**Fig. 12-6**). Fluorescein angiograms demonstrate retinal pigment epithelial transmission defects adjacent to present areas of atrophy that correspond to future regions where the atrophy will extend (**Fig. 12-7**).[69] The choroidal atrophic areas are associated with dense peripheral scotomata (**Figs. 12-1 to 12-5**). Relative loss of retinal sensitivity accompanies the regions of retinal pigment epithelial changes seen on fluorescein angiogram.[13,69] As the areas of atrophy enlarge, they coalesce and extend toward the posterior pole, eventually resulting in generalized constriction of peripheral visual fields (**Figs. 12-1 to 12-5**).

COMPOSITE PICTURE

GYRATE ATROPHY OF THE CHOROID AND RETINA

Gyrate atrophy accounts for approximately 1.4% of RP and allied disorders (9 of 630) in the Registry of the Retinitis Pigmentosa Center of Oregon, but the true incidence is much lower since most cases were spe-

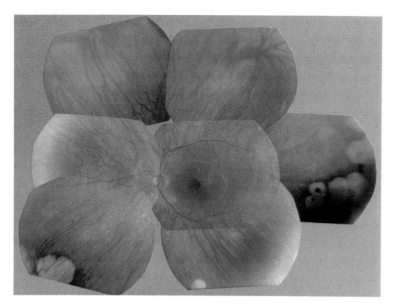

A

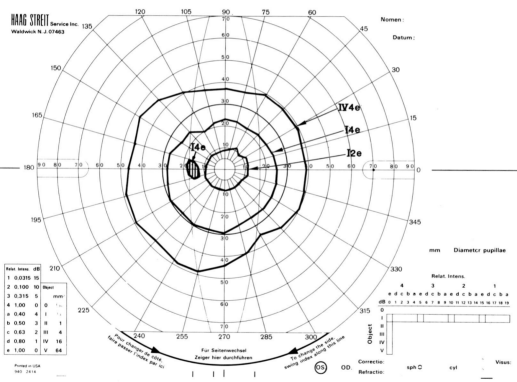

B

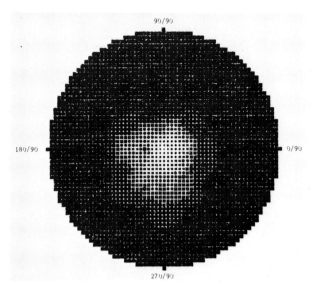

90/90

180/90

0/90

270/90

Symb.	⠿	⠿	⠿	⠿	⠿	⠿	⠿	⠿	■
dB	51–36	35–31	30–26	25–21	20–16	15–11	10–6	5–1	0
asb	0,008–0,25	0,31–0,8	1–2,5	3,1–8	10–25	31–80	100–250	315–800	1000

1 asb = 0,318 cd/m²

C

FIG. 12-1. The fundus appearance (*A*) and Goldmann kinetic (*B*) and Octopus static (combined programs 23 and 34) (*C*) perimetric visual fields of left eye of a 15-year-old girl with B₆-nonresponsive gyrate atrophy. *A* demonstrates circular and irregular discrete areas of total vascular atrophy of the choroid and retina in the periphery. Fundus involvement was symmetrical bilaterally. Note that the diagnosis could not be established from frames taken of either the posterior pole or certain other regions where extensive areas of choroid and retina are preserved. Note also that for this patient the visual fields show greater constriction of peripheral vision than would be anticipated on the basis of the fundus appearance alone. Compare these visual fields with those shown in Figure 12-4. Note the gradual slope or reduction of retinal sensitivity going from the central to peripheral field. Visual acuity was 20/30 in each eye with a moderately high myopic correction (−6.00 +2.00 × 90° in each eye). The maximal scotopic ERG measured 19 μV (normal, 501–777 μV); the photopic ERG was 17 μV at 44.4 msec (normal, 153–351 μV at 25.9–30.7 msec).[84] EOG ratios were 1.04 OD and 1.12 OS.

cifically referred. Gyrate atrophy can be subclassified into vitamin B₆-responsive and nonresponsive forms on the basis of biochemical studies. The age of our gyrate atrophy patients at the time of their first diagnostic evaluation averaged 40 years but varied from 12 to 90 years. Most gave the history of myopia from early childhood and limitation of side vision and defective night vision from the second to third decade of life. The mean visual acuity was 20/50, but the range was from 20/20 to no light perception. The average spherical equivalent refractive error was −5.50 D with a range of −1.88 to −16 D; two patients were aphakic. Reduction of visual acuity resulted from cystoid macular edema, cataracts, preretinal macular fibrosis, or degenerative maculopathy. In gyrate atrophy, the

ERG and EOG are usually severely to profoundly abnormal except in very early disease and in vitamin B₆-responsive patients. The ERG was small but measurable (15 to 150 μV) in five patients, three of whom were B₆-responsive. Dark adaptometry demonstrated normal or abnormal cone and/or rod segments of the full curve. On fundus examination, all patients showed areas of atrophy of choroid and retina in the periphery with associated loss of visual field. All patients have had elevated serum or plasma ornithine levels; most have had subnormal lysine levels. Ornithine aminotransferase (OAT) has been found to be deficient in all cells so studied.

(*Text continues on p. 208*)

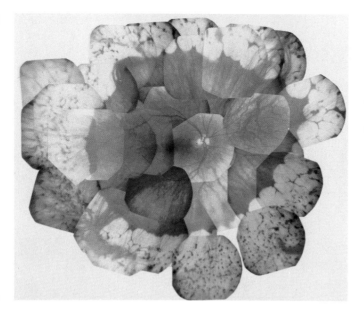

FIG. 12-2. The fundus appearance *(A, B)* and kinetic visual fields *(C)* of a 28-year-old woman with B₆-responsive gyrate atrophy (patient 1, references 37, 86, and 88 and Figs. 12-10 and 12-11). Note the classic scalloped or gyrate appearance of the border between atrophic peripheral and more intact posterior choroid and retina. Note that the patient's visual fields closely correspond to the retinal appearance. Visual acuity was 20/30 in each eye with a high myopic correction.

A

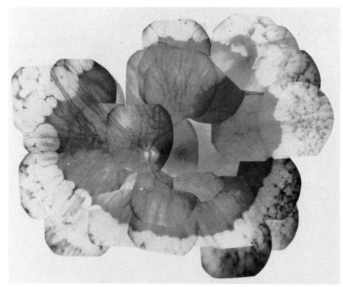

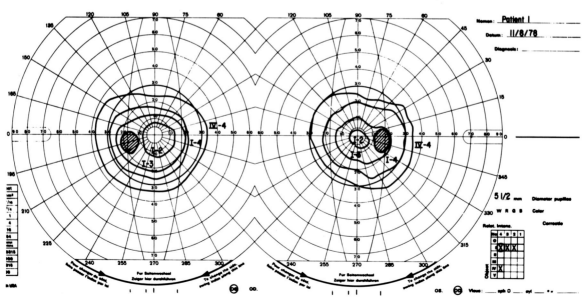

C

FIG. 12-3. Fundus appearance *(A, B)* and visual fields *(C)* of the 30-year-old sister (patient 2, references 37, 86, and 88 and Figs. 12-10, 12-11, and 12-12) of the patient in Fig. 12-2. Note that visual field defects in the periphery are not confluent and roughly correspond with the degree of peripheral involvement. Visual acuity with a moderate myopic correction was 20/20 in each eye.

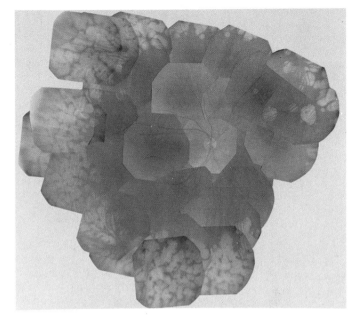

A

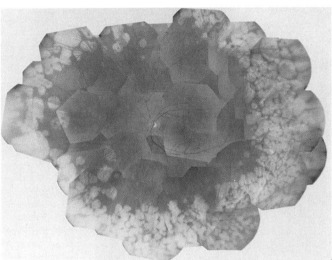

B

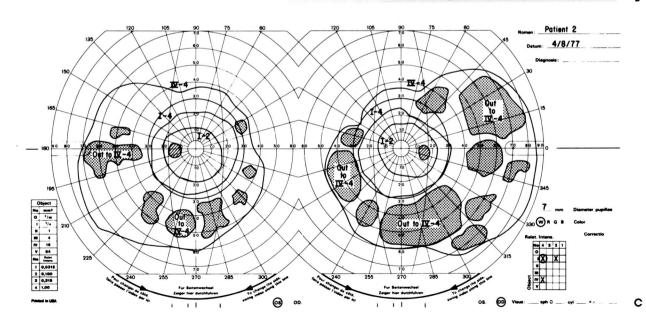

C

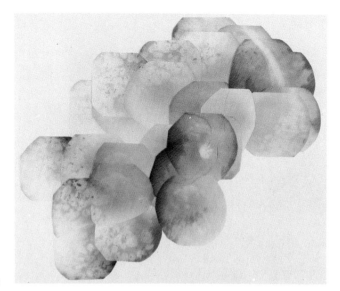

A

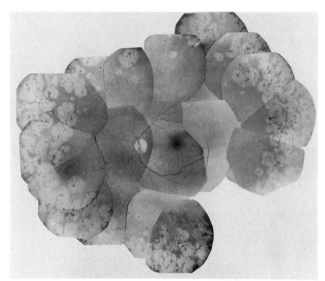

B

FIG. 12-4. Fundus appearance *(A, B)* and kinetic visual fields *(C)* of a 37-year-old woman with B₆-responsive gyrate atrophy (patient 3, references 37, 86, and 88 and Figs. 12-7, 12-10, and 12-11). Note vitreous veil in superior nasal periphery of right fundus. Detail is blurred in the right eye because of a posterior subcapsular cataract. Goldmann kinetic *(D)* and Octopus static (combined programs 23 and 34) *(E)* visual fields of left eye 6½ years after visual field depicted in *C*, demonstrated no significant worsening of visual field during this period; the visual field in the right eye has decreased, but this is mostly from increase in dense cataract. Note relatively sharp slope to retinal sensitivity to peripheral nonseeing areas for left eye. Visual acuity with a mild myopic correction was 20/400 in right eye and 20/20 in left eye.

C

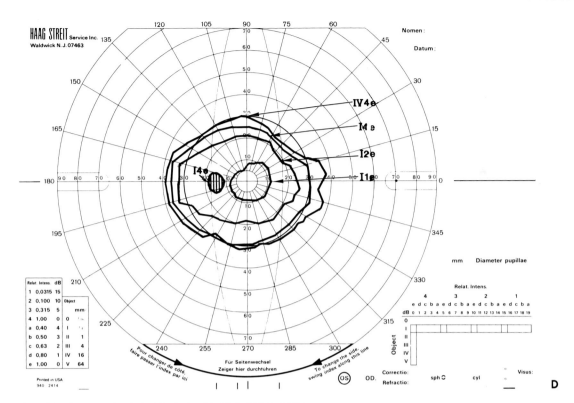

HAAG STREIT Service Inc.
Waldwick N. J. 07463

D

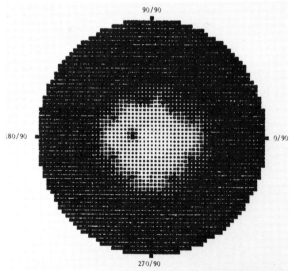

Symb.	⠿	⠿	⠿	⠿	⠿	⠿	⠿	⠿	■
dB	51−36	35−31	30−26	25−21	20−16	15−11	10−6	5−1	0
asb	0,008−0,25	0,31−0,8	1−2,5	3,1−8	10−25	31−80	100−250	315−800	1000

1 asb = 0,318 cd/m²

E

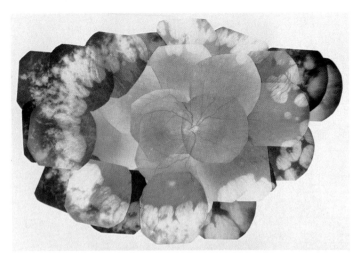

A

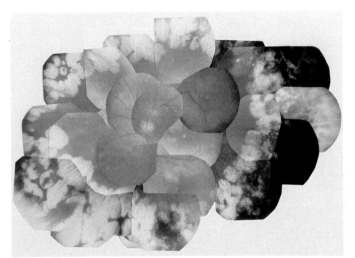

B

FIG. 12-5. Fundus appearance *(A, B)* and visual fields *(C)* of a 40-year-old man with B₆-nonresponsive gyrate atrophy (patient 4, references 37, 86, 88 and Figs. 12-8, 12-10, 12-11, and 12-13). Note accumulation of dense brown-black pigment in regions of total vascular choroidal and retinal atrophy in far periphery. Visual acuity was 20/40, right eye, and 20/200, left eye, from mild to moderate posterior subcapsular cataracts and maculopathy (see Fig. 12-8), both worse in left eye.

C

FIG. 12-6. Fundus appearance at right *(A)* and left *(B)* fundi and fluorescein angiogram *(C)* of a 28-year-old woman with B₆-nonresponsive gyrate atrophy (patient 7, reference 88). Note vitreous veil and preretinal membrane in region temporal to the right macula. Note also darker maroon color of retina adjacent to regions of atrophy. Visual acuity was 20/200 in each eye.

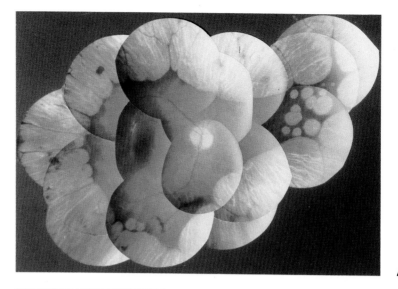

A

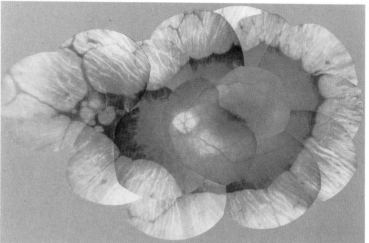

B

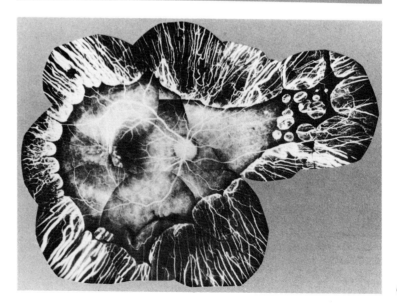

C

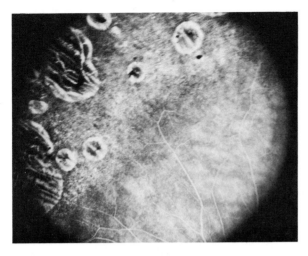
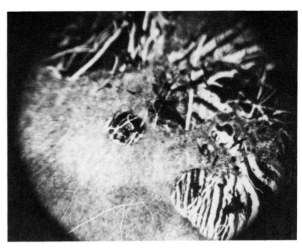

A

B

FIG. 12-7. Fluorescein angiogram *(A, B)* of scalloped border between atrophic and more intact retina and choroid in gyrate atrophy. The RPE adjacent to the atrophic regions shows a zone of patchy, diffuse transmission defects, indicating where future atrophy will extend. Left eye of patient shown in Figure 12-4.

Usually, central visual acuity is retained in one or both eyes with gyrate atrophy until midlife. However, cataracts, usually posterior subcapsular, are frequent, and occasionally can contribute to significant reduction of visual acuity early in life.[31,69] Color vision is usually preserved unless visual acuity is moderately decreased. Macular edema, macular degenerative changes, and retinal vascular leakage can further reduce visual function (**Fig. 12-8**). Preretinal and vitreous membranes and veils can occur (**Figs. 12-4 and 12-6**). Night vision is variably affected and can range from normal to markedly abnormal.

Moderate to high progressive axial myopia is almost universal in gyrate atrophy. In patients nonresponsive to B₆, especially those of Finnish extraction, atrophy of choroid and retina within the posterior pole, either peripapillary or perimacular, may occur relatively early in the disorder (**Fig. 12-6**).[35,69,74] Usually, constriction of visual field, or in a smaller group loss of central acuity, results in legal blindness status by the fourth to fifth decade of life. More severe losses of vision to counting fingers, detection of hand motion only, or even no light perception have been reported.[69,74] The B₆-responsive patients with gyrate atrophy appear to have a milder disease and usually retain better visual fields and visual acuity into midlife and later years.[34,88]

Although only a few patients have had mild muscle weakness, many patients, when tested, have abnormal electromyography.[30,62] The most common findings are a myopathic pattern of short duration, low-amplitude motor unit action potentials, and increased polyphasic potentials.[62] Muscle biopsies in all patients examined have shown atrophy of type 2 muscle fiber with subsarcolemmal inclusions that appear as tubular aggregates on electron microscopy (**Fig. 12-9A & B**).[37,46,62] These abnormalities in muscle may relate to local deficiency of creatine phosphate as a secondary manifestation of end-product inhibition of creatine synthesis through the arginine–glycine transamidinase pathway (see also Biochemical Considerations, Pathogenesis, and Approaches to Therapy).[60] Although not associated with clinically significant heart disease, the electrocardiogram has been abnormal in a number of patients. T-wave flattening, broad P waves, or prolonged QT interval was found in 11 of 17 patients and prolongation of systolic time in 3 of 11 patients.[62] Several patients have had abnormal electroencephalography or a history of seizures.[30,34,35,37,44–46,65,69,73,79] Mentation usually appears to be normal, although uncommon cases with mild mental retardation or subnormal intelligence quotients (IQs) have been reported.[45,46,65,69,73] Saito reported delayed language

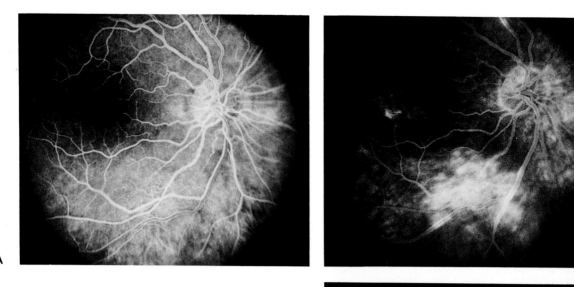

A

B

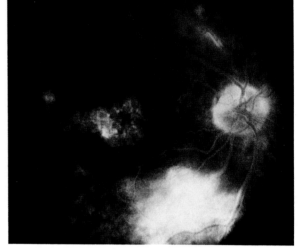

C

FIG. 12-8. Fluorescein angiogram *(A–C)* of right fundus of same patient as in Figure 12-5, demonstrating diffuse and focal retinal vascular leakage, especially along inferior temporal vessel, and macular edema. Similar vascular leakage can be seen in RP. Note the cuff-like staining along the superior artery and inferior temporal vein. The visual acuity in this eye was 20/40.

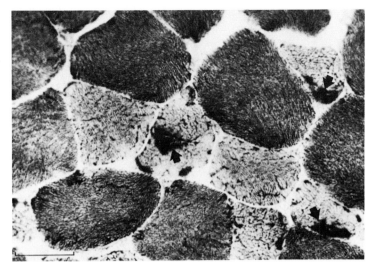

A

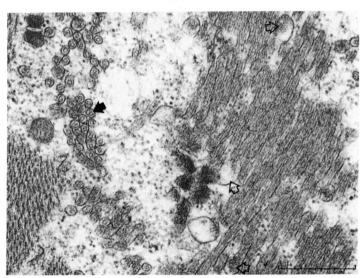

B

FIG. 12-9. Muscle biopsy from a patient with gyrate atrophy (same patient as in Fig. 12-3). Subsarcolemmal inclusions *(solid arrows)* are evident in type 2 muscle fibers on light microscopy (NADH-tetrazolium reductase stain) *(A).* (Calibration bar is 20 μm.) These appear as tubular aggregates *(solid arrows)* on electron microscopy *(B).* Note dilated saccules with granular contents *(open arrows)* on longitudinal section. (Calibration bar is 0.5 μm.) (Reproduced with permission from Kennaway NG, Weleber RG, Buist NRM: Gyrate atrophy of the choroid and retina with hyperornithinemia: Biochemical and histological studies and response to vitamin B_6. Am J Hum Genet 32: 529–541, 1980).

development, and this could account for the subnormal IQs reported in some children.[54] Abnormal mitochondria have been reported on liver biopsy of patients with gyrate atrophy, but no clinically significant hepatic dysfunction has been found.[2,45]

ELECTROPHYSIOLOGIC AND PSYCHOPHYSICAL FINDINGS

The electroretinogram (ERG) is severely to profoundly abnormal in patients with gyrate atrophy, even in childhood.[8,33,65,69,86] The B_6- responsive form of gyrate atrophy appears to be milder in severity and is usually associated with a larger residual ERG response at a given age.[86,88] Both rod- and cone-dominated ERG responses are subnormal, with perhaps better relative preservation of cone-mediated responses when disease is primarily peripheral.[8,86] The subnormalities involve both responses mediated by photoreceptors (a-waves) and responses mediated by middle and inner retinal neurons and Müller cells (corneal positive peaks) **(Figs. 12-10 and 12-11)**. Unlike patients with typical RP with markedly subnormal but recordable ERGs, the oscillatory potentials of ERGs from patients with B_6-responsive gyrate atrophy may appear relatively preserved. The implicit times for both rod- and cone-mediated responses appear to be either normal or mildly prolonged.[8,86]

DARK-ADAPTED RESPONSES

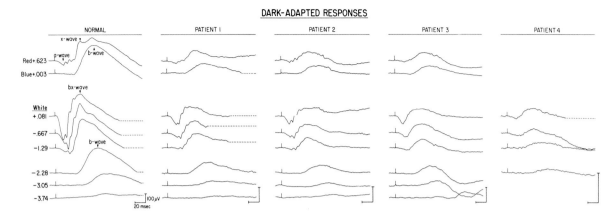

FIG. 12-10. Averaged dark-adapted ERGs from three patients with B₆-responsive gyrate atrophy (patients 1–3) and one B₆-nonresponsive patient (patient 4).[37,86,88] (The calibration scale indicates 100 μV vertically and 20 msec horizontally for all tracings.) The numbers to the left side of the normal tracings indicate the stimulus intensity in log foot-lambert-seconds for white flashes and log μJoule/cm²-steradian for the red and blue stimuli. Note relatively good oscillatory potentials on ascending limb of b-wave for patient 2. (Reproduced from Weleber RG, Kennaway NG: Clinical trial of vitamin B₆ for gyrate atrophy of the choroid and retina. Ophthalmology 88:316–324, 1981)

CONE-MEDIATED RESPONSES

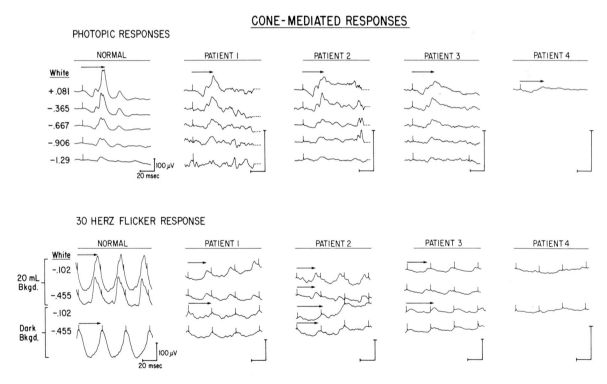

FIG 12-11. Average light-adapted and 30-Hz flicker ERGs from the same patients as shown in Figure 12-10. (The calibration scale indicates 100 μV vertically and 20 msec horizontally.) For certain of the 30-Hz flicker responses, patients 2 and 3 gave implicit times that were significantly prolonged. For the great majority of B₆-nonresponsive gyrate atrophy patients, the ERGs, either scotopic or photopic, are not discernible from noise (i.e., <10 μV) unless averaged over many iterations. (Reproduced from Weleber RG, Kennaway NG: Clinical trial of vitamin B₆ for gyrate atrophy of the choroid and retina. Ophthalmology 88:316–324, 1981)

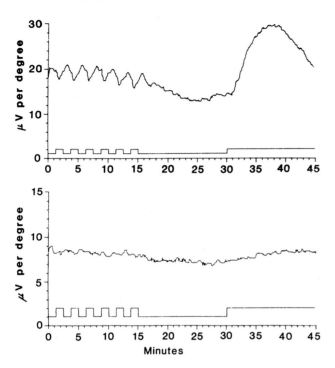

FIG. 12-12. The electro-oculogram from a normal subject (light-to-dark ratio, 2.26), above, and a patient with B₆- responsive gyrate atrophy (same patient as in Fig. 12-3) (light-to-dark ratio, 1.25; normal, >1.85), below. Note that although profoundly subnormal, a light-induced rise of the resting potential was recordable. The line below each graph indicates the status of the background light (20 ft-L): *up* indicates the background light was on, *down* indicates the background light was off. During the first 15 minutes of testing, the light was alternated off and on for 75-sec intervals to elicit fast oscillations of the resting potential. Note different vertical scale for each graph.

The electro-oculogram (EOG) is also severely abnormal in most patients with gyrate atrophy (**Fig. 12-12**).[69,88] In very early disease or in B₆- responsive patients, the EOG light-induced rise of the resting potential, as indicated by the light-to-dark ratio, may be either normal or only mildly subnormal.[33,86,88] The resting potential of the eye, as indicated by the dark trough of the EOG, appears to become severely subnormal in advanced gyrate atrophy of the choroid and retina similar to advanced RP.*

Patients with gyrate atrophy may complain of difficulty with either night vision or adjusting from light to dark. The full dark adaptation curve may be normal in very early disease or may show elevation of either the cone or the rod segments of the curve, or both, indicating elevation of either cone or rod retinal sensitivity thresholds (**Fig. 12-13**). The cone-rod break may be mildly prolonged. Compared with nonresponders, patients who are vitamin B₆-responsive usually have lesser elevations of dark adaptation thresholds.[88]

*R. Weleber, unpublished observations.

Color vision may remain normal as long as central acuity is good. When the visual acuity reaches 20/40, a significant color vision defect usually can be demonstrated. This may be tritan in nature or a more generalized diffuse disturbance in hue discrimination.[69]

DIFFERENTIAL DIAGNOSIS OF GYRATE ATROPHY

The major differential diagnosis for gyrate atrophy rests with choroideremia and other forms of choroidal atrophy.[70,83] Both gyrate atrophy and choroideremia are classified as diffuse total atrophies of the choroid and retina.[39] Gyrate atrophy is often confused with choroideremia, although differentiation should be readily achieved in all but the most advanced cases by attention to fundus findings.[69,70] In early choroideremia, the choroidal atrophy involves first the choriocapillaris and small choroidal vessels. In gyrate atrophy, the earliest findings are thinning and focal defects in the retinal pigment epithelium (RPE).[33,69] When choroidal atrophy becomes appar-

FIG. 12-13. Full dark adaptometry curves from a patient with gyrate atrophy, demonstrating mild elevation of the final rod threshold in right eye and marked elevation of both the cone and rod parts of the curve for the left eye (same patient as in Fig. 12-5)

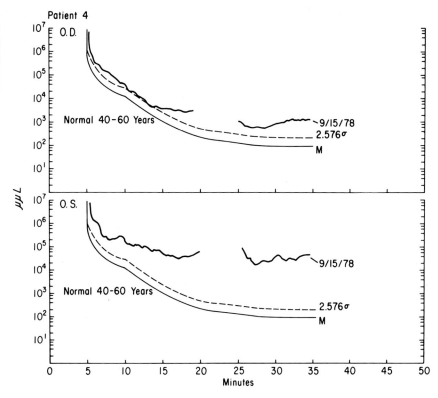

ent, typically in the mid- and far periphery, the vascular atrophy is near total in gyrate atrophy. In choroideremia, one does not see as sharp a demarcation between total vascular atrophy and more intact retina and choroid as is seen in gyrate atrophy. Also, although circular and irregular areas of more complete loss of RPE and choriocapillaris occur characteristically within the first two decades of life, in choroideremia the pattern and distribution of choroidal atrophy is more diffuse and spread throughout the fundus (**Fig. 12-14** and illustrations in Chapter 10, Choroideremia). Choroideremia usually produces more severe distrubance of color vision and dark adaptation earlier in the disease. The cone-mediated ERG b-wave implicit time is usually markedly prolonged in choroideremia, whereas in gyrate atrophy the cone-mediated b-wave implicit time is usually either normal or only mildly prolonged, especially in B_6- responsive patients.[8,83,86] In B_6-nonresponsive gyrate atrophy, the cone-mediated b-wave implicit time may be markedly prolonged (e.g., this was the case for the patient shown in Fig. 12-1).

Choroideremia is an X-linked recessive disorder, and family investigation and examination of women for the carrier findings (see Chapter 10, Choroideremia) will often help to establish the correct diagnosis.

Peripheral choroidal atrophies that can mimic the appearance of gyrate atrophy do exist (**Fig. 12-15**). When tested, these individuals invariably have normal serum levels of ornithine and lysine. Moreover, all of these individuals have been past middle age when diagnosed, and on retinal evaluation have had less severe disturbances of function than gyrate atrophy with hyperornithinemia. OAT was normal in three patients.* If one is in doubt about the diagnosis, serum or plasma ornithine determination will, in all cases, settle the issue.

A minority of older individuals with high myopia may have myopic retinal degeneration with confluent scalloped loss of RPE similar to gyrate atrophy.[22] The atrophy is not as total nor as extensive as

*R. Weleber, N. Kennaway, G. Fishman, unpublished observation

(*Text continues on p. 216*)

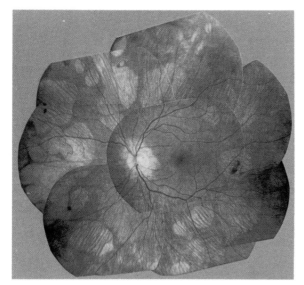

A

FIG. 12-14. Fundus appearance *(A)*, fluorescein angiogram *(B)*, and Octopus static visual field *(C)* of left eye of a 15-year-old boy with choroideremia. Areas of diffuse, patchy atrophy of choroid and retina are interspersed with areas of circular or irregular-shaped loss of RPE and choriocapillaris. The depression of retinal sensitivity on static perimetry closely corresponds to the regions of RPE loss. Indeed, this patient was initially considered by a competent retinal surgeon as having gyrate atrophy. Serum ornithine was normal; the patient's maternal grandfather went blind in midlife, and both his mother and sister showed typical fundus findings of choroideremia carrier state. Visual acuity was 20/20 in each eye. ERG and EOG were severely abnormal.

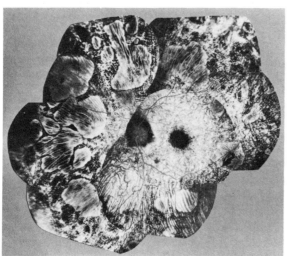

B

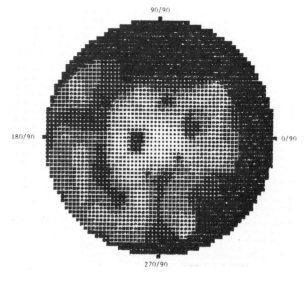

C

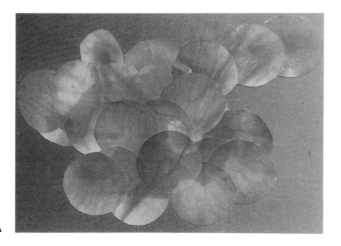

A

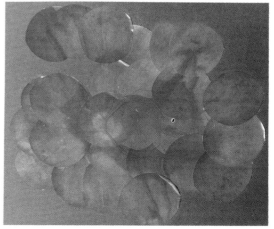

B

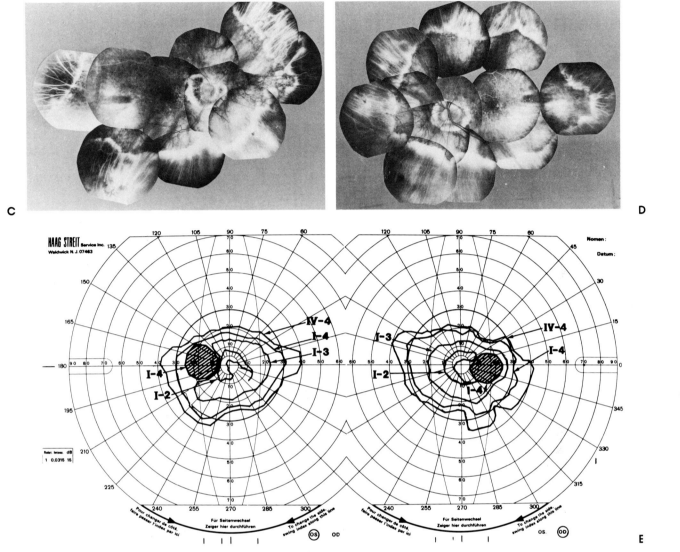

FIG. 12-15. Fundus appearance *(A, B)*, fluorescein angiogram *(C, D)*, and kinetic visual fields *(E)* of an 81-year-old man with peripheral atrophy, suggesting the diagnosis of gyrate atrophy. Visual acuity with a small refractive error was 20/50, right eye, and 20/70, left eye, mostly as a result of nuclear sclerotic cataracts. Note that the vascular atrophy is not total but does involve much of the fine and medium choroidal vessels. The ERG was subnormal for age (maximal scotopic response, 59 μV—normal, 372–647 μV; maximal photopic response, 25 μV at 32.2 msec—normal, 48–246 μV at 25.9–30.7 msec) but not nearly as abnormal as seen in most patients with gyrate atrophy. The electro-oculogram gave subnormal light-to-dark ratios (1.26, right eye; 1.16, left eye). A moderate tritan color vision defect was present in each eye. The visual fields were constricted similarly to that seen with gyrate atrophy. The serum ornithine and lysine levels were normal, and OAT activity in cultured skin fibroblasts was normal. Disease in patients such as this should not be called gyrate atrophy unless ornithine is elevated (and, if measured, OAT is deficient).

is typical for gyrate atrophy; often only one or two quadrants show involvement. Plasma ornithine levels are either normal or only minimally elevated (some values reported have not been obtained from fasting blood samples and hence may not be significantly elevated). We believe these patients may represent variations of paving-stone peripheral retinal degeneration.

Gyrate atrophy has been confused with atypical RP, but in most cases, careful ophthalmological examination will enable the correct diagnosis to be made. Occasionally, RP may be associated with moderate to marked cobblestone or paving-stone peripheral retinal degeneration, leading the examiner to consider the diagnosis as gyrate atrophy of the choroid and retina. RP usually presents with defective night vision and loss of side vision, symptoms that also can be seen in moderately advanced gyrate atrophy. Bone spicule formation, which characteristically

occurs in the midperiphery in RP, is not usually seen within the more intact retina in gyrate atrophy. Pigmentation does occur in moderately late stages of gyrate atrophy, but its distribution is much different. Dense clumps of brown to black pigment appear within the areas of total vascular choroidal atrophy, especially in the far periphery (**Figs. 12-1 to 12-6**).[69,87]

BIOCHEMICAL CONSIDERATIONS, PATHOGENESIS, AND APPROACHES TO THERAPY

Ornithine is not directly incorporated into protein and is not an essential dietary amino acid. However, ornithine plays important roles in intermediary metabolism, as substrate or product for reactions in the urea cycle, in the production of polyamines, and in the synthesis of glutamate and proline (**Fig. 12-16**).

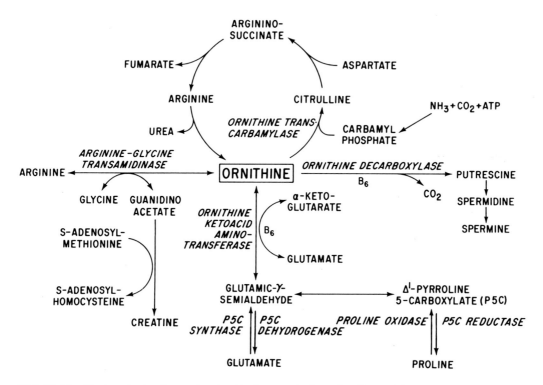

FIG. 12-16. Biochemical pathways involved in the metabolism of ornithine. (Modified from Weleber RG, Kennaway NG, Buist NRM: Gyrate atrophy of the choroid and retina: Approaches to therapy. Int Ophthalmol 4:12–32, 1981)

It is also an end-product inhibitor of the first step of creatine synthesis. Ornithine is transported into the mitochondria by a specific transport protein.

Ornithine is both produced by and consumed within the urea cycle, so that excess ornithine does not accumulate. Arginine in the diet can be converted to ornithine by either the enzyme arginase, which has moderately high activity in the retina,[18] or through the arginine–glycine transamidinase reaction, the first step in the production of creatine. Two enzymes involving reactions that consume excess ornithine are ornithine-δ-aminotransferase (OAT) and ornithine decarboxylase. Ornithine decarboxylase is involved in the synthesis of putresine and other polyamines; however, these compounds are not consistently elevated in gyrate atrophy, and it is highly unlikely that much excess ornithine is consumed through this pathway in nondividing, differentiated tissues such as the neuroretina and RPE.[37]

OAT is a pyridoxal phosphate-dependent mitochondrial enzyme that converts α-ketoglutarate and ornithine to glutamate and glutamate-γ-semialdehyde (**Fig. 12-16**). Glutamate, by dehydrogenation or transamination to α-ketoglutarate, can enter the tricarboxylic acid cycle. Glutamate-γ-semialdehyde is in nonenzymatic equilibrium with Δ[1]-pyrroline-5-carboxylate (P5C), an intermediate in the synthesis of both glutamate and proline, the former through P5C dehydrogenase and the latter through the enzyme P5C reductase. OAT is present in high activity in the retina,[21] liver, and kidney. In liver, OAT is induced by protein and probably functions to regulate ornithine levels required for urea synthesis.[42,55,82] In kidney, OAT may function to remove excess ornithine generated by the arginine glycine transamidinase reaction in the synthesis of creatine.[55] The role of OAT in the retina is not at present understood. The equilibrium constant of the OAT reaction strongly favors the formation of P5C and hence the synthesis of glutamate and/or proline.[66] Indeed, ornithine has been shown to be an important precursor of proline in cultured mammalian cells.[64] Proline oxidase is lacking in RPE, choroid, and neuroretina.[18] P5C dehydrogenase activity is low, but P5C reductase activity is high in the retina.[18] Thus the overall cooperative action of OAT and P5C reductase in the retina appears to favor the formation of proline.

The precise pathophysiology of gyrate atrophy is not known. The existence of another disorder, hyperornithemia, hyperammonemia, and homocitrullinuria (HHH),[58] which is not associated with either choroidal or retinal degeneration or an abnormal ERG,[5] has been used as evidence that the elevation of ornithine itself cannot be toxic.[5] However, HHH is believed due to a specific defect in the transport of ornithine into mitochondria, resulting in elevation of serum or tissue ornithine levels but presumably normal or low levels within the mitochondria.[25] The concept that ornithine may be toxic if it accumulates within the mitochondria is supported by the finding of swollen mitochondria on liver biospy[2,45] and iridectomy specimens[81] from patients with gyrate atrophy.

Ornithine, but not arginine, is toxic to the retina and choroid when injected intravitreally in rat and monkey. It produces a degeneration of RPE and ultimately the entire retina, reported to resemble that of gyrate atrophy.[40] However, intravitreal injection of other unrelated amino acids (glutamate, glycine, and L-cysteine) also produces retinal degeneration.[38,50,51] Several other studies support the concept that ornithine is toxic to the choroid and retina. Ornithine in levels above 10 mM have been shown to be toxic to cultured keratocytes and skin fibroblasts.[76] Ornithine, in levels found in gyrate atrophy, suppresses retinal protein synthesis in vitro.[24] At concentrations as low as 1 mM, ornithine is toxic to cultured RPE.[11] This latter concentration approaches the level of ornithine in the plasma or cerebrospinal fluid of patients with gyrate atrophy. Thus the RPE appears to be more sensitive than other tissues to the toxic effect of ornithine.

Deficiencies of either proline or creatine have been proposed as the mechanism of chorioretinal damage in patients with gyrate atrophy. Although creatine deficiency may play a role in the abnormalities seen in muscle, where creatine phosphate is a major source of energy, little is known about the role of creatine phosphate as an energy store in the retina. Arginine glycine transamidinase, the enzyme which catalyzes the first step in the synthesis of creatine, appears to be lacking in the retina.[52] A mechanism more likely contributing to the pathogenesis of gyrate atrophy is a localized defect of proline synthesis in the retina.[52] OAT may provide an important pathway for the synthesis of proline in retina since proline appears to be very poorly transported across the blood–brain barrier, and hence presumably also the blood–retinal barrier.[49] Thus a defect in endogenous proline synthesis may be more detrimental to the retina than to other tissues. High levels of ornithine also appear to inhibit the alternate pathway of proline synthesis, the formation of P5C from glutamate by P5C synthase in cultured cells.[41] Although P5C synthase is not present in retina, its activity in RPE has not been determined.[28,43] Thus OAT deficiency may lead to local deficiency of proline by two distinct mechanisms. Proline is incorporated into collagen, but the role of localized proline deficiency in progressive myopia is not established.

TREATMENT REGIMENS

Several approaches have been tried in an attempt to alleviate the metabolic, structural, or physiologic abnormalities in gyrate atrophy. These have included administration of coenzyme (pyridoxine or vitamin B_6),[6,9,19,85,86] restriction of dietary arginine through the use of low-protein diets,[4,6,9,29,44,79,80] and supplementation of the diet with lysine,[17,65,90] proline,[19,67] or creatine.[61] Vitamin B_6 in doses of 20 to 500 mg per day, lowers the serum ornithine levels by approximately 50% and normalizes the serum lysine levels in the few patients (approximately 6% of cases) who appear to be B_6-responsive.[8,19,37,85] Short-term, mild improvement of ERG responsiveness was

reported in two patients.[86] Neither double-blind studies nor long-term follow-up have been presented, and it may be very difficult to prove (or disprove) benefit of vitamin B_6 administration in those patients who appear to respond biochemically. Even a modest slowing of the expected rate of progression would be valuable but difficult to document using current techniques. Protein restriction must be severe (<15 gm per day) in order to lower serum ornithine appreciably but, when this has been accomplished, short-term improvements in retinal function have been reported.[29,32,44] It must be emphasized that the protein restriction is not without risk. Significant hyperammonemia and negative nitrogen balance may occur, especially in children.[17,44] Supplementation of nonessential nitrogen and essential amino acids is important in maintaining nitrogen balance. Patients should not be placed on severe protein restriction except when nitrogen balance and metabolic needs can be assessed adequately, preferably as part of a research study, since the long-term efficacy and safety of such diets are not known. Administration of lysine supplementation in conjunction with protein restriction has been used to lower serum ornithine and normalize serum lysine levels, but long-term efficacy in alleviating the disease has not been shown.[17,23,90] Long-term stability of retinal lesions has been claimed with the use of dietary supplements of 3 gm proline per day.[19,67] Administration of creatine supplements appears to decrease the frequency of atrophy of type 2 muscle fibers, but does not appear to influence the ocular manifestations in any measurable way.[61]

REFERENCES

1. Akiya S, Ohsawa M, Ogata T: Gyrate atrophy of the choroid and retina: The long-term observation of two brothers with gyrate atrophy of the choroid and retina with hyperornithinemia. Acta Soc Ophthalmol Jpn 81:310–322, 1977
2. Arshinoff SA, McCulloch JC, Matuk Y et al: Amino-acid metabolism and liver ultrastructure in hyperornithinemia with gyrate atrophy of the choroid and retina. Metabolism 28:979–988, 1979
3. Botermans CHG: Neuroretinal degenerations. In Vinken PJ, Bruyn GW (eds): Handbook of Clinical Neurology, vol 13, p 256. Amsterdam, North Holland Publishing, 1972
4. Bell L, McInnes RR, Arshinoff SA et al: Dietary treatment of hyperornithinemia in gyrate atrophy. J Am Diet Assoc 79:139–145, 1981
5. Berson EL: Discussion of paper by Takki K, Simell O: Gyrate atrophy of the choroid and retina with hyperornithinemia (HOGA). Birth Defects Original Article Series. 12:373–384 and discussion 401–408, 1976
6. Berson EL, Hanson AH III, Rosner B et al: A two-year trial of low protein, low arginine diets or vitamin B_6 for patients with gyrate atrophy. Birth Defects 18:209–218, 1982
7. Berson EL, Schmidt SY, Rabin AR: Plasma amino acids in hereditary retinal disease. Br J Ophthalmol 60:142–147, 1976
8. Berson EL, Schmidt SY, Shih VE: Ocular and biochemical abnormalities in gyrate atrophy of the choroid and retina. Ophthalmology 85:1018–1027, 1978
9. Berson EL, Shih VE: Ocular findings in patients with gyrate atrophy on pyridoxine and low-protein, low-arginine diets. Ophthalmology 88:311–315, 1981
10. Cutler CW: Drei ungewöhnliche Fälle von Retino-Chorioideal-Degeneration. Arch Augenheilkd 30:117–122, 1895

11. Del Monte MA, Hu DN, Maumenee IH et al: Selective ornithine toxicity to cultured human retinal pigment epithelium (abstr). Invest Ophthalmol Vis Sci (ARVO suppl) 22:173, 1982

12. Deutman AF, Sengers RCA, Trybels JMF: Gyrate atrophy of the choroid and retina with reticular pigment dystrophy and ornithine–ketoacid–transaminase deficiency. Int Ophthalmol Clin 1:49–56, 1978

13. Enoch JM, O'Donnell J, Williams RA et al: Retinal boundaries and visual function in gyrate atrophy. Arch Ophthalmol 102:1314–1316, 1984

14. François J: Gyrate atrophy of the choroid and retina. Ophthalmologica 178:311–320, 1979

15. François J, Barbier F, de Rouch A: Les conducteurs du gene de l'atrophia gyrata chorioideae et retinae de Fuchs (anomalie d'Adler). Acta Genet med Gemellol (Roma) 9:74–91, 1960

16. Fuchs E: Ueber zwer der Retinitis pigmentosa verwandte Krankheiten (Retinitis punctata albescens und ·atrophia gyrata choroideae et retinae). Arch Augenheilkd 32:111–116, 1896

17. Giordano C, De Santo NG, Pluvio M et al: Lysine in treatment of hyperornithinemia. Nephron 22:97–106, 1978

18. Hayasaka S, Matsuzawa T, Shiono T et al: Enzymes metabolizing ornithine–proline pathways in the bovine eye. Exp Eye Res 34:635–638, 1982

19. Hayasaka S, Saito T, Nakajima H et al: Clinical trials of vitamin B_6 and proline supplementation for gyrate atrophy of the choroid and retina. Br J Ophthalmol 69:283–290, 1985

20. Hayasaka S, Saito T, Nakajima H et al: Gyrate atrophy with hyperornithinemia: Different types of responsiveness to vitamin B_6. Br J Ophthalmol 65:478–483, 1981

21. Hayasaka S, Shiono T, Takaku Y et al: Ornithine ketoacid aminotransferase in the bovine eye. Invest Ophthalmol Vis Sci 19:1457–1460, 1980

22. Heckenlively J: Possible syndrome of high myopia with retinal degeneration, cataract, manic depression, and elevated plasma amino acids. Metabol Pediatr Ophthalmol 4:155–160, 1980

23. Hodes DT, Oberholzer VG, Mushin AS et al: Hyperornithinaemia with gyrate atrophy of the choroid and retina in two siblings. J R Soc Med 73:588–591, 1980

24. Hollyfield JG: Simulation of the conditions of gyrate atrophy *in vitro* suppresses retinal protein synthesis. Trans Ophthalmol Soc UK 103:385–389, 1983

25. Hommes FA, Ho CK, Roesel RA et al: Decreased transport of ornithine across the inner mitochondrial membrane as a cause of hyperornithinaemia. J Int Metabol Dis 5:41–47, 1982

26. Inana G, Totsuka S, Redmond M et al: Molecular cloning of human ornithine aminotransferase mRNA. Proc Natl Acad Sci USA 83:1203–1207, 1986

27. Jacobsohn E: Ein fall von retinitis pigmentosa atypıca. Klin Monatsbl Augenheilkd 26:202–206, 1888

28. Jones ME: Conversion of glutamate to ornithine and proline: Pyrroline-5-carboxylate, a possible modulator of arginine requirements. J Nutr 115:509–515, 1985

29. Kaiser-Kupfer MI, de Monasterio FM, Valle D et al: Gyrate atrophy of the choroid and retina: Improved visual function following reduction of plasma ornithine by diet. Science 210:1128–1131, 1980

30. Kaiser-Kupfer MI, Kuwabara T, Askansas V et al: Systematic manifestations of gyrate atrophy of the choroid and retina. Ophthalmology 88:302–306, 1981

31. Kaiser-Kupfer MI, Kuwabara T, Uga S et al: Cataract in gyrate atrophy: Clinical and morphologic studies. Invest Ophthalmol Vis Sci 24:432–436, 1983

32. Kaiser-Kupfer MI, de Monasterio F, Valle D et al: Visual results of a long-term trial of a low-arginine diet in gyrate atrophy of choroid and retina. Ophthalmology 88:307–310, 1981

33. Kaiser-Kupfer MI, Ludwig IH, de Monasterio FM et al: Gyrate atrophy of the choroid and retina: Early findings. Ophthalmology 92:394–410, 1985

34. Kaiser-Kupfer MI, Valle D, Bron AJ: Clinical and biochemical heterogeneity in gyrate atrophy. Am J Ophthalmol 89:219–222, 1980

35. Kaiser-Kupfer MI, Valle D, Del Valle LA: A specific enzyme defect in gyrate atrophy. Am J Ophthalmol 85:200–204, 1978

36. Kennaway NG, Weleber RG, Buist NRM: Gyrate atrophy of the choroid and retina: Deficient activity of ornithine ketoacid aminotransferase in cultured skin fibroblasts. N Engl J Med 297:1190, 1977

37. Kennaway NG, Weleber RG, Buist NRM: Gyrate atrophy of the choroid and retina with hyperornithinemia: Biochemical and histologic studies and response to vitamin B_6. Am J Hum Genet 32:529–541, 1980

38. Korol S, Leuenberger PM, Englert U et al: *In vivo* effects of glycine on retinal ultrastructure and averaged electroretinogram. Brain Res 97:235–251, 1975

39. Krill AE: Diffuse choroidal atrophies. Krill AE (ed). Krill's Hereditary Retinal and Choroidal Diseases, Vol II, Clinical Characteristics, pp 979–1041, Harper & Row, Hagerstown 1977

40. Kuwabara T, Ishikawa Y, Kaiser-Kupfer MI: Experimental model of gyrate atrophy in animals. Ophthalmology 88:331–334, 1981

41. Lodato RF, Smith RJ, Valle D et al: Regulation of proline biosynthesis: The inhibition of pyrroline-5-carboxylate synthase activity by ornithine. Metabolism 30:908–913, 1981

42. Lyons RT, Pitot HC: Hormonal regulation of ornithine aminotransferase biosynthesis in rat liver and kidney. Arch Biochem Biophys 180:472–479, 1977

43. Matsuzawa T: Diseases of the ornithine-proline pathway. Δ^1-Pyrroline-5-carboxylate reductase deficiency in the retina of retinal degeneration mice. Metabol Pediatr Syst Ophthalmol 6:123–128, 1982

44. McInnes RR, Arshinoff SA, Bell L et al: Hyperornithinaemia and gyrate atrophy of the retina: improvement of vision during treatment with a low-arginine diet. Lancet 1:513–517, 1981

45. McCulloch JC, Arshinoff SA, Marliss EB et al: Hyperornithinemia and gyrate atrophy of the choroid and retina. Ophthalmology 85:918–928, 1978

46. McCulloch C, Marliss EB: Gyrate atrophy of the choroid and retina with hyperornithinemia. Am J Ophthalmol 80:1047–1057, 1975

47. O'Donnell JJ, Sandman RP, Martin SR: Deficient L-ornithine:2-oxoacid aminotransferase activity in cultured fibroblasts from a patient with gyrate atrophy of the retina. Biochem Biophys Res Commun 79:396–399, 1977

48. O'Donnell J, Cox D, Shows T: The ornithine aminotransferase gene is on human chromosome 10 [Abstr.]. Invest Ophthalmol Vis Sci (ARVO Suppl.) 26(3):128, 1985

49. Oldendorf WH: Brain uptake of radiolabeled amino acids, amines, and hexoses after arterial injection. Am J Physiol 221:1629–1639, 1971

50. Pedersen OØ, Karlsen RL: The toxic effect of L-cysteine on the rat retina: a morphological and biochemical study. Invest Ophthalmol Vis Sci 19:886–892, 1980

51. Potts AM, Modrell KW, Kingsbury C: Permanent fractionation of the electroretinogram by sodium glutamate. Am J Ophthalmol 50:900–907, 1960

52. Rao GN, Cotlier E: Ornithine δ-aminotransferase activity

in retina and other tissues. Neurochem Res 9:555–562, 1984

53. Rinaldi E, Stoppolori GP, Savastano S et al: Gyrate atrophy of choroid associated with hyperornithinaemia: Report of the first case in Italy. J Pediatr Ophthalmol Strabismus 16:133–135, 1979

54. Saito T, Omura K, Hayasaka S et al: Hyperornithinemia with gyrate atrophy of the choroid and retina: a disturbance in de novo formation of proline. Tohuku J Exp Med 135:395–402, 1981

55. Sanada Y, Suemori I, Katunuma N: Properties of ornithine aminotransferase from rat liver, kidney and small intestine. Biochim Biophys Act 20:42–50, 1970

56. Sengers RCA, Trijbels JMF, Brussaart JH et al: Gyrate atrophy of the choroid and retina and ornithine- ketoacid aminotransferase deficiency [Abstr.]. Pediatr Res 10:894, 1976

57. Shih VE, Berson EL, Mandel R et al: Ornithine ketoacid transaminase deficiency in gyrate atrophy of the choroid and retina. Am J Hum Genet 30:174–179, 1978

58. Shih VE, Efron ML, Moser WH: Hyperornithinemia, hyperammonemia, and homocitrullinuria: a new disorder of amino acid metabolism associated with myoclonic seizures and mental retardation. Am J Dis Child 117:83–92, 1969

59. Shih VE, Mandell R, Jacoby LB et al: Genetic complementation analysis in fibroblasts from gyrate atrophy and the syndrome of hyperornithinemia, hyperammonemia and homocitrullinuria [Abstr.]. Pediatr Res 15:569, 1982

60. Sipilä I: Inhibition of arginine-glycine amidinotransferase by ornithine: a possible mechanism for the muscular and chorioretinal atrophies in gyrate atrophy of the choroid and retina with hyperornithinemia. Biochim Biophys Acta 613:79–84, 1980

61. Sipilä I, Rapola J, Simell O et al: Supplementary creatine as a treatment for gyrate atrophy of the choroid and retina. N Engl J Med 304:867–870, 1981

62. Sipilä I, Simell O, Rapola J. et al: Gyrate atrophy of the choroid and retina with hyperornithinemia: tubular aggregates and type 2 fiber atrophy in muscle. Neurology 29:996–1005, 1979

63. Simmel O, Takki K: Raised plasma-ornithine and gyrate atrophy of the choroid and retina. Lancet 2:1031–1033, 1973

64. Smith RJ, Phang JM: The importance of ornithine as a precursor for proline in mammalian cells. J Cell Physiol 98:475–482, 1979

65. Stoppoloni G, Prisco F, Santinelli R et al: Hyperornithinemia and gyrate atrophy of choroid and retina; report of a case. Helv Paediatr Acta 33:429–433, 1978

66. Strecker HJ: Purification and properties of rat liver ornithine δ-transaminase. J Biol Chem 240:1225–1230, 1965

67. Tada K, Saito T, Hayasaka S et al: Hyperornithinemia with gyrate atrophy: pathophysiology and treatment. J Inher Metab Dis 2:105–106, 1983

68. Tada K, Saito T, Omura K et al: Hyperornithinaemia associated with gyrate atrophy of the choroid and retina: *in vivo* and *in vitro* response to vitamin B₆. J Inher Metab Dis 4:61–62, 1981

69. Takki K: Gyrate atrophy of the choroid and retina associated with hyperornithinaemia. Br J Ophthalmol 58:3–23, 1974

70. Takki K: Differential diagnosis between the primary total choroidal vascular atrophies. Br J Ophthalmol 58:24–35, 1974

71. Takki K: Gyrate atrophy of the choroid and retina asso-

ciated with hyperornithinemia. Thesis, University of Helsinki, Helsinki, 1975

72. Takki K, Simmel O: Genetic aspects in gyrate atrophy of the choroid and retina with hyperornithinemia. Br J Ophthalmol 58:907–916, 1974

73. Takki K, Simell O: Gyrate atrophy of the choroid and retina with hyperornithinemia (HOGA). Birth Defects: Original Article Series 12:373–384 and discussion 401–408, 1976

74. Takki KK, Milton RC: the natural history of gyrate atrophy of the choroid and retina. Ophthalmol 88:292–301, 1981

75. Trijbels JMF, Sengers RCA, Bakkeren JAJM et al: L-ornithine–ketoacid–transaminase deficiency in cultured fibroblasts of a patient with hyperornithinaemia and gyrate atrophy of the choroid and retina. Clin Chim Acta 79:371–377, 1977

76. Valle D, Boison AP, Kaiser-Kupfer MI: Increased sensitivity of gyrate atrophy fibroblasts to ornithine toxicity. Pediatr Res 13:426, 1979

77. Valle D, Kaiser-Kupfer MI, Del Valle LA: Gyrate atrophy of the choroid and retina: deficiency of ornithine aminotransferase in transformed lymphocytes. Proc Natl Acad Sci USA 74:5159–5161, 1977

78. Valle D, Simell O: The hyperornithinemias. In Stanbury JB, Wyngaarden JB, Fredrickson DS, Goldstein JL, Brown MS (eds): The Metabolic Basis of Inherited Disease, ed. 5, pp 382–401, New York, McGraw-Hill, 1983

79. Valle D, Walser M, Brusilow SW et al: Gyrate atrophy of the choroid and retina: amino acid metabolism and correction of hyperornithinemia with an arginine-deficient diet. J Clin Invest 65:371–378, 1980

80. Valle D, Walser M, Brusilow S et al: Gyrate atrophy of the choroid and retina: biochemical considerations and experience with an arginine-restricted diet. Ophthalmology 88:325–330, 1981

81. Vannas-Sulonen K, Vannas A, O'Donnell JJ et al: Pathology of iridectomy specimens in gyrate atrophy of the retina and choroid. Acta Ophthalmol 61:9–19, 1983

82. Volpe P, Sawamura R, Strecker HJ: Control of ornithine δ-transaminase in rat liver and kidney. J Biol Chem 244:719–726, 1969

83. Weleber RG: Hereditary dystrophies of the choroid and retina. Perspect Ophthalmol 3:37–43, 1979

84. Weleber RG: The effect of age on human cone and rod ganzfeld electroretinograms. Invest Ophthalmol Vis Sci 20:392–399, 1981

85. Weleber RG, Kennaway NG, Buist NRM: Vitamin B₆ in management of gyrate atrophy of choroid and retina. Lancet 2:1213, 1978

86. Weleber RG, Kennaway NG: Clinical trial of vitamin B₆ for gyrate atrophy of the choroid and retina. Ophthalmology 88:316–324, 1981

87. Weleber RG, Kennaway NG, Buist NRM: Gyrate atrophy of the choroid and retina: approaches to therapy. Int Ophthalmol 4:23–32, 1981

88. Weleber RG, Wirtz MK, Kennaway NG: Gyrate atrophy of the choroid and retina: Clinical and biochemical heterogeneity and response to vitamin B₆. Birth Defects: Original Article Series 18:219–230, 1982

89. Wirtz MK, Kennaway NG, Weleber RG: Heterogeneity and complementation analysis of vitamin B₆ responsive and non-responsive patients with gyrate atrophy of the choroid and retina. J Inher Metab Dis 8:71–74, 1985

90. Yatziv S, Statter M, Merin S: Metabolic studies in two families with hyperornithinemia and gyrate atrophy of the choroid and retina. J Lab Clin Med 93:749–757, 1979

13

RP Syndromes

JOHN R. HECKENLIVELY

To this point, the text has focused on ocular-only forms of retinitis pigmentosa (RP). There are numerous systemic diseases, some well defined and many not at all understood, which are associated with a pigmentary retinopathy. It should be noted that the term "pigmentary retinopathy" is used by authors in a variety of ways, usually indicating disease affecting the retinal pigment epithelium (RPE) from typical "bone spicule" pigmentary deposits to atrophic nonpigmented changes of the RPE. Some of these diseases are definitely heritable, others may be inherited. Those common pigmentary retinopathies known to be secondary to infectious or toxic origin are reviewed in Chapter 11.

USHER'S SYNDROME

Usher's syndrome is used to describe patients with *congenital* neurosensory hearing loss and RP; Usher's syndrome patients should not be confused with those RP patients who develop an adult-onset partial deafness. Early diagnosis is particularly beneficial to profoundly deaf patients and their families, since these patients have special educational, rehabilitative, and emotional needs.

Usher's syndrome is the most common RP syndrome constituting between 6% and 10% of RP patients. It is estimated that the incidence of Usher's syndrome is 4.4 per 100,000 in the general population,[1,2] and within the deaf population the prevalence rate has been found to range from 3% to 6%.[1] However, a pigmentary retinopathy associated with deafness occurs in other syndromes, and Usher's syndrome must be differentiated from these diseases; this differential is reviewed at the end of this section.

The first publication describing an association of RP and deafness was by Von Graefe in 1858,[3] and Liebreich in 1861 commented on a relatively high frequency of the two problems in Jews in Berlin.[4] However, it was the British ophthalmologist C. H. Usher, who emphasized the hereditary nature of the disease. He demonstrated that 11 of his 69 RP patients were deaf and that this was consistent within families. Various reports by Lindenov, Kloepfer, Nuutila, and Amman have reemphasized the hereditary nature of Usher's syndrome.[5-8] The most definitive early RP study which included Usher's syndrome was by Julia Bell, who found a 10% incidence of Usher's syndrome in a population of 919 patients with RP.[9]

It is important to distinguish RP patients with congenital deafness from those RP patients who later develop some degree of hearing loss during their adult years. Determining whether the patient's hearing loss is congenital or early onset is usually fairly simple (e.g., if the patient has total hearing loss from infancy). A situation that may be more difficult to sort out involves patients who present with congenital partial hearing loss; some patients may not be aware of their problem or may not associate their hearing loss with their eye symptoms, and will fail to mention it when the medical history is obtained. These patients invariably have a nasal quality or identifiable impediment to their speech unless they had intensive speech therapy as children.

Many authors have included cataract formation as an essential part of Usher's syndrome, although there is no evidence that this is a direct gene effect. At UCLA only 42% of Usher's syndrome patients were found to have posterior subcapsular cataracts,[10] while in a study of 48 consecutive Usher's syndrome patients with both complete and partial hearing loss, Fishman found that 50% had no lens opacity. Furthermore, 44% showed either atrophic or cystic-appearing bilateral foveal changes.[11] Of those patients with cystic foveal lesions, six had cystoid edema on fluorescein angiography, while one patient had no leakage and partial-thickness holes on biomicroscopy with contact lens. This latter finding has been seen several times in Usher's syndrome patients at UCLA (see case 2, type I below). Fishman found that most of his patients maintained visual acuity of 20/60 or better until their midthirties.

COMPOSITE PICTURE

USHER'S SYNDROME

The average age of the patient at time of testing was 24.8 years, with a 14-year history of symptoms. Approximately 10% of RP patients seen at UCLA have Usher's syndrome with an even split between types I and II. The mean visual acuity was 20/40. The mean

refraction was -1.09 $+1.12$ $\times 97$. Forty-two percent of patients had posterior subcapsular cataracts. On electroretinographic testing, 7 of 24 had some aspect of the ERG which was recordable. On evaluation of fundus photographs, 78% had nerve fiber layer dropout, with a mean cup-to-disc ratio of 0.15. Fluorescein angiography studies show that 29% had a macular window defect, while 14% had a paramacular window defect. Parapapillary edema occurred in 42%, vascular arcade edema in 33%, temporal optic nervehead atrophy in 21%, telangiectasia in 29%, and macular hypofluorescence in 58%.

Usher's syndrome comprises a heterogeneous set of diseases; however, all forms of Usher's syndrome have had pedigrees consistent with autosomal recessive inheritance.[12] Whether all forms of Usher's syndrome are allelic genes, different gene loci, or variable expression of the same gene (the latter is thought unlikely) is not known. Boughman's analysis of two separate Usher's syndrome populations found segregation ratios consistent with autosomal recessive inheritance, but, interestingly, there was a slight excess of males in both groups.[1]

While several authors have designed classification schemes for Usher's syndrome,[13-15] this chapter will present the Merin classification.[16]

MERIN CLASSIFICATION OF USHER'S SYNDROME

Merin and co-workers presented data from 35 patients with RP and deafness belonging to 20 families

TABLE 13-1
USHER'S SYNDROME (Merin classification)[16]

Type I, pigmentary retinopathy, congenital total deafness, no vestibular function

Type II, pigmentary retinopathy, partial congenital deafness, normal vestibular function

Type III pigmentary retinopathy, congenital deafness, vestibulocerebellar ataxia, psychoses (Hallgren's syndrome)

Type IV pigmentary retinopathy, congenital total deafness, and mental retardation (see also phytanic acid storage disease)

TABLE 13-2

CHARACTERISTICS OF USHER'S SYNDROME TYPES I AND II

CHARACTERISTICS	TYPE I	TYPE II
Onset of nyctalopia	Within first or beginning of second decade	Latter part of second or beginning of third decade
Visual field loss	Marked, often within first decade	Variable field loss, from normal to marked
Central vision	Variable: 20/20 to 20/200 or less	Variable: 20/20 to 20/200 or less
Extent of pigmentary retinopathy	Intrafamilial similarity is the rule	Intrafamilial variability may be apparent
Electroretinogram	Nondetectable	Variable, from nondetectable to subnormal scotopic
Hearing impairment	Profound; similar within same family	Moderate to profound; intrafamilial variability may be apparent
Speech	Unintelligible*	Intelligible
Vestibular responses	Areflexic or marked hypoactivity	Vestibular sensitivity is normal; testing may show decruitment or hyperactivity
Ataxia	May be clinically apparent, reports vary as to frequency	Rarely apparent
Mental retardation	Has been reported in some series	Not a feature of type
Psychosis	Reported in some series; part of the genetic syndrome (?)	Not a feature of type
Electroencephalogram	Abnormalities have been reported	Abnormalities not present as a feature of type

* Unless patient receives intense speech therapy
(Modified from Fishman GA: Arch Ophthalmol 101:1373, 1983; published by permission)

who underwent clinical, genetic, audiologic, and electroretinographic studies. They were able to distinguish four clinical types of Usher's syndrome which they felt represented at least two genetic types (Table 13-1). Fishman and co-workers had further defined types I and II in their patient population.[11,15] A summary of their findings is found in Table 13-2.

USHER'S TYPE I

Type I patients have RP, congenital complete deafness, minimal to no vestibular response to caloric or rotatory excitation, and normal mental development without any neurologic deficit. The retinal changes are typical of RP; the earliest change may be a grayish tapetal reflex, which may have yellow dots or lesions resembling retinitis punctata albescens. Pigmentary stippling and, later, bone spicule-

like deposits are seen. Posterior subcapsular cataracts which may progress to mature cataracts may be seen, but are not a consistent feature of the syndrome (see cataract section, Chapter 5). No patients are born blind.

Visual acuities range from 20/20 to 20/30 in younger patients in the first two decades, and 20/50 to 20/70 is typical for patients in their twenties and thirties. By the early forties, most patients are severely affected, with count-finger to hand-motion vision.

By the time it is performed, the electroretinogram (ERG) in most cases is nondetectable; onset of nyctalopia typically is noted early and in all patients by the second decade. Visual field loss is usually seen within the first decade, and ring scotomata and progressive peripheral visual field loss are seen over time.

Neuro-otologic evaluation reveals profound hearing loss, with some patients occasionally having residual (<10%) hearing at lower frequencies. Vestibular function by caloric and rotatory testing typically shows nonresponsiveness although a few patients demonstrate a hypoactive response.[15] All Merin's patients had normal mental and motor development, and no neurologic deficiencies were detected.

Robbins and colleagues studied lymphoblastoid lines from nine Usher's syndrome patients representing eight kindreds, and found a statistically significant hypersensitivity to the lethal effects of x-rays when compared with normal fibroblast lines.[17] They believe that defective DNA repair mechanisms may be involved in the pathogenesis, but this hypothesis has not been adequately studied.

CASE STUDIES

Case 1 A young white woman was first seen at age 18 with type I Usher's syndrome. She reported night blindness from birth and loss of peripheral vision over the 4 previous years. She had complete deafness since birth and has no recognizable speech. She is otherwise in good health. The only other affected family member is her brother (case 2).

Her presenting visual acuity was OD 20/40, OS 20/60. On biomicroscopy there was no evidence of cataract, but there were pigmented flecks in the anterior vitreous. Funduscopy revealed diffuse atrophy of the RPE with pigmented bone spicule-like deposits in the equatorial regions **(Fig. 13-1)**, retinal vessel attenua-

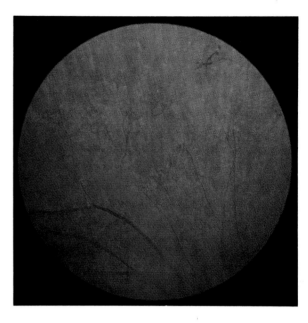

FIG. 13-1. Fundus photography of an 18-year-old female Usher's I patient (case 1) showing diffuse retinal atrophy and early pigmentary changes in the equatorial region.

tion, surface wrinkling, and retinal pigment epithelial abnormalites in the macular area **(stereo Fig. 13-2)**. A few vitreous-condensates were present near the retina and optic nervehead **(Fig. 13-3)**. Moderate pigmented deposits were present in the equator and anterior retina. The fluorescein angiogram at that time did not reveal window defects or cystoid edema.

The ERG was nonrecordable, and with a 1° test object at 12° above fixation after 40 minutes dark adaptation, the patient had a 3.35-log unit elevation

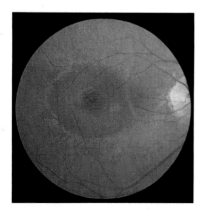
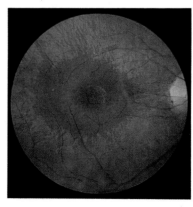

FIG. 13-2. Stereographic fundus photographs, case 1 with Usher's I, macular right eye, with inner limiting membrane wrinkling, RPE as weol as macular retinal abnormalities. Retinal vessels are attenuated.

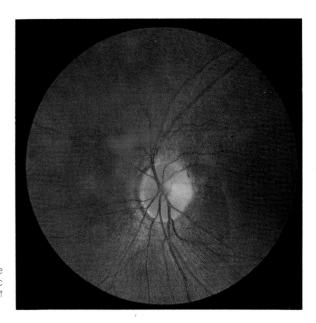

FIG. 13-3. Fundus photograph, case 1 at age 18, with diffuse retinal atrophy nasally, vessel attenuation, with pink optic nervehead. Vitreal opacities are seen nasally and adjacent to disc.

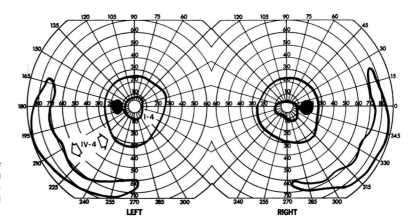

FIG. 13-4. Goldmann visual field, case 1, showing advanced ring scotomata process (i.e., a small area of central vision with a larger peripheral temporal island OU).

of the final rod threshold. Goldmann visual field was approximately 25° centrally with temporal islands with the IV-4 and 8° with I-4 isopter OU **(Fig. 13-4).**

Four years later, on a return examination, the patient complained of further distortion of her vision; the visual acuity was OD 20/80, OS 20/100. There was no evidence of cataract formation, but on direct ophthalmoscopy, macular multilobulated cysts could be seen in each macula *(stereo Fig. 13-5)* although they were somewhat obscured by overlying vitreal condensates which, on indirect ophthalmoscopy,

looked like amorphous white masses in the mid-vitreous **(stereo Fig. 13-6).** Fluorescein angiography, however, showed no evidence of cystoid edema **(Fig. 13-7).** The patient's final rod threshold worsened to 4.4 log units of elevation, but the visual field remained relatively stable, with the IV-4 averaging about 23° and the I-4 7° OU.

Case 2 The 20-year-old brother of case 1, who on presentation had no complaints of night blindness. However, he had noticed alterations in his peripheral

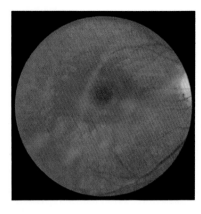
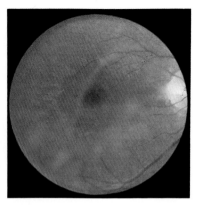

FIG. 13-5. Stereographic fundus photographs of case 1, 4 years after Figure 13-2, demonstrating multiobulated cyst-like lesions in the macular area. Vitreal condensates overlie posterior pole.

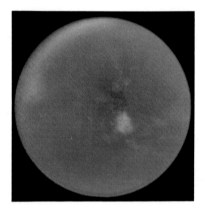
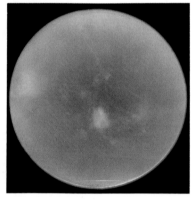

FIG. 13-6. Stereographic fundus photographs of vitreal condensates in case 1 which also occurred in a similar fashion in the patient's older brother, case 2.

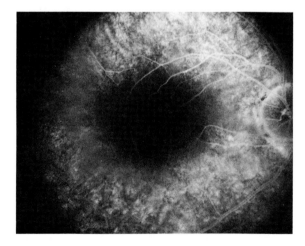

FIG. 13-7. Fluorescein angiogram, right eye, case 1 at age 22, with Usher's I, posterior pole shows no evidence of macular edema or window defects despite abnormalities seen on color photographs.

vision starting at age 17. Other than complete congenital deafness, the medical history was noncontributory, with no history of diabetes, polydactyly, or neurological problems. No family members other than his sister had eye or hearing problems.

On examination, the visual acuity was OD 20/50, OS 20/40. Biomicroscopy showed 1-mm posterior subcapsular cataracts OU, with pigmented flecks in the anterior vitreous. Direct ophthalmoscopy revealed surface wrinkling but no major abnormalities of the macula. Indirect ophthalmoscopy showed a diffuse retinal atrophy with bone spicule formation.

Electrophysiological testing revealed a nonrecordable ERG, and the electro-oculogram (EOG) light peak-to-dark trough ratio was OD 125%, OS 137%. The final rod threshold with a 1° target at 12° above fixation was .30 log units elevated (normal). At 20° it was 3.45 and at 30° 4.30 log units elevated. This cor-

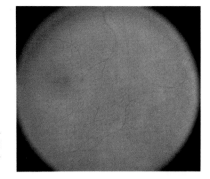
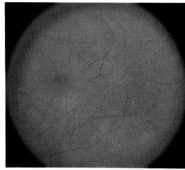

FIG. 13-8. Stereographic fundus photographs, case 2, left eye, with Usher's I syndrome, showing early macular cyst-like lesions.

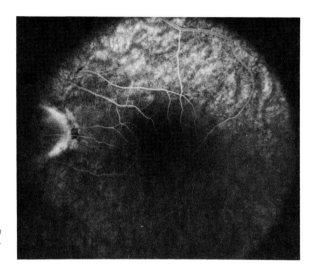

FIG. 13-9. Fluorescein angiogram of case 2 which shows no evidence of dye accumulation in cyst-like lesions in left macula.

related with the Goldmann visual field which was about 20° with the IV-4 isopter.

The patient returned 2 years later complaining of visual loss. The visual acuity was OD 20/200, OS 20/50. On direct ophthalmoscopy, a large cyst was seen in the right fovea, and irregularities were visualized in the left **(stereo Fig. 13-8)**. Fluorescein angiography did not show any leakage of dye **(Fig. 13-9)**.

USHER'S TYPE II

This group consists of patients with RP, congenital partial hearing loss, and normal vestibular function in most cases, with normal mentation and neurologic clinical findings. Merin originally reported that type II patients had progressive hearing loss, but Fishman found no subjective or objective progressive loss in his 46 patients[15]; this also has been our experience at UCLA. However, rare cases of progressive hearing loss in association with RP have been reported.[14]

It is likely that Usher's type II is more common than realized, and the patient's nasal or speech impediment is frequently ignored. However, these patients often can greatly benefit from hearing aids, so audiometric evaluations should be arranged for any RP patient who is suspected of having hearing loss, whether congenital or of later onset.

The audiogram in type II patients typically demonstrates an oblique, almost straight-line drop-off, with lower frequencies showing less loss than higher frequencies **(Fig. 13-10)**. Patients with type II have intelligible speech, although it may have a nasal quality.

Type II inheritance also is autosomal recessive,

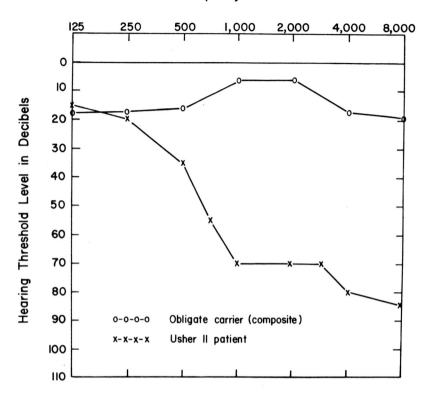

Frequency in Hertz

o-o-o-o   Obligate carrier (composite)

x-x-x-x   Usher II patient

FIG. 13-10. Audiogram, Usher's II patient, showing oblique increasing dropoff of function from middle to high frequencies in both ears.

but it is thought to be a different gene than the one for type I. The partial or complete hearing loss is consistent within families, and there are no reports where both types have been found in the same family.

Fishman, as well as Davenport, found that type II patients' ocular symptoms develop around puberty, generally later than in type I. Vestibular function was normal to hyperactive. ERG responses in most patients were nondetectable although a few patients were recordable.

Bloom, Fishman, and Mafee evaluated 12 Usher's syndrome patients, 2 with type I and 10 with type II Usher's syndrome, with conventional and dynamic computed tomography (CT).[18] All type II patients demonstrated either cerebellar and occipital atrophy by conventional CT (**Fig. 13-11**) or focal areas of delayed or diminished circulation (**Fig. 13-12**). One

type I patient was normal, and the other showed focal areas of diminished circulation of the left cerebellar hemisphere.

CASE STUDIES

Case 3 A 32-year-old woman presented with a 9-year history of night blindness and characterized her side vision problems as occurring over a "long time." She had a congenital partial sensorineural hearing loss with poor speech discrimination ability, resulting in a nasal quality to her speech. There was no history of polydactyly, diabetes mellitus, nor any family history of deafness or visual problems. Results of a phytanic acid plasma test were normal.

On examination, the best corrected visual acuity was OD 20/30 − 2, OS 20/20 − 1. There were small pos-

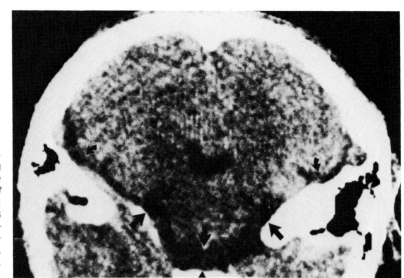

FIG. 13-11. Horizontal section of posterior fossa of Usher's II patient, showing wide prepontine and cerebellopontine cisterns *(dark areas outlined by straight arrows)* indicative of brain stem atrophy. Note atrophy along the lateral aspects of cerebellar hemispheres *(curved arrows)*, the left greater than the right. (Reproduced by permission, Retina 3:110, 1983. Photograph courtesy of Gerald A. Fishman, M.D.)

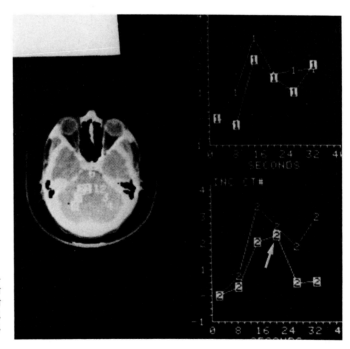

FIG. 13-12. Graphic display of the hindbrain circulation in a patient with Usher's II. Note that the transit time is delayed (20 sec) on the right side, lower right *(arrow)*. (Reproduced by permission, Retina 3:110, 1983. Photograph courtesy of Gerald A. Fishman, M.D.)

terior subcapsular opacities, and funduscopy showed moderately heavy pigmentary (bone spicule) deposition with diffuse RPE loss. The area temporal to the macula had a "lobule" mottled pattern of degeneration **(Fig. 13-13)**. Goldmann visual fields over 6 years have demonstrated loss of peripheral field with the IV-4 isopter **(Fig. 13-14A&B)**.

The fluorescein angiogram demonstrated diffuse staining of the RPE, but there was no evidence of posterior pole dropout of RPE or choriocapillaris **(Fig. 13-15)**. Late phases demonstrated peripapillary and vascular arcade staining.

Case 4 The patient is a 31-year-old white male with a 17-year history of night blindness and a 3-year history of noting difficulty with his side vision. He notes

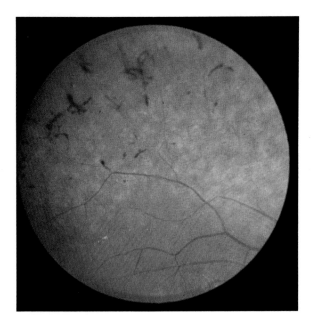

FIG. 13-13. Fundus photograph, case 3 with Usher's II, showing superior temporal area to macula OD; mottled "lobule" pattern of RPE degeneration is typical of many types of RP.

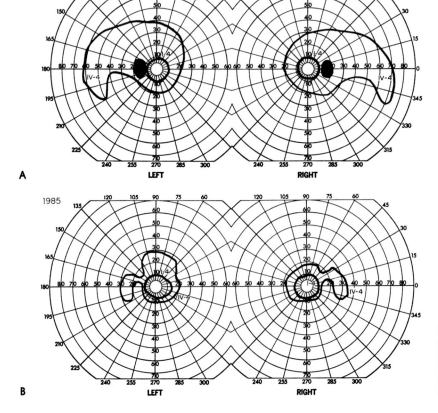

FIG 13-14. Goldmann visual fields case 3, (*A*) upper fields from 1979, while (*B*) lower set of fields are from 1985. Marked loss of field is seen with the IV-4 isopter, while the I-4 isopter, seen in the macular region, is unchanged.

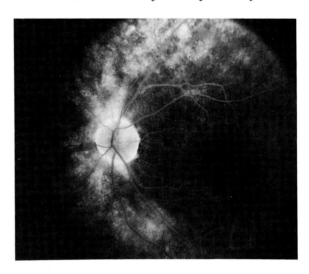

FIG. 13-15. Fluorescein angiogram, case 3 in late venous phase. RPE has granular appearance with focal areas of hypofluorescence. The choriocapillaris is patent. Disc staining is present.

flashes and rolling waves of light "constantly" and has occasional headaches. His family history is negative, and the medical history was noncontributory with no polydactyly, kidney problems, or skin problems. The patient has been partially deaf since early childhood and has a nasal quality to his speech. Audiologic evaluation found a sensorineural hearing loss with a

mild to profound sloping deficit from 250 to 8000 hertz **(Fig. 13-16).**

Funduscopy revealed a blond fundus, resulting in part from diffuse atrophy or depigmentation of the RPE, with minimal pigment deposition and slight pallor of the optic nerve **(Fig. 13-17).** Fluorescein angiography revealed a granularity to the RPE of the pos-

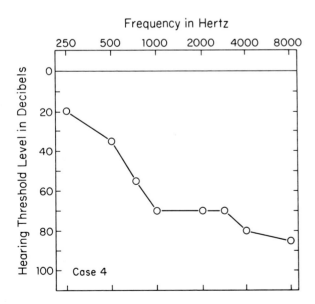

FIG. 13-16. Audiogram, case 4 with congenital partial hearing loss and RP. There is an oblique dropoff in function from low to high frequencies; this type of loss is typical of patients with Usher's II.

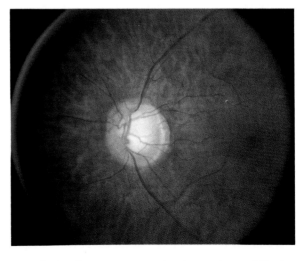

FIG. 13-17. Fundus photograph, left eye of case 4. Depigmentation of RPE gives generalized blond appearance to the retina; there was minimal deposition of pigment in periphery (not shown). Mild pallor of the optic nervehead is present.

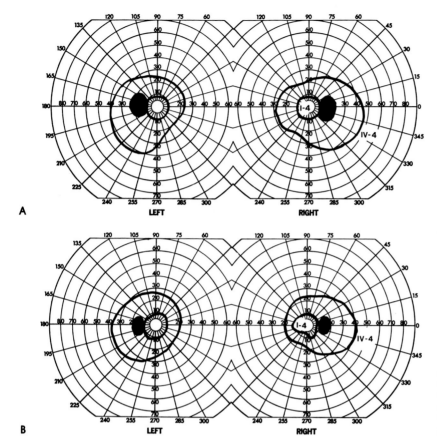

FIG. 13-18. Goldmann visual field, case 4, with Usher's II syndrome over a 7-year period; upper fields were recorded in 1979, while lower set were tested in 1986. The visual fields show little change over this time.

terior pole, and the macular area was more hypofluorescent than usual compared with the surrounding retina. Goldmann visual fields over the last 7 years have demonstrated little progression (**Fig. 13-18** *A&B*).

USHER'S TYPE III (HALLGREN'S SYNDROME)

Hallgren's syndrome, or Merin Usher's type III, consists of RP with complete deafness and vestibular ataxia, which may present in a swinging gait and a tendency to fall to one side when walking with closed eyes. (Some type I patients may also tend to be clumsy and fall to one side as above, but they never develop true ataxia.) Merin suggests that type III also can be called Hallgren's syndrome since 90% of Hallgren's patients in his large Swedish study were of this type. Psychoses, mainly schizophrenia, were found in over 20% of Hallgren's cases, a finding

confirmed by Nuutila.[19] However, it is not clear whether the psychoses may be environmental and social manifestations of living where there is proportionately less sunlight compared with many other countries, or whether the mental problems are directly related to gene expression. Also, it is not known whether type III is a genetic variant of type I. Type III is not commonly seen outside of Scandinavia.

At UCLA we have examined a set of fraternal twins, a brother and sister, with type I Usher's syndrome, both of whom otherwise developed normally until the father in the family died when the twins were age 18. At that time, the sister had a mental breakdown which was described as a schizophrenia variety, but her brother is free of mental health problems and is quite intelligent. While the sister has recovered from the acute episode, she appears retarded compared with her brother; on examination, her dullness was observed to be loss of affect rather than intelligence.

USHER'S TYPE IV

Usher's type IV consists of RP, congenital complete deafness, and mental retardation. Twenty percent of Hallgren's original group of patients were also mentally retarded, so the characteristics and validity of types III and IV are less well understood.

Weleber recently defined the ophthalmic manifestations of *infantile phytanic acid storage disease*[20]; these infants are hypotonic, have severe hearing impairment, and are developmentally delayed. They have a pigmentary retinopathy and very abnormal ERGs. Serum phytanic acid levels are elevated, although not to the same levels as in Refsum's disease. These patients meet the basic criteria for Merin type IV and may represent the same entity previously described.

CARRIER MANIFESTATIONS OF USHER'S SYNDROME

The carrier frequency is calculated to be between 1 in 100 and 1 in 200.[1] Studies by De Haas and colleagues in Rotterdam of 13 heterozygotes showed that 8 of 13 had abnormal dark adaptation, 5 of which were 1 or more log units elevated. About half of their patients also had abnormal EOG light peak-to-dark trough ratios.[21] Sondheimer and colleagues were unable to confirm abnormal dark adaptation values or to find any ophthalmoscopic changes in 14 heterozygous carriers of Usher's syndrome.[22] Currently, there is no test other than pedigree analysis for determining Usher carrier state.

REHABILITATION

Karp and Santore published recommendations for rehabilitation in Usher's syndrome patients emphasizing educational and vocational psychosocial counseling and genetic counseling. Hearing aids may benefit selected patients, and lip-reading is useful unless macular atrophy and/or retinal degeneration is advanced. In the latter case, sign language and tactile communication must be used.[23]

Vernon and colleagues have also written on strategies for dealing with some of the clinical problems displayed by Usher's syndrome patients.[24] Patients may need extensive counseling and information, since the trauma of coping with eventual deaf–blindness is severe. Gallaudet College offers an educational publication entitled "Living with Deaf–Blindness—nine profiles" for readers interested in learning about deaf–blind persons.[25]

Agencies which offer services to the deaf–blind are listed in the Appendix of Chapter 6.

COUNSELING AND SPECIAL EDUCATION FOR THE DEAF–BLIND PATIENT

Of all the forms of RP, the deaf child has the greatest handicap. With rare exception, these patients have normal intelligence and little time to complete their education before their vision deteriorates. Suggestions for developing special academic programs for Usher's syndrome patients have been published.[26] Management of RP patients can be found in Chapter 6.

DIFFERENTIAL DIAGNOSIS

While Usher's syndrome is the most common form of retinal degeneration and deafness, the differential diagnosis is extensive, consisting mainly of rarely seen entities, but the alternatives still must be considered (Table 13-3). The diseases which are the most similar to Usher's syndrome include Alstrom's syndrome, Refsum's disease, phytanic acid storage disease (above), Flynn-Aird syndrome, Cockayne's syndrome, and osteopetrosis (Albers-Schönberg disease). Other hereditary diseases with deafness and retinal abnormalities include Alport's syndrome, spondyloepiphyseal dysplasia congenita, Friederich's ataxia, Hurler's syndrome (MPS-I), and Waardenburg's syndrome. Bateman documented nine cases of retinal degeneration with hearing impairment, including two cases with enamel dysplasia which are interesting, but this association needs further investigation.[27] Konigsmark and Gorlin reviewed a number of diseases with genetic hearing loss associated with eye disease in their text.[28]

TABLE 13-3

RETINAL DEGENERATION AND DEAFNESS

Alport's Syndrome

Nephropathy, deafness, myopia, cataract, retinal detachment, autosomal dominant

Alstrom's Syndrome

Atypical pigmentary retinal degeneration, deafness, obesity, diabetes mellitus, nephropathy, acanthosis nigricans, autosomal recessive

Cockayne's Syndrome

Pigmentary retinal degeneration, optic atrophy, deafness, cachectic dwarfism, characteristic facies, mental retardation, autosomal recessive

Dysplasia Spondyloepiphysaria Congenita

Dwarfism, mild deafness, cleft palate, congenital high myopia with associated retinal degeneration, cataracts, glaucoma, autosomal dominant

Flynn-Aird Syndrome

Atypical pigmentary retinopathy, cataract, myopia, nerve deafness, ataxia, skin atrophy, baldness, cystic bone changes, autosomal dominant

Friedreich Ataxia

Spinocerebellar degeneration, limb incoordination, nerve deafness, retinal degeneration, optic atrophy, autosomal recessive

Hallgren Syndrome (See Usher's Type III)

Hurler's Syndrome (MPS-I)

Early corneal clouding, gargoyle facies, deafness, mental retardation, dwarfism, skeletal abnormalities, hepatosplenomegaly, subnormal ERG, optic atrophy, autosomal recessive

Marshall Syndrome

Myopia, cataract, saddle nose, and sensorineural hearing loss, probably autosomal dominant

Myopia, Blue Sclerae, Marfanoid Habitus, and Sensorineural Deafness[24]

Osteopetrosis (Albers-Schonberg Disease)

Defective resorption of immature bone, macrocephaly, progressive deafness, hepatosplenomegaly, anemia, retinal degeneration, abnormal or extinguished ERG, autosomal recessive

Phytanic Acid Storage Disease

Hypotonic as infant, severe hearing impairment, developmental delay, pigmentary retinopathy, abnormal ERG. Serum phytanic acid levels are elevated, although not in the same range as in Refsum's disease.

Pigmentary Retinopathy, Hearing Loss, and Enamel Dysplasia[23]

Progressive External Ophthalmoplegia, Ptosis, Pigmentary Retinopathy, Mixed Hearing Loss, Heart Conduction Defects (Kearns-Sayre Syndrome)

Refsum's Disease

Elevations of phytanic acid, pigmentary retinopathy, partial deafness, cerebellar ataxia, ichthyosis.

TABLE 13-3 (*continued*)
RETINAL DEGENERATION AND DEAFNESS

Usher's Syndrome (Merin Classification)

Type I. Pigmentary retinopathy, congenital total deafness, no vestibular function

Type II. Pigmentary retinopathy, partial deafness, normal vestibular function

Type III. Pigmentary retinopathy, congenital deafness, vestibulocerebellar ataxia, psychoses (variable), autosomal recessive (Hallgren syndrome)

Type IV. Pigmentary retinopathy, congenital total deafness and mental retardation (see also phytanic storage disease)

Waardenburg's Syndrome

Hypertelorism, wide bridge of nose, ochlear deafness, white forelock, heterochromia iridis, poliosis, pigment disturbance of RPE, normal to subnormal ERG

ALSTROM'S SYNDROME

In l959, Alstrom described three individuals with atypical pigmentary retinal degeneration, sensorineural deafness, obesity, diabetes mellitus, and normal intelligence.[29] Klein and Ammann, in reviewing Bardet-Biedl syndrome and related disorders, presented two additional cases of Alstrom's disease. They added acanthosis nigricans and male hypogenitalism as findings in this syndrome.[30] Goldstein and Fialkow noted baldness and hypertriglyceridemia as well as renal disease in their cases.[31] A summary of this syndrome with two new cases and a follow-up on Goldstein and Fialkow's cases has been published.[32] In the two new cases, unique retinal findings were noted; the maculae demonstrated RPE atrophy and wrinkling, and the retinal vessels were ghost-like (**Fig. 13-19**). This latter finding may be related to the patients' hyperlipidemic state.

COCKAYNE'S SYNDROME

Cockayne's syndrome, first described by Cockayne in 1936, is characterized by an arrest of development in a previously normal child during his or her second year, followed by a progressive mental and physical deterioration.[33] By the teenage years, a cachectic dwarfism with a senile or progeric appearance is present. The hearing loss is moderate to severe, developing during childhood. The major ocular feature is pigmentary degeneration of the retina with optic atrophy.[34] Because of overlapping features, plasma phytanic acid levels should be checked to rule out infantile phytanic acid storage disease.[20]

EDWARDS' SYNDROME

Edwards and colleagues reported three siblings with RP, deafness, small testes, gynecomastia, mental retardation, and diabetes mellitus.[35] They differentiate their patients from Alstrom's syndrome patients by their mental retardation.

FLYNN-AIRD SYNDROME

Flynn and Aird described an autosomal dominant syndrome of atypical pigmentary retinopathy, cataract, myopia, neurosensory deafness, ataxia, peripheral neuritis, epilepsy, skin atrophy, baldness, dental caries, cystic bone changes, and joint stiffness.[36]

OSTEOPETROSIS (ALBERS-SCHÖNBERG DISEASE)

Osteopetrosis is an autosomal recessive disease characterized by progressive deafness, pigmentary retinopathy with optic atrophy, macrocephaly, hepatosplenomegaly, anemia, and defective resorption of immature bone with increased density of all bones.[37] Variable findings include growth retardation, osteomyelitis of jaw as a complication of tooth extraction, fractures, and mental retardation.

REFSUM'S DISEASE (HEREDOPATHIA ATACTICA POLYNEURITIFORMIS)

Heredopathia atactica polyneuritiformis or Refsum's disease was first described in 1945[38]; the characteristic findings in this disease are RP, hearing loss, chronic polyneuritis with progressive paresis of distal parts of extremities, dry skin, elevated cerebrospinal fluid protein levels, and ataxia and other cerebellar signs. On occasion, anosmia, pupillary abnormalites, cataracts, alteration of the electroencephalogram, and skeletal abnormalites may be seen. Nyctalopia is the most common initial ocular symptom which usually occurs before the third decade.

Ataxia and weakness are generally noted in childhood or early adult life. Other common findings include paresthesia, ichthyosis, spondylitis, exostoses, and kyphoscoliosis.[39] Hearing loss may be asymmetric.

An abnormal long-chain fatty acid has been detected in the serum, urine, kidney, and liver of a patient with Refsum's disease.[40] It may be that competitive inhibition of palmitic acid,[41] found in its esterified form in high concentration in the normal retina, interferes with the incorporation of palmitic acid into the vitamin A ester of the rhodopsin cycle.

In an ocular pathology study, Toussaint and Danis found lipid material throughout all layers of the eye, including the RPE.[43]

A low-phytanic acid diet may be useful in treating this disorder, and patients with severe neurological problems on such a diet have been reported improved.[42,44]

Recently, Weleber reported the ocular findings in *phytanic acid storage disease syndrome* (see discussion, Usher's type IV), which is characterized by infantile onset, deafness, RP, short stature, hepatosplenomegaly, and usually mental deficit.[20]

Because there are so many RP syndromes, only the most commonly encountered or well-defined ones will be reviewed in this chapter. A summary description of other RP syndromes is included for quick reference.

ALAGILLE SYNDROME

Arteriohepatic dysplasia, a familial intrahepatic cholestatic disease, presents with neonatal jaundice or failure to thrive, but unlike most intrahepatic cholestatic syndromes, the outlook is relatively good, since the cholestasis improves with age.[45] Cholestasis causes poor intestinal absorption of vitamins A and E because of abnormally low concentrations of intraluminal bile acid. Four main clinical findings have been reported: (1) peripheral neuropathy, (2) cerebellar dysfunction, (3) eye movement abnormalities, including limitation in upward gaze, decreased adduction, oculomotor apraxia, and absence of optokinetic nystagmus, and (4) retinal degeneration. Electrophysiological studies suggest that these patients may not be as severely affected as typical RP patients. Posterior embryotoxon has been noted and may be an additional principal ocular feature.[46] Treatment of the vitamin deficiency is the definite therapy.

BASSEN-KORNZWEIG SYNDROME

In 1950, Bassen and Kornzweig described two children of a consanguineous marriage who had atypical RP with macular involvement, central nervous system findings similar to Friedreich's ataxia, and crenated red blood cells.[47] In another patient, Salt and associates established the absence of β-lipoproteins.[48] Later studies revealed the metabolic abnormalities to be more widespread, with low serum fats and cholesterol, and a concomitant lowering of fat-soluble vitamins, particulary vitamins A and E.[49] Acanthocytes are a reliable sign of the disease and may represent up to 70% of the circulating red blood cells.[50]

Infants with the disease are usually asymptomatic during the neonatal period, but after a few months develop steatorrhea, abdominal distention and growth retardation. Fat vacuoles in hepatocytes and jejunum villi are reported to be striking.[48,50] Progressive ataxia, distal muscle weakness, and wasting occur in childhood, and the pigmentary retinopathy may occur as early as 2 years, but typically is diagnosed in the second decade. Vitamin A supplements sufficient to raise serum vitamin A levels to normal restore normal dark adaptation thresholds and ERG values.[51] Judisch reported an unusual case of abetalipoproteinemia in a 13-month-old male infant whose ERG improved from a nonrecordable state to 30% of normal following vitamin supplementation and dietary modification.[52] Abetalipoproteinemia is currently one of the few treatable forms of RP (see also Fig. 9-9).

BARDET-BIEDL SYNDROME

In 1920, Bardet defined a syndrome characterized by RP, polydactyly, and obesity,[53] and Biedl in 1922 added mental retardation and hypogenitalism as additional features.[54] Solis-Cohen and Weiss[55] connected the Bardet-Biedl syndrome to a report by Laurence and Moon cited by Hutchinson.[56] It is still unclear whether the Laurence-Moon and Bardet-Biedl syndromes are separate entities or part of a spectrum of disease. The most notable features from the ophthalmologist's point of view are the pigmentary retinopathy with macular degeneration (**Fig. 13-19**), polydactyly (**Fig. 13-20**), and obesity. The syndrome is consistent with autosomal recessive inheritance, which is further supported by an incidence of 23.4% of parental consanguinity reported by Bell.[57]

Schachat and Maumenee reported an unusual case with features similar to the Bardet-Biedl syndrome and summarized the features of related syn-

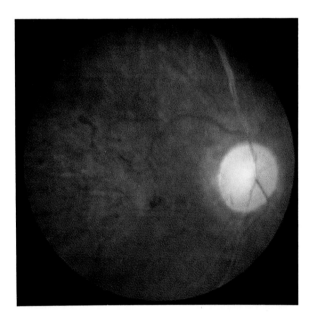

FIG. 13-19. Alstrom's syndrome. Posterior pole of a 23-year-old man of consanguineous marriage, who developed a pigmentary retinopathy by 6 months; diabetes mellitus with hyperlipidemia was diagnosed at age 20. The patient was of short stature and moderately obese, and had above-normal intelligence. Fundus photograph shows large circumscribed area of macular RPE atrophy with retinal vessels that are ghost-like and attenuated.

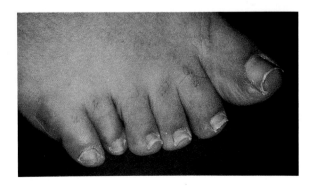

FIG. 13-20. Polydactyly in a 24-year-old man with Bardet-Biedl syndrome.

dromes (Table 13-4); they argued that these syndromes are separate entities.[58] It should be noted that Carpenter's syndrome, with a clinical picture of obesity, mental deficiency, hypogenitalism, and polydactyly, is similar to the ocular syndromes in Table 13-4 but has neither RP nor deafness.[59] Edward reported three siblings with RP, hypogonadism, gynecomastia, mental retardation, deafness, diabetes mellitus, and minor pyramidal tract abnormalites; these patients may represent a variant of Alstrom's syndrome.[35]

Reflecting the heterogeneity of these clinical features, various surveys have compared the frequency of cardinal features of the Bardet-Biedl syndrome[60] (Table 13-5). The discrepancy in the frequency of hypogenitalism between men and women is not totally explained by the easier diagnosis in men, since there are also endocrine and physiological differ-

ences. While Bardet-Biedl female patients have borne children, no affected male patient has yet been reported to have become a father. At UCLA we have seen one female patient with Bardet-Biedl syndrome with a negative family history for eye disease who delivered a child with retinoblastoma.[64]

Patients with Bardet-Biedl syndrome have a much higher incidence of early macular degeneration. In early stages, the macula may demonstrate a fine granularity, retinal wrinkling, and a slight golden sheen (**Figure 13-21A&B**). As the degeneration progresses, paramacular atrophy and thickening or hyperpigmentation of foveal RPE are common (**Fig. 13-22A–C**). In advanced stages, pigmentary deposits and atrophy in the macula are often seen (**Fig. 13-23A&B**).

Some patients may present with diffuse retinal atrophy and macular degeneration without pigmentary deposits (retinitis pigmentosa sine pigmento),

TABLE 13-4

CLASSIFICATION OF CLINICAL SYNDROMES WITH VARIOUS COMBINATIONS OF OCULAR DEFECT, MENTAL RETARDATION, GENITAL HYPOPLASIA, OBESITY, AND DIGITAL ANOMALY*

FEATURE	LAURENCE-MOON	BARDET-BIEDL	WEISS[17]	ALSTROM[18]	BIEMOND II[19]	SCHACHAT-MAUMENEE[14]
Pigmentary retinopathy	+	+	−	+	−	−
Congenital cataracts	−	−	−	−	−	+
Iris coloboma	−	−	−	−	+	−
Nerve deafness	−	−	+	+	−	−
Mental retardation	+	+	+	−	+	+
Spastic paraplegia	+	−	−	−	−	−
Obesity	−	+	+	+	+	+
Hypogenitalism	+	+	+	+/−	+	+
Diabetes mellitus	−	−	−	+	−	−
Polydactyly	−	+	−	+/−	+	+
Short stature	+	+	+	−	−	+

* +, present; −, absent.

*See discussion in Usher's section

(Schachat, Maumenee: Arch Ophthalmol 100:286, 1982; published by permission)

TABLE 13-5

FREQUENCY OF THE DIFFERENT CARDINAL SYMPTOMS OF BARDET-BIEDL SYNDROME*

CLINICAL FEATURE	KLEIN[65]		BELL[13]	
	Men	Women	Men	Women
Retinitis pigmentosa	(24)86%	(20)100%	(152)95%	(103)91%
Obesity	(26)93%	(20)100%	(142)89%	(106)94%
Mental defect	(24)86%	(14)70%	(139)87%	(99)88%
Mild retardation	(13)54%	(8)57%		
Moderate retardation	(4)17%	(3)21%		
Severe retardation	(3)12%	(2)14%		
Dyslexic	(2)8%			
Retardation, degree unknown	(2)8%	'(1)7%		
Polydactyly/syndactyly	(23)82%	(17)85%	(120)75%	(81)72%
Hypogenitalism	(24)86%	(9)45%	(119)74%	(60)53%

* Number of cases are in parentheses.

(Klein, Ammann: J Neurol Sci 9:484–491, 1969)

although pigment deposits eventually develop. Most patients with recordable ERGs have a rod-cone pattern of loss, but occasional patients will have a cone-rod pattern. At UCLA we evaluated two male siblings with Bardet-Biedl syndrome, one aged 14, severely affected on visual field testing with a rod-cone ERG pattern, and his brother, aged 16, who was mildly affected on visual field testing and had an ERG with a cone-rod pattern.[66]

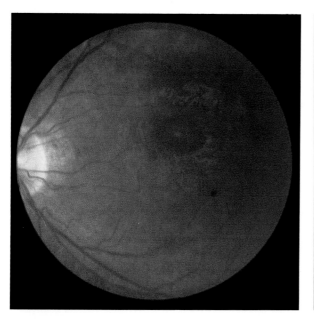 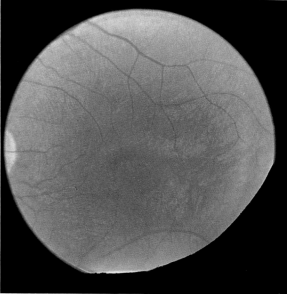

A   B

FIG. 13-21. Bardet-Biedl syndrome, early macular changes. *(A)* A 17-year-old woman with vision of 20/100 OD and *(B)* a 14-year-old boy whose vision is 20/80 – 2 OS, both of whom show early atrophic macular changes with granularity and wrinkling of the retina. A slight golden sheen is present in the fovea.

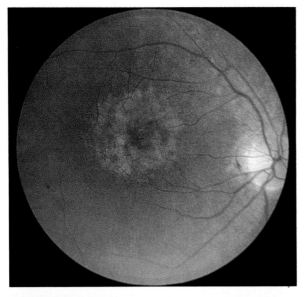

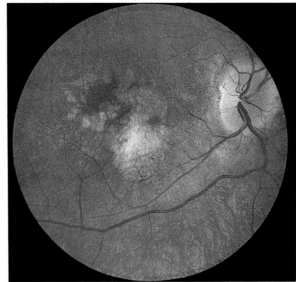

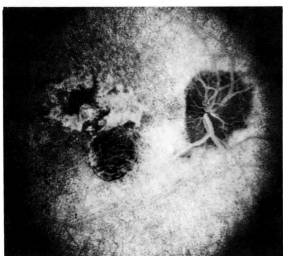

FIG. 13-22. Bardet-Biedl syndrome, middle stage of macular degeneration. *(A)* A 17-year-old patient with count finger vision and *(B)* a 21-year-old women with 20/300 vision, showing thickened hyperpigmented foveas, paramacular retinal atrophy. *(C)* Fluorescein angiogram of same area; hypofluorescent fovea is surrounded by hyperfluorescent-staining RPE, with an adjacent circumscribed area of atrophy. Background RPE shows salt-and-pepper-like pigmentation.

FIG. 13-23. Bardet-Biedl syndrome, advanced stage. *(A)* A 22-year-old-woman with 20/300 vision and *(B)* a 24-year-old man with light perception vision. Both show advanced macular atrophy.

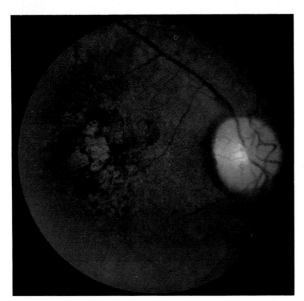

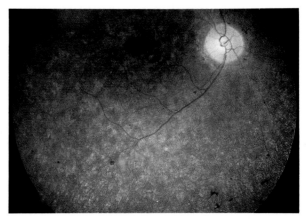

BATTEN'S DISEASE(S)

Four diseases, often called Batten's disease, ceroid lipofuscinosis, or formerly "amaurotic idiocy," are now clearly recognized on the basis of clinical features and electron microscopic pathologic changes[67] (**Fig. 13-24**); these include Haltia-Santavuori disease, Jansky-Bielschowsky disease, Spielmeyer-Vogt disease, and Kufs' disease. All varieties are autosomal recessive. The relatively benign Kufs' disease is not associated with retinal degeneration. All these disorders may be specifically diagnosed through electron microscopic examination of white blood cells, conjunctiva, or neuronal-containing tissue.

Haltia-Santavuori disease patients have the earliest onset, with decreasing vision at age 2 to 3 months. Microcephaly is common, and affected individuals follow a rapid downhill course with mental retardation, hypotonia, ataxia, and a generalized retinal degeneration.

Jansky-Bielschowsky disease is a late infantile variety, with onset at age 2 to 4 years, and is associated with a rapid systemic and retinal deterioration. After about the age of 2 years, the child fails to develop and shows clear neurologic regression; poor vision may precede any clear systemic finding. The ERG usually is poorly recordable. Fundus examination shows diffuse retinal and optic atrophy. The foveal area often looks hyperpigmented in comparison with the rest of the retina (**Fig. 13-25**).

Spielmeyer-Vogt disease has an onset at age 6 to 8 years and has a more slowly progressive systemic course with a generalized retinal degeneration.

Batten's original case report (below) of what to-

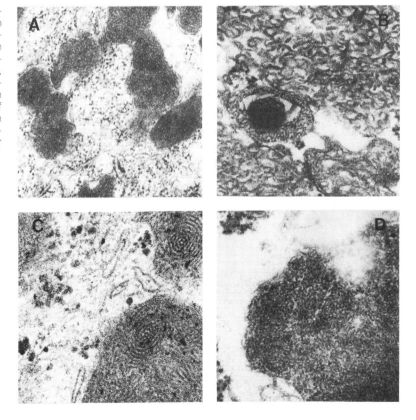

FIG. 13-24. Ultrastructure of membrane-bound neuronal ceroid bodies in different types of neuronal ceroid-lipofuscinosis (all ×60,000). *(A)* Bodies with finely granular matrix, formed in Haltia-Santavuori type. *(B)* Curvilinear bodies, usually seen in neurons in Jansky-Bielschowsky type. *(C)* Ceroid bodies with fingerprint pattern, characteristic of Spielmeyer-Vogt variety. *(D)* Bodies with granular matrix seen in Kufs' type. (Electron micrographs courtesy of Professor Wolfgang Zeman.)

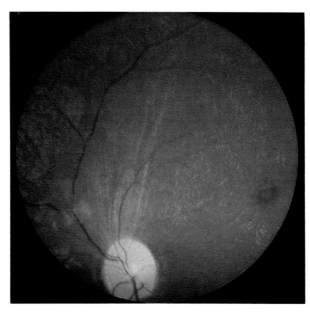

FIG. 13-25. Jansky-Bielschowsky disease. Fundus photograph of a 7-year-old boy, showing diffuse retinal and optic nervehead atrophy, nerve fiber layer dropout, and hyperpigmentation of fovea.

day would be called Spielmeyer-Vogt disease is still instructive, since it accurately portrays the clinical course and findings.

CASE REPORT[68] (edited)

"R.B., age 7 years, was a healthy child until about 12 months ago. She learnt to talk and walk early, but was never good at her lessons. Twelve months ago she became spiteful at school, had attacks of violent temper, and about that time it was noticed that her sight was failing, and she 'looked out of the corners of her eyes to see an object.'

"The family history revealed seven children, the first, age 15, boy, is healthy; the 2nd, girl, age 13, is in Darenth Asylum; 3rd, boy, died of convulsions at 2 1/2, 4th, the patient, and three others who are healthy.

"The physical condition of the child was good. She walked well, and found her way about the ward. She was extremely irritable at times and would shout and scream for hours, but complained of no headache. She talked well, could count beads, and tell their colour. Knee-jerks were obtained with difficulty and the plantar reflex tended to give an extensor response.

"While the vision was extremely defective, she seemed to see fairly well with the periphery of the field of vision. There was occasional fine nystagmus. The pupils were equal, reacted poorly to light, and did not maintain their contraction well. The discs were slightly pale, but not markedly atrophic. There were peppered pigmentary changes all over the retina, and at each macula there was a reddish-black spot, larger and more defined in the left than right eye. The shape was irregular and not round, and the margin was not very sharply defined. The adjacent area was paler than the rest of the fundus, and more atrophic-looking. Retinal vessels were on the 'small side' but not markedly so."

The association of a pigmentary retinopathy with other hereditary disorders is frequently encountered; some of these disorders have RP or a pigmentary retinopathy as a regular feature; the main ones are listed in Table 13-6.

INCONTINENTIA PIGMENTI

Bloch-Sulzberger syndrome or incontinentia pigmenti has an inheritance pattern that is consistent with X-linked dominant disease in which there is prenatal lethality to affected males. The female-to-

TABLE 13-6

SECONDARY PIGMENTARY RETINOPATHIES (ASSOCIATED WITH SYSTEMIC DISORDERS)

Autosomal Dominant

CHARCOT-MARIE-TOOTH[85,86]

Pigmentary retinopathy, degeneration lateral horn spinal cord, optic atrophy

FLYNN-AIRD SYNDROME[87]

Atypical pigmentary retinopathy, cataract, myopia, neurosensory deafness, ataxia, skin atrophy, baldness, cystic bone changes

MYOTONIC DYSTROPHY (STEINERT DISEASE)[80,88]

Muscle wasting, "Christmas tree" cataract, retinal degeneration, possible pigment deposits, ERG subnormal to abnormal.

OCULODENTODIGITAL DYSPLASIA SYNDROME[89]

Thin nose with hypoplastic alae, narrow nostrils, abnormality of fourth and fifth fingers, hypoplastic dental enamel, congenital cataract, colobomata

OLIVOPONTOCEREBELLAR ATROPHY[90]

Retinal degeneration (peripheral and/or macular), cerebellar ataxia, possible external ophthalmoplegia

PAGET'S DISEASE[91]

Occasionally, angioid streaks, one pedigree of retinopathy

PIERRE-MARIE SYNDROME[92]

Cone-rod degeneration, bitemporal hemianopsia, choked disc, disturbed hair growth, pachyacria

STICKLER SYNDROME (ARTHRO-OPHTHALMOPATHY)[93,94]

Progressive myopia with myopic retinal degeneration, joint hypermobility, and arthritis. Cleft palate and retinal detachment common; micrognathia and neurosensory deafness less common. ERG subnormal to abnormal, visual field changes consistent with myopia, occasional pigmented paravenous retinal degeneration pattern or pigment deposits.

WAGNER HEREDITARY VITREORETINAL DEGENERATION[95]

Narrowed and sheathed retinal vessels, pigmented spots in the retinal periphery and along retinal vessels, choroidal atrophy and optic atrophy, extensive liquefaction and membranous condensation of vitreous, retinal detachments common, subnormal ERG, overlapping features with Stickler syndrome.

WAARDENBURG'S SYNDROME[96]

Hypertelorism, wide bridge of nose, cochlear deafness, white forelock, heterochromia iridis, poliosis, pigmentary disturbance of RPE, normal to subnormal ERG

Autosomal Recessive Pigmentary Retinopathies

ABETALIPOPROTEINEMIA (BASSEN-KORNZWEIG SYNDROME)

Vitamin A deficiency due to deficiency in beta portion of lipoprotein carrier; acanthocytosis, anemia (see text)

BATTEN'S DISEASE

Haltia-Santavuori, occurs in infancy with rapid deterioration, fine granular inclusions
Jansky-Bielschowsky, onset 2–4 years, rapid central nervous system deterioration, curvilinear body inclusions
Spielmeyer-Vogt, onset 6–8 years, slowly progressive, fingerprint inclusions
Kuf's, adult form not known to have retinopathy

BARDET-BEIDL (LAURENCE-MOON)

Pigmentary retinopathy, mild mental retardation, polydactyly, obesity, hypogenitalism, barely recordable to nonrecordable ERG, progressive visual field loss, macular lesions common (more details in text)

CAROTINEMIA (FAMILIAL)

Retinal degeneration from vitamin A deficiency; failure of cleavage of beta-carotene

TABLE 13-6 (*continued*)

SECONDARY PIGMENTARY RETINOPATHIES (ASSOCIATED WITH SYSTEMIC DISORDERS)

CEREBROHEPATORENAL (ZELLWEGER) SYNDROME[97]

Muscular hypotonia, high forehead, hypertelorism, hepatomegaly, deficient cerebral myelination, nystagmus, cataract, microphthalmia, retinal degeneration, optic atrophy, nonrecordable ERG. Survival rarely more than a few months, often mistaken for Down's syndrome.

CYSTINOSIS[98]

Pigmentary retinopathy, occasional macular lesions, crystalline deposits in conjunctiva, cornea, iris, retinal pigment epithelium, nephropathy

DIABETES MELLITUS, JUVENILE ONSET; OPTIC ATROPHY (WOLFRAM SYNDROME)[99]

Diabetes mellitus, optic atrophy, neurosensory hearing loss, diabetes insipidus, hyperalanineuria, cone-rod degeneration

FRIEDREICH'S ATAXIA[100]

Spinocerebellar degeneration, limb incoordination, nerve deafness, retinal degeneration, optic atrophy

HOMOCYSTINURIA[101]

Fine pigmentary or cystic degeneration of retina, marfanoid habitus, myopia, subluxation or dislocated lenses, cardiovascular abnormalities, glaucoma, mental retardation, subnormal ERG

MANNOSIDOSIS[102]

Resembles Hurler's syndrome; macroglossia, flat nose, large head and ears, skeletal abnormalities, possible hepatosplenomegaly, storage material in retina

MUCOPOLYSACCHARIDOSIS I (HURLER'S SYNDROME)[103]

Early corneal clouding, gargoyle facies, deafness, mental retardation, dwarfism, skeletal abnormalities, hepatosplenomegaly, subnormal ERG, optic atrophy

MUCOPOLYSACCHARIDOSIS IS (SCHEIE'S SYNDROME)[74]

Coarse facies, aortic regurgitation, stiff joints, early clouding of cornea, normal life span, normal intellect, occasional pigmentary retinopathy, normal ERG

MUCOPOLYSACCHARIDOSIS III (SANFILIPPO'S SYNDROME)[103]

Severe mental retardation, little corneal clouding, pigmentary retinopathy, optic atrophy, retinal vascular narrowing, subnormal to nonrecordable ERG

OSTEOPETROSIS (ALBERS-SCHÖNBERG DISEASE)[104]

Defective resorption of immature bone, macrocephaly, progressive deafness, hepatosplenomegaly, anemia, retinal degeneration, cataract, abnormal to extinguished ERG

PALLIDAL DEGENERATION AND RP[105]

Progressive pigmentary retinopathy, extrapyramidal rigidity, dysarthria; destruction of pallida and substantia nigra

POLYCYSTIC KIDNEY, CATARACT, CONGENITAL BLINDNESS (SENIOR-LOKEN, SALDINO-MAINZER SYNDROMES)[106]

Short stature, early retinal degeneration, cataracts, nephropathy (see text, Usher's section differential). It is not clear whether Senior-Loken and Saldino-Mainzer syndromes are genetically different (see Chapter 7).

PROGRESSIVE EXTERNAL OPHTHALMOPLEGIA, PTOSIS, PIGMENTARY RETINOPATHY, HEART BLOCK, MIXED HEARING LOSS (KEARNS-SAYRE SYNDROME)

See text

REFSUM'S DISEASE

Plasma elevations of phytanic acid, pigmentary retinopathy, partial deafness, cerebellar ataxia, ichthyosis (see Usher's syndrome differential section)

RENAL DYSPLASIA AND RETINAL APLASIA

Congenital blindness, kidney developmental abnormalities; probably the same as Senior-Loken syndrome

TABLE 13-6 (*continued*)

SECONDARY PIGMENTARY RETINOPATHIES (ASSOCIATED WITH SYSTEMIC DISORDERS)

X-Linked Recessive Pigmentary Retinopathies

INCONTINENTIA PIGMENTI (BLOCH-SULZBERGER SYNDROME)

Skin pigmentation in lines and whorls, alopecia, dental anomalies, optic atrophy, falciform folds, cataract, nystagmus, strabismus, patchy mottling of fundi, conjunctival pigmentation (see text)

MUCOPOLYSACCHARIDOSIS II (HUNTER'S SYNDROME)

Little corneal clouding, mild clinical course, mental retardation, some retinal arteriole narrowing, subnormal to normal ERG[107]

PELZAEUS-MEIZBACHER DISEASE

Infantile progressive leukodystrophy, cerebellar ataxia, limb spasticity, mental retardation, possible pigmentary retinopathy with absent foveal reflex

Inheritance Mode Unknown

CHORIORETINOPATHY AND PITUITARY DYSFUNCTION (CPD)[108]

The CPD syndrome is characterized by severe early-onset chorioretinopathy resembling choroideremia, trichosis, evidence of pituitary dysfunction, including dwarfism, sparse scalp hair, hypothyroidism, sexual infantilism.

Acquired (Nonhereditary) Pigmented Retinopathies

See Chapter 11, pseudo-RP

---

male ratio has been reported to be from 231:13 to 653:16.[69] Evidence for X-linked dominant inheritance with a prenatal lethal effect in males includes a report by Kuster in which an affected woman, who had 12 children, had 1 normal son and 6 affected daughters.[70]

Systemic abnormalities include congenital onset of skin lesions resulting in patchy, streaky, or whorled chocolate brown skin pigmentations on the trunk and extremities. Variable findings include alopecia, dental and bony abnormalities, and anomalies of the central nervous system.

Ocular associated findings may be seen in up to 20% of cases and may include a wide spectrum of anomalies, including falciform folds, pseudoglioma, cataract, nystagmus, strabismus, and pigmentation of conjunctiva. Retinal findings may include patchy mottling of RPE, abnormal arteriovenous connections, avascular areas, and vascular anomalies.[71] François reported two cases in which the ERG was extin-

guished in one patient and moderately attenuated in the other.[69]

KEARNS-SAYRE SYNDROME

The hallmarks of Kearns-Sayre syndrome include ptosis, progressive external ophthalmoplegia, heart block, and atypical retinal degeneration. The pigment deposits appear subretinal and have a "salt-and-pepper" quality similar to that seen in measles retinopathy. ERG and visual field tests demonstrate mild abnormalities in most cases. There is a wide spectrum of expressivity, including some infantile cases in which multiple neurologic abnormalities are found in association with the progressive external ophthalmoplegia, ptosis, heart block, ragged red fibers on muscle biopsy, and RP. The cause of Kearns-Sayre syndrome is unknown although mitochondrial abnormalites have been reported on electron microscopy[72] (see also Chapter 4).

CASE STUDY

KEARNS-SAYRE SYNDROME (MILDER FORM)

Case 5 The patient is a 20-year-old woman who has had blepharoptosis from age 11. When progression of the lid droop was noted, she visited her ophthalmologist, who found a pigmentary retinopathy. Because of the possibility of Kearns-Sayre syndrome, she was referred to a cardiologist for evaluation. A bifascicular block was noted on her electrocardiogram. By age 20, she had undergone four operations for ptosis. She related no problems of visual field or dark adaptation. The family history was noncontributory with no similarly affected individual on either side of the family going back two generations.

On examination, the visual acuity was 20/50 OU with correction OD −1.75 +.50 ×90 and OS −2.50 +.50 ×85, and the patient had restricted versions in all fields. Biomicroscopy revealed mild keratopathy from inability to blink fully. Funduscopy revealed a diffuse fine hyperpigmentation at the level of the RPE **(Fig. 13-26***A&B*) similar to the salt-and-pepper appearance seen in rubella. There were no bone spicules or sign of retinal atrophy.

The patient's photopic ERG was abnormal with a b-wave amplitude OD 50uV, OS 60 uV with 40 msec latency (normal mean 160 uV, 32 msec). The rod-mediated ERG showed b-wave amplitudes of 180 uV with 96 msec latencies (normal mean 440 uV, 69 msec). Final rod thresholds showed a 1.1-log unit elevation at 12°, 20°, and 30° above fixation. Goldmann visual fields showed a 50° field with an I-4 isopter OU.

If an electroretinography classification were to be made in this case, the patient would be stated to have a cone-rod degeneration; the final rod threshold is consistent with this finding. The atypical pigmentary retinopathy is similar to that in other reports.[73]

MUCOPOLYSACCHARIDE (MPS) DISORDERS

Four of the MPS disorders are known to have a pigmentary retinopathy in association with this lysosomal storage disease; these include MPS I-H (Hurler's syndrome), MPS I-S (Scheie's syndrome), MPS II (Hunter's syndrome), and MPS III (Sanfilippo's syndrome). Patient cooperation and corneal clouding may make ophthalmoscopy difficult. The retinal degeneration is usually evident by the teenage years.

One of the early reviews of the ocular findings in

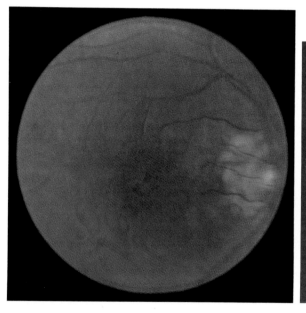
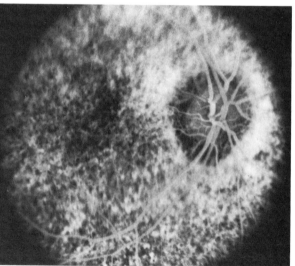

FIG. 13-26. Kearns-Sayre syndrome. *(A)* Fundus photograph, right eye, case 13-5. Mottling and fine pigment deposition is seen at level of RPE. *(B)* Fluorescein angiogram of same area emphasizes the fine pigmentary mottling occurring throughout the retina.

MPS was authored by Gills, who correlated retinal and electroretinographic findings in five types of MPS.[74] Leung examined 13 additional patients, further confirming the retinal involvement of MPS I.

Abraham tested two siblings with Hunter's syndrome (MPS II) and found that the ERGs were moderately abnormal and the final rod threshold was elevated slightly more than 1 log unit.[75] Patients with Morquio syndrome (MPS IV) have essentially normal findings electrophysiologically.[76] Since mucopolysaccharides have been found in the interstitial matrix of photoreceptor outer segments,[77] abnormalities of mucopolysaccharide metabolism may also directly affect the retina.

MYOTONIC DYSTROPHY

This autosomal dominant neuromuscular disorder is characterized by muscular atrophy, myotonia of voluntary movements, and other systemic manifestations.[78] Ocular findings include lenticular changes (focal refractile crystalline areas), extraocular muscle abnormalities, and hypotony. Macular and peripheral pigmentary changes have been reported infrequently.[79,80] The ERG may be mildly to severely abnormal, and elevated final rod thresholds are found.[35]

REFSUM'S DISEASE

See discussion in Usher's syndrome section.

VASCULAR ANOMALIES AND RP (COATS' DISEASE, VON HIPPEL TUMORS, AND STURGE-WEBER SYNDROME)

While rare, there are reports of RP in association with vascular abnormalites, such as RP and Coats' disease, RP and von Hippel tumors, RP and Sturge-Weber syndrome, RP and peripheral vascular anomalies, and RP and neovascularization,[80a] that raise the possibility that these vascular anomalies may occur more than by chance. Yet this coincidence does not necessarily mean that they are specific genetic entities or new forms of RP; they may be multiple gene expression or variable gene expression.

An example of variable or multiple expressivity which could be mistakenly called a new type of RP is exemplified by two Navajo sisters with autosomal recessive RP who were found to have uniocular neovascularization and a hemangioma of the von Hippel type (**Fig. 13-27A&B**); however, on inspection of 40 other autosomal recessive Navajo RP patients, many

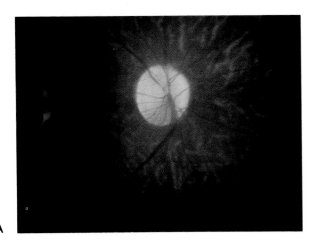 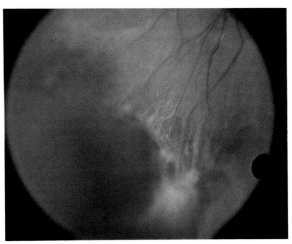

A **B**

FIG. 13-27. von Hippel-Lindau–like tumor and RP. *(A)* Posterior pole, right eye of a 18-year-old Navajo woman with autosomal recessive RP and *(B)* von Hippel-Lindau–like retinal tumor inferior to disc. Note asymmetry of retinal vasculature at disc with increase in size of the inferior retinal vessels, and afferent and efferent vessels to vascular tumor. RP patients with Coats' reaction or vascular tumors show asymmetry of vessel size at the disc of the involved eye.

blood relatives of the patients with the vascular abnormalites, no other cases of retinal neovascularization were found.[81] Most cases with vascular anomalies and RP, however, have been "simplex" or "multiplex" events in which no mendelian pattern of inheritance of the associated vascular finding is present. Kollarits reported another such example in which three siblings were found to have von Hippel tumors and early-onset RP.[82]

Two concurrent disease states occasionally can be documented and may explain associated findings with RP.

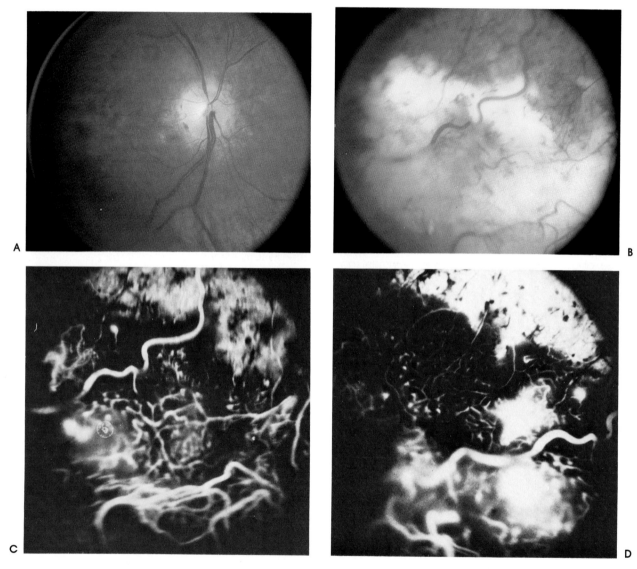

FIG 13-28. RP and Coats' disease. (*A*) Posterior pole, right eye, case 6, a 32-year-old woman with advanced simplex RP and thalassemia minor, who developed a Coats'-like exudative reaction. Note asymmetry of vessel sizes at disc. (*B*) Fundus photograph, Coats'-like reaction inferior retina. (*C*) Fluorescein angiogram of exudative area inferiorly showing a bed of capillary telangiectasia. (*D*) Fluorescein angiogram of Coats'-like exudation reaction demonstrating telangiectasia of overlying vessels and several focal areas of neovascularization. Photocoagulation dried up the area of exudation for about 1 year, after which neovascularization and severe proliferative retinopathy recurred at the edge of treatment.

CASE STUDY

Case 6[83] A 32-year-old woman had known RP and nyctylopia from age 16 and severe deterioration of vision at age 29. No family history of RP or other ocular problems was found. For many years she had been told that she was anemic, and her lowest documented hemoglobin was 9.0 gm% at age 23.

At age 30, she was found to have asymmetry of retinal vessels at the disc in the right eye **(Fig. 13-28***A*) and large retinal vessels coursing inferiorly, where there was a large area of subretinal and intraretinal exudation with overlying telangiectasia **(Fig. 13-28***B– D*), and the diagnosis of Coats' disease was made. Hematologic tests during her evaluation for Coats' disease revealed a 4.4% A2 and 2.9% fetal hemoglobin, consistent with the diagnosis of thalassemia minor.

Approximately 2 years later, when the patient had a visual acuity of 5/200 and 3° fields, she developed neovascular fronds at the edge of the involved area. Xenon photocoagulation was performed surrounding the area, and regression of the exudates and neovascularization occurred. The patient noted a fairly severe postphotocoagulation visual loss, from which she took 6 weeks to recover.

When the neovascularization recurred in the right eye about 1 year later, argon laser treatment and cryotherapy to the area of neovasculariation were employed rather than xenon photocoagulation, because of the previous visual loss associated with xenon. However, the patient had severe recurrent vitreous hemorrhages and developed severe vitreal

proliferative changes. When the patient was 35 years old, the left eye developed diffuse retinal telangiectasia as well as subretinal neovascularization in the equatorial region, without exudates. This condition regressed with argon panretinal photocoagulation. The patient was treated OS even though she had advanced RP with light perception vision, because of the potential sequelae of vitreous hemorrhage and proliferative organization, as well as possible rubeotic glaucoma, all of which could cause her to lose the eye.

The neovascularization occurring in cases of Coats' disease is interesting because both retinal and choroidal neovascularization have been documented. Fogle and associates reported histopathologic evidence of a choroidal origin for neovascularization in their case.[84] Of interest in the above case is that neovascularization in the right eye was retinal, while it was choroidal (subretinal) in the left eye.

In order better to understand the heterogeneity within specific disease states, it will be increasingly important to identify secondary factors which influence the course of the disease. Finding and understanding these factors will help to identify those diseases which are the result of single gene defects and eventually will lead to better classification and determination of their pathogenetic mechanisms.

REFERENCES

1. Vernon M: Usher's syndrome-deafness and progressive blindness. Clinical cases, prevention, theory and literature survey. J Chron Dis 22:133–151, 1969
2. Boughman JA, Vernon M, Shaver KA: Usher syndrome: Definition and estimate of prevalence from two high-risk populations. J Chron Dis 36:595–603, 1983
3. Von Graefe A: Exceptionelles Verhalten des Gesichtsfeldes bei Pigmententartung der nefshaut. Graefes Arch Clin Exp Ophthalmol 4:250–253, 1858
4. Liebreich R: Abkunft aus Ehen unter Blutsverwandten als Grund von Retinitis pigmentosa. Dtsch Klin 13:53, 1861
5. Lindenov H: The etiology of deaf-mutism with special reference to heredity. Op Ex Domo Biol Hered Hum Univ Hafniensis 8:1–268, 1945
6. Kloepfer HW, Laguaite JK, McLaurin JW: The hereditary syndrome of congenital deafness and retinitis pigmentosa: (Usher's syndrome). Laryngoscope 76:850–862, 1966
7. Nuutila A: Dystrophia retinae pigmentosa-dysacusis syndrome (DRD): Study of the Usher or Hallgren syndrome. J Hum Genet 18:57–88, 1970
8. Amman F, Klein D, Franceschetti A: Genetic and epidemiological investigations on pigmentary degeneration of the retina and allied disorders in Switzerland. J Neurol Sci 2:183–196, 1965
9. Bell J: Retinitis pigmentosa and allied diseases. In: The Treasury of Human Inheritance. London, Cambridge University Press, 1933
10. Heckenlively JR: The frequency of posterior subcapsular cataract in the hereditary retinal degenerations. Am J Ophthalmol 93:733–738, 1982
11. Fishman G, Vasquez V, Fishman M et al: Visual loss and foveal lesions in Usher's syndrome. Br J Ophthalmol 63:484–488, 1979
12. McKusick VA: Mendelian Inheritance in Man, 5th ed, pp 694–695. Baltimore, The Johns Hopkins University Press, 1978
13. Davenport, SLH, Omeann CS: The heterogeneity of

Usher Syndrome (abstract 215). Fifth International Conference on Birth Defects, Montreal, Aug 21–27, 1977

14. Gorlin RJ, Tilsner TJ, Feinstein S et al: Usher's syndrome type III. Arch Otolaryngol 105:353–354, 1979
15. Fishman GA, Kumar A, Joseph ME et al: Usher's syndrome: Ophthalmic and neuro-otologic findings suggesting genetic heterogeneity. Arch Ophthalmol 101:1367–1374, 1983
16. Merin S, Abraham FA, Auerbach E: Usher's and Hallgren's syndromes. Acta Genet Med— Gemellol— 23:49–55, 1974
17. Robbins JH, Scudiero DA, Otsuka F et al: Hypersensitivity to DNA-damaging agents in cultured cells from patients with Usher's syndrome and Duchenne muscular dystrophy. J Neurol Neurosurg Psychiatry 47:391–398, 1984
18. Bloom TD, Fishman GA, Mafee MF: Usher's syndrome: CNS defects determined by computed tomography. Retina 3:108–113, 1983
19. Nuutila A: Retinitis pigmentosa dysacusis syndrome. Preliminary report. Acta Neurol Scand 43(suppl 31):68–69, 1967
20. Weleber RG, Tongue AC, Kennaway NG et al: Ophthalmic manifestations of infantile phytanic acid storage disease. Arch Ophthalmol 102:1317–1321, 1984
21. De Haas EBH, Van Lith GHM, Rijnders J et al: Usher's syndrome with special reference to heterozygous manifestations. Doc Ophthalmol 28:166–190, 1970
22. Sondheimer S, Fishman GA, Young RS et al: Dark adaptation testing in heterozygotes of Usher's syndrome. Br J Ophthalmol 63:547–550, 1979
23. Karp A, Santore F: Retinitis pigmentosa and progressive hearing loss. J Speech Hear Disord 48:308–314, 1983
24. Vernon M, Boughman JA, Annala L: Considerations in diagnosing Usher's syndrome: RP and hearing loss. Visual Impair Blind 258–261, September 1982
25. Yoken C: Living with Deaf–Blindness—Nine Profiles. Washington, DC, The National Academy of Gallaudet College, 1979
26. Hicks WM, Hicks DE: The Usher's syndrome adolescent: Programming implications for school administrators, teachers, and residential advisors. Am Ann Deaf 126:422–431, 1981
27. Bateman JB, Riedner ED, Levin LS et al: Heterogeneity of retinal degeneration and hearing impairment syndromes. Am J Ophthalmol 90:755–767, 1980
28. Konigsmark BW, Gorlin RJ: Genetic and Metabolic Deafness, pp 74–134. Philadelphia, WB Saunders, 1976
29. Alström CH, Hallgren B, Nilsson LB et al: Retinal degeneration combined with obesity, diabetes mellitus and neurogenous deafness: A specific syndrome (not hitherto described) distinct from the Laurence-Moon-Bardet-Biedl syndrome. Acta Psychiatr Neurol Scand 34(suppl 129):1–35, 1959
30. Klein D, Ammann F: The syndrome of Laurence-Moon-Bardet-Biedl and allied diseases in Switzerland: Clinical, genetic, and epidemiological studies. J Neurol Sci 9:479–513, 1969
31. Goldstein JL, Fialkow PJ: The Alstrom syndrome. Medicine 52:53–71, 1973
32. Millay RH, Weleber RG, Heckenlively JR: Alstrom's disease; ophthalmologic and systemic manifestations. Am J Ophthalmol (in press)
33. Cockayne EA: Dwarfism with retinal atrophy and deafness. Arch Dis Child 11:1–8, 1936
34. Pearce WG: Ocular and genetic features of Cockayne's syndrome. Can J Ophthalmol 7:435–444, 1972
35. Edwards JA, Sethi PK, Scoma AJ et al: A new familial syndrome characterized by pigmentary retinopathy, hypogonadism, mental retardation, nerve deafness, and glucose intolerance. Am J Med 60:23–32, 1976
36. Flynn P, Aird RB: A neuroectodermal syndrome of dominant inheritance. J Neurol Sci 2:161–182, 1965
37. Keith CG: Retinal atrophy in osteopetrosis. Arch Ophthalmol 79:234–241, 1968
38. Refsum S: Heredopathia atactica polyneuritiformis. Acta Psychiatr Neurol Scand (Suppl) 38:1–303, 1946
39. Richterich R, Moser H, Rossi E: Refsum's disease (heredopathia atactica polyneuritiformis). Humangenetik 1:322–323, 1965
40. Richterich R, Kahlke W, van Mechelen P et al: Refsum's syndrome: Ein angeborener Defekt im Lipid-Stoffwechsel mit Speicherung von 3,7,11,15-tetramethylhexadecansaure. Klin Wochenschr 41:800–801, 1963
41. Baum J, Tannenbaum M, Kolodny E: Refsum's syndrome with corneal involvement. Am J Ophthalmol 60:699–708, 1965
42. Eldjarn L, Try K, Stokke O et al: Dietary effects on serum phytanic acid levels and on clinical manifestations in heredopathia atactica polyneuritiformis. Lancet 1:691–693, 1966
43. Toussaint D, Danis P: An ocular pathologic study of Refsum's syndrome. Am J Ophthalmol 72:342–347, 1971
44. Eldjarn L, Try K, Stokke O et al: Dietary effects on serum-phytanic-acid levels and on clinical manifestations in heredopathia atactica polyneuritiformis. Lancet 1:691–693, 1966
45. Alvarez F, Landrieu P, Laget P et al: Nervous and ocular disorders in children with cholestasis and vitamin A and E deficiencies. Hepatology 3:410–414, 1983
46. Puklin JE, Riely CA, Simon RM et al: Anterior segment and retinal pigmentary abnormalities in arteriohepatic dysplasia. Ophthalmology 88:337–347, 1981
47. Bassen F, Kornzweig A: Malformation of the erythrocytes in a case of atypical retinitis pigmentosa. Blood 5:381–387, 1950
48. Salt H, Wolfe O, Lloyd J et al: On having no beta-lipoprotein. A syndrome comprising abeta-lipoproteinemia, acanthocytosis, and steatorrhoea. Lancet ii:325, 1960
49. Ways P, Reed CF, Hanahan DJ: Red-cell and plasma lipids in acanthocytosis. J Clin Invest 42:1248–1260, 1963
50. Kornzweig A: Bassen-Kornzweig syndrome, present status. J Med Genet 7:271–276, 1970
51. Gouras P, Carr RE, Gunkel RD: Retinitis pigmentosa in abetalipoproteinemia: Effects of vitamin A. Invest Ophthalmol 10:784–793, 1971
52. Judisch GF, Rhead WJ, Miller DK: Abetalipoproteinemia: Report of an unusual patient. Ophthalmologica 189:73–79, 1984
53. Bardet G: Sur un syndrome d'obsit infantile avec polydactylie et rétinite pigmentaire (Contribution l'étude des formes cliniques de l'obsit hypophysair). Thesis 479, Paris, 1920
54. Biedl A: Ein Geschwisterpaar mit adiposogenitaler dystrophie. Dtsch Med Wochenschr 48:1630, 1922
55. Solis-Cohen S, Weiss E: Dystrophia adiposogenitalis, with atypical retinitis pigmentosa and mental deficiency: The Laurence-Biedl syndrome: A report of four cases in one family. Am J Med Sci 169:489–505, 1925
56. Hutchinson J: On retinitis pigmentosa and allied affections, as illustrating the laws of heredity. Ophthalmol Rev 1:2–7, 26–30, 1900
57. Bell J: The Laurence-Moon syndrome. In Penrose LS (ed): The Treasury of Human Inheritance, vol 5, part 3, pp 51–96. London, Cambridge University Press, 1958

58. Schachat AP, Maumenee IH: Bardet-Biedl syndrome and related disorders. Arch Ophthalmol 100:285–288, 1982

59. Temtamy SA: Carpenter's syndrome: Acrocephalopolysyndactyly: An autosomal recessive syndrome. J Pediatr 69:111–120, 1966

60. Ehrenfold EN, Rowe H, Auerbach E: Laurence-moon-Bardet-Biedl syndrome in Israel. Am J Ophthalmol 70:524–532, 1970

61. Weiss E: Cerebral adiposity with nerve deafness, mental deficiency and genital dystrophy: Variant of the Laurence-Biedl syndrome. Am J Med Sci 183:268–272, 1932

62. Alström CH, Hallgren B, Nilsson LB et al: Retinal degeneration combined with obesity, diabetes mellitus, and neurogenous deafness. Acta Psychiatr Scand 34(suppl 129):1–35, 1959

63. Biemond A: Het syndrome van Laurence-Biedl en een niew aanverwant syndroom. Ned Tijdschr Geneeskd 78:180l–1809, 1934

64. O'Donnell J: Personal communication

65. Klein D, Ammann F: The syndrome of Laurence-Moon-Bardet-Biedl and allied diseases in Switzerland. Clinical, genetic and epidemiological studies. J Neurol Sci 9:479–513, 1969

66. Unpublished data (Cowan & Heckenlively)

67. Zeman W: Batten disease: Ocular features, differential diagnosis and diagnosis by enzyme analysis. In Bergsma D, Bron AJ, Cotlier E (eds): The Eye and Inborn Errors of Metabolism, pp 441–453. AR Liss, 1976

68. Batten FE: Cerebral degeneration with symmetrical changes in the maculae in two members of a family. Trans Ophthalmol Soc UK 23:386–387, 1903

69. François J: Incontinentia pigmenti (Bloch-Sulzberger syndrome) and retinal changes. Br J Ophthalmol 68:19–25, 1984

70. Kuster F, Olbing H: Incontinentia pigmenti. Bericht ueber neun Erkrankunger in einer Familie und einem Obduktions befund. Ann Pediatr 202:92–100, 1964

71. Watzke RC, Stevens TS, Carney RG: Retinal vascular changes of incontinentia pigmenti. Arch Ophthalmol 94:743–746, 1976

72. Eagle RC, Hedges TR, Yanoff M: The Kearns-Sayre syndrome. A light and electron microscopic study. Trans Am Ophthalmol Soc 80:218–234, 1982

73. Steindler P, Tormene AP, Micaglio GF et al: Correlation of ERG and pigment epithelium changes in external progressive ophthalmoplegia (EPO). Doc Ophthalmol 60:421–426, 1985

74. Gills JP, Hobson R, Hanley WB et al: Electroretinography and fundus oculi findings in Hurler's disease and allied mucopolysaccharidoses. Arch Ophthalmol 74:596–603, 1965

75. Abraham FA, Yatziv S, Alexander R et al: Electrophysiological and psychophysical findings in Hunter syndrome. Arch Ophthalmol 91:181–186, 1974

76. Abraham FA, Yatziv S, Russell A et al: A family with two siblings affected by Morquio Syndrome (MPS IV). Arch Ophthalmol 91:265–269, 1974

77. Sidman RL: Histochemical studies on photoreceptor cells. NY Acad Sci 72:1; 62, 1958

78. Steinert H: Myopathologische Beitrage. I. Ueber das klinische und amatomische Bild des Muskelschwunds der Myotoniker. Dtsch Z Nervenheilkd 37:58–104, 1909

79. Betten MG, Bilchik RC, Smith ME: Pigmentary retinopathy of myotonic dystrophy. Am J Ophthalmol 72:720–723, 1971

80. Burian HM, Burns CA: Ocular changes in myotonic dystrophy. Am J Ophthalmol 63:22–34, 1967

80a. Uliss AE, Gregor ZJ, Bird AC: Retinitis pigmentosa and retinal neovascularization. Ophthalmology 93:1599–1603, 1986

81. Heckenlively JR, Friedereich R, Frason C et al: Retinitis pigmentosa in the Navajo. Metab Pediatr Syst Ophthalmol 5:201–206, 1981

82. Kollarits CR, Mehelas TJ, Shealy TR et al: Von Hippel tumors in siblings with retinitis pigmentosa. Ann Ophthalmol 14:256–259, 1982

83. Heckenlively J. Retinitis pigmentosa, unilateral Coats's disease and thalassemia minor—a case report. Metab Pediatr Syst Ophthalmol 5:67–72, 1981

84. Fogle JA, Welch RB, Green WR: Retinitis pigmentosa and exudative vasculopathy. Arch Ophthal 96:696–702, 1978

85. Charcot JM, Marie P. Sur une forme particuliere d'atrophie musculaire progressive, souvent familiale debutant par les pieds et les jambes et atteignant plus tard les mains. Rev Med 6:97–132, 1886

86. Brody IA, Wilkins RH: Charcot-Marie-Tooth disease. Arch Neurol 17:552–553, 1967

87. Flynn P, Aird RB: A neuroectodermal syndrome of dominant inheritance. J Neurol Sci 2:161–182, 1965

88. Betten MG, Bilchik RC, Smith ME: Pigmentary retinopathy of myotonic dystrophy. Am J Ophthalmol 72:720–723, 1971

89. Gillespie FD: Hereditary dysplasia oculodentodigitalis. Arch Ophthalmol 71:187–192, 1964

90. Böjrk A, Lindblom U, Wadensten L: Retinal degeneration in hereditary ataxia. J Neurol Neurosurg Psychiatry 19:186–193, 1956

91. van Bogaert L: Uber eine hereditare und familiare Form der Pagetschen Ostitis deformans mit Chorioretinitis pigmentosa. Zentralbl Gesamte Neurol Psychiatr 147:327–345, 1933

92. Deutman AF: Hereditary diseases and syndromes with retinal, choroidal, or optic nerve abnormalities. In: Krill's Hereditary Retinal and Choroidal Diseases, p 1326. Hagerstown, Harper & Row, 1977

93. Stickler GB, Belau PG, Farrell FJ et al: Hereditary progressive arthro-ophthalmopathy. Mayo Clin Proc 40:433–455, 1965

94. Hagler WS, Crosswell HH: Radial perivascular chorioretinal degeneration and retinal detachment. Trans Am Acad Ophthalmol Otolaryngol 72:203–216, 1968

95. Maumenee IH, Stoll HU, Mets MB: The Wagner syndrome versus hereditary arthroophthalmopathy. Trans Am Ophthalmol Soc 80:349–365, 1982

96. Goldberg MF. Waardenburg's syndrome with fundus and other anomalies. Arch Ophthalmol 76:797–810, 1966

97. Moser AE, Singh I, Brown FR et al: The cerebrohepatorenal (Zellweger) syndrome. N Engl J Med 3l0:1114–1146, 1984

98. Sanderson PO, Kuwabara T, Start WJ et al: A clinical, histopathologic, and ultrastructural study. Arch Ophthalmol 91:270–274, 1974

99. Niemeyer G, Marquardt JL: Retinal function in an unique syndrome of optic atrophy, juvenile diabetes mellitus, diabetes insipidus, neurosensory hearing loss, autonomic dysfunction, and hyperalanineuria. Invest Ophthalmol 11:612–624, 1972

100. Alfano JE, Berger JP: Retinitis pigmentosa, ophthalmoplegia and spastic quadriplegia. Am J Ophthalmol 43:231–240, 1957

101. Personal observation

102. Kjellmann B, Gamstorp I, Brun A et al: A clinical and histopathologic study. J Pediatr 75:366–373, 1969

103. Leung LE, Weinstein GW, Hobson RR: Further electro-

retinographic studies of patients with mucopolysaccharidoses. Birth Defects Original Article Series March of Dimes, vol VII, no. 3, pp 32–40, 1971

104. Keith CG: Retinal atrophy in osteopetrosis. Arch Ophthalmol 79:324–341, 1968
105. Winkelman NW: Progressive pallidal degeneration. Arch Neurol Psychiatr 27:1–21, 1932
106. Ellis DS, Heckenlively JR, Martin CL et al: Leber's congenital amaurosis associated with familial juvenile nephronophthisis and cone-shaped epiphyses of the hands (The Saldino-Mainzer Syndrome). Am J Ophthalmol 97:233–239, 1984
107. Abraham FA, Yatziv S, Russell A et al: Electrophysiological and psychophysical findings in Hunter syndrome. Arch Ophthalmol 91:181–186, 1974
108. Judisch GF, Lowry RB, Hanson JW et al: Chorioretinopathy and pituitary dysfunction; the CPD syndrome. Arch Ophthalmol 99:253–356, 1981

Index

The letter *f* after a page number indicates a figure; *t* following a page number indicates tabular material.